METHODS IN MOLECULAR BIOLOGY

For further volumes:
http://www.springer.com/series/7651

For over 35 years, biological scientists have come to rely on the research protocols and methodologies in the critically acclaimed *Methods in Molecular Biology* series. The series was the first to introduce the step-by-step protocols approach that has become the standard in all biomedical protocol publishing. Each protocol is provided in readily-reproducible step-by-step fashion, opening with an introductory overview, a list of the materials and reagents needed to complete the experiment, and followed by a detailed procedure that is supported with a helpful notes section offering tips and tricks of the trade as well as troubleshooting advice. These hallmark features were introduced by series editor Dr. John Walker and constitute the key ingredient in each and every volume of the *Methods in Molecular Biology* series. Tested and trusted, comprehensive and reliable, all protocols from the series are indexed in PubMed.

Nipah Virus

Methods and Protocols

Edited by

Alexander N. Freiberg

Department of Pathology, University of Texas Medical Branch, Galveston, TX, USA

Barry Rockx

Wageningen Bioveterinary Institute, Lelystad and Department of Viroscience, Erasmus University Medical Center Rotterdam, Rotterdam, The Netherlands

Humana Press

Editors
Alexander N. Freiberg
Department of Pathology
University of Texas Medical Branch
Galveston, TX, USA

Barry Rockx
Wageningen Bioveterinary Institute, Lelystad and Department of Viroscience
Erasmus University Medical Center Rotterdam
Rotterdam, The Netherlands

ISSN 1064-3745 ISSN 1940-6029 (electronic)
Methods in Molecular Biology
ISBN 978-1-0716-3282-6 ISBN 978-1-0716-3283-3 (eBook)
https://doi.org/10.1007/978-1-0716-3283-3

This Humana imprint is published by the registered company Springer Science+Business Media, LLC, part of Springer Nature.
The registered company address is: 1 New York Plaza, New York, NY 10004, U.S.A.

Preface

This book summarizes key methods that have been developed over the past 28 years and supported advancements in the field of henipavirus molecular biology. As emerging bat-borne paramyxoviruses, there is an increased need not only to better understand the pathogenicity caused by Nipah and Hendra viruses, but also to further develop diagnostics, antiviral therapeutics, and vaccines.

This comprehensive volume consists of 20 chapters and covers various aspects of henipavirus research, including biochemical, cell-based, and in vivo models. Current protocols are provided in great detail with the intention to equip researchers with state-of-the-art protocols of widely used techniques and to further broaden the repertoire of experienced virologists by adding most recently developed technologies.

Chapters 1, 2, 3, 4, 5, 6, 7, 8 and 9 describe protocols for different in vitro assays to detect henipavirus infection, study the virus-host interactions, and provide tools for antiviral screenings. In Chaps. 10, 11, 12, 13, 14, 15 and 16 different animal models of henipavirus infection are described, as well as their use in studying the pathogenesis and for preclinical evaluation of intervention strategies. Finally, in Chaps. 17, 18, 19, and 20 protocols are provided to characterize the host (immune) response following henipavirus infection.

We would like to thank all the contributors to this book.

Galveston, TX, USA *Alexander N. Freiberg*
Rotterdam, The Netherlands *Barry Rockx*

Contents

Contributors

HECTOR C. AGUILAR • *Department of Microbiology and Immunology, College of Veterinary Medicine, Cornell University, Ithaca, NY, USA*
MOUSHIMI AMAYA • *Department of Microbiology and Immunology, Uniformed Services University, Bethesda, MD, USA*
DANIELLE E. ANDERSON • *Programme in Emerging Infectious Diseases, Duke-NUS Medical School, Singapore, Singapore; Victorian Infectious Diseases Reference Laboratory, The Peter Doherty Institute for Infection and Immunity, Melbourne, VIC, Australia; Department of Microbiology and Immunology, The University of Melbourne, Melbourne, VIC, Australia*
STÉPHANE BARRON • *INSERM-Laboratory P4 Jean Mérieux, Lyon, France*
ANDREW G. D. BEAN • *CSIRO Australian Animal Health Laboratory, Health & Biosecurity, Geelong, VIC, Australia*
J. KYLE BOHANNON • *NIAID Integrated Research Facility, Ft. Detrick, Frederick, MD, USA*
CHRISTOPHER C. BRODER • *Department of Microbiology and Immunology, Uniformed Services University, Bethesda, MD, USA*
YINGYUN CAI • *NIAID Integrated Research Facility, Ft. Detrick, Frederick, MD, USA*
YEE-PENG CHAN • *Department of Microbiology and Immunology, Uniformed Services University, Bethesda, MD, USA*
YU CONG • *NIAID Integrated Research Facility, Ft. Detrick, Frederick, MD, USA*
CHRISTOPHER COWLED • *CSIRO Australian Animal Health Laboratory, Health & Biosecurity, Geelong, VIC, Australia*
SUDEEP DAHAL • *CSIRO Australian Animal Health Laboratory, Health & Biosecurity, Geelong, VIC, Australia*
AURÉLIE DUTHEY • *INSERM-Laboratory P4 Jean Mérieux, Lyon, France*
MAREIKE ELVERT • *Institute of Virology, Philipps University Marburg, Marburg, Germany*
OLIVIER ESCAFFRE • *Department of Pathology, University of Texas Medical Branch, Galveston, TX, USA*
RYAN J. FARR • *CSIRO Australian Animal Health Laboratory, Health & Biosecurity, Geelong, VIC, Australia*
ALEXANDER N. FREIBERG • *Department of Pathology, University of Texas Medical Branch, Galveston, TX, USA*
DEBORAH L. FUSCO • *Department of Microbiology and Immunology, Uniformed Services University, Bethesda, MD, USA*
THOMAS W. GEISBERT • *Galveston National Laboratory, University of Texas Medical Branch, Galveston, TX, USA; Department of Microbiology and Immunology, University of Texas Medical Branch, Galveston, TX, USA*
MICHAEL R. HOLBROOK • *NIAID Integrated Research Facility, Ft. Detrick, Frederick, MD, USA*
BRANKA HORVAT • *Immunobiology of Viral Infections, International Center for Infectiology Research-CIRI, INSERM U1111, CNRS UMR5308, University Lyon 1, ENS de Lyon, Lyon, France*
MATHIEU IAMPIETRO • *Immunobiology of Viral Infections, International Center for Infectiology Research-CIRI, INSERM U1111, CNRS UMR5308, University Lyon 1, ENS de Lyon, Lyon, France*

KENDRA JOHNSON • *Department of Microbiology and Immunology, University of Texas Medical Branch, Galveston, TX, USA*
TERRY JUELICH • *Department of Pathology, University of Texas Medical Branch, Galveston, TX, USA*
A. A. KELVIN • *Department of Microbiology and Immunology, Dalhousie University, Halifax, NS, Canada*
DAVID J. KELVIN • *Department of Microbiology and Immunology, Dalhousie University, Halifax, NS, Canada*
JOHN KLENA • *Viral Special Pathogens Branch, Centers for Disease Control and Prevention, Atlanta, GA, USA*
MATTHEW G. LACKEMEYER • *NIAID Integrated Research Facility, Ft. Detrick, Frederick, MD, USA*
ERIC D. LAING • *Department of Microbiology and Immunology, Uniformed Services University, Bethesda, MD, USA*
BENHUR LEE • *Department of Microbiology, Icahn School of Medicine at Mount Sinai, New York, NY, USA*
JANIE LIANG • *NIAID Integrated Research Facility, Ft. Detrick, Frederick, MD, USA*
MICHAEL K. LO • *Viral Special Pathogens Branch, Centers for Disease Control and Prevention, Atlanta, GA, USA*
ANDREA MAISNER • *Institute of Virology, Philipps University Marburg, Marburg, Germany*
SHAILENDRA MANI • *Programme in Emerging Infectious Diseases, Duke-NUS Medical School, Singapore, Singapore; NCR Biotech Science Cluster, Translational Health Science and Technology Institute, Faridabad, Haryana, India*
CHAD E. MIRE • *Galveston National Laboratory, University of Texas Medical Branch, Galveston, TX, USA; Department of Microbiology and Immunology, University of Texas Medical Branch, Galveston, TX, USA; National Bio- and Agro-defense Facility, Agricultural Research Services, United States Department of Agriculture, Manhattan, NY, USA*
I. ABRREY MONREAL • *Department of Microbiology and Immunology, College of Veterinary Medicine, Cornell University, Ithaca, NY, USA*
BRUCE A. MUNGALL • *Australian Animal Health Laboratory, CSIRO Livestock Industries, Geelong, VIC, Australia; GlaxoSmithKline Vaccines, Seoul, South Korea; Vaccines and Immune Therapies, Astra Zeneca, Singapore, Singapore*
MEHMET HAKAN OZDENER • *Monell Chemical Senses Center, Philadelphia, PA, USA*
KETAN PATEL • *Viral Special Pathogens Branch, Centers for Disease Control and Prevention, Atlanta, GA, USA*
ELENA POSTNIKOVA • *NIAID Integrated Research Facility, Ft. Detrick, Frederick, MD, USA*
NANCY E. RAWSON • *Monell Chemical Senses Center, Philadelphia, PA, USA*
BARRY ROCKX • *Wageningen Bioveterinary Institute, Lelystad and Department of Viroscience, Erasmus University Medical Center, Rotterdam, The Netherlands*
BENJAMIN A. SATTERFIELD • *Department of Cardiovascular Medicine, Mayo Clinic, Rochester, MN, USA*
LUCIE SAUERHERING • *Institute of Virology, Philipps University Marburg, Marburg, Germany*
JENNIFER SMITH • *Department of Pathology, University of Texas Medical Branch, Galveston, TX, USA*

SPENCER L. STERLING • *Department of Microbiology and Immunology, Uniformed Services University, Bethesda, MD, USA*
CAMERON R. STEWART • *CSIRO Australian Animal Health Laboratory, Health & Biosecurity, Geelong, VIC, Australia*
CHEE WAH TAN • *Programme in Emerging Infectious Diseases, Duke-NUS Medical School, Singapore, Singapore*
LEON TRIBOLET • *CSIRO Australian Animal Health Laboratory, Health & Biosecurity, Geelong, VIC, Australia*
GUSTAVO VALBUENA • *UC Berkeley-UCSF Joint Medical Program, Berkeley, CA, USA*
LIN-FA WANG • *Programme in Emerging Infectious Diseases, Duke-NUS Medical School, Singapore, Singapore*
KAI XU • *Department of Veterinary Biosciences, College of Veterinary Medicine, The Ohio State University, Columbus, OH, USA; Center for Retrovirus Research, The Ohio State University, Columbus, OH, USA*
LIANYING YAN • *Department of Microbiology and Immunology, Uniformed Services University, Bethesda, MD, USA*
D. S. YANG • *Department of Microbiology and Immunology, Dalhousie University, Halifax, NS, Canada*
SHUIQING YU • *NIAID Integrated Research Facility, Ft. Detrick, Frederick, MD, USA*
TIAN S. ZENG • *Department of Microbiology and Immunology, Dalhousie University, Halifax, NS, Canada*

Chapter 1

Overview of Experimental Vaccines and Antiviral Therapeutics for Henipavirus Infection

Benjamin A. Satterfield, Chad E. Mire, and Thomas W. Geisbert

Abstract

Hendra virus (HeV) and Nipah virus (NiV) are highly pathogenic paramyxoviruses, which have emerged in recent decades and cause sporadic outbreaks of respiratory and encephalitic disease in Australia and Southeast Asia, respectively. Over two billion people currently live in regions potentially at risk due to the wide range of the Pteropus fruit bat reservoir, yet there are no approved vaccines or therapeutics to protect against or treat henipavirus disease. In recent years, significant progress has been made toward developing various experimental vaccine platforms and therapeutics. Here, we describe these advances for both human and livestock vaccine candidates and discuss the numerous preclinical studies and the few that have progressed to human phase 1 clinical trial and the one approved veterinary vaccine.

Key words Nipah, Hendra, Henipavirus, Virus, Vaccine, Therapeutics

1 Introduction

The paramyxovirus genus henipavirus contains two known human pathogens, Hendra virus (HeV) and Nipah virus (NiV). These two pathogenic henipaviruses cause similar medical syndromes in humans including severe respiratory disease, meningoencephalitis, and systemic vasculitis [1]. Both viruses are transmitted by their host reservoir of fruit bats belonging to the genus *Pteropus*, commonly called flying foxes [2–4].

HeV has caused sporadic outbreaks in Australian horse populations with subsequent spillover transmission to humans [5–9]. NiV has caused outbreaks in Malaysia [10], Singapore [11], Bangladesh [12–19], India [20–22], and the Philippines [23], sometimes through livestock intermediaries such as swine [10, 24] and horses [23] and at other times through consumption of contaminated date palm sap [17, 19, 25]. The strain of NiV that has caused repeated outbreaks in Bangladesh and India is designated $NiV_{Bangladesh}$ (NiV_B) and has been reported to be more virulent in both humans [26] and the African green monkey (AGM) animal

Alexander N. Freiberg and Barry Rockx (eds.), *Nipah Virus: Methods and Protocols*, Methods in Molecular Biology, vol. 2682, https://doi.org/10.1007/978-1-0716-3283-3_1, © Springer Science+Business Media, LLC, part of Springer Nature 2023

model [27] than the strain of NiV that caused the initial outbreak in Malaysia and Singapore designated $NiV_{Malaysia}$ (NiV_M). Some outbreaks have had case fatality rates approaching 100% [28] motivating research into developing vaccines and therapeutics that can prevent or treat henipavirus infection in humans [29–36]. The urgent need for such vaccines and therapeutics has been highlighted by the current coronavirus disease 2019 (COVID-19) pandemic caused by severe acute respiratory syndrome coronavirus 2 (SARS-CoV-2) [37]. In fact, the Coalition for Epidemic Preparedness Innovations (CEPI) has declared NiV as one of their six priority pathogens for vaccine development in the near future [38, 39]. The financial and technical feasibility of developing henipavirus vaccines is discussed elsewhere [29], while here we discuss the progress that has been made in developing experimental henipavirus vaccines and therapeutics.

Various animal models have been used to study henipavirus pathogenesis and to test experimental vaccines and therapeutics. These include Syrian golden hamsters, ferrets, cats, swine, horses, ponies, and AGMs as described below. In some cases, mice have been used to study the innate and adaptive immune responses to vaccination, although wild-type mice are not susceptible to henipavirus infection. Ideally, strong vaccine candidates will prove protective in multiple animal models with the AGM being the gold standard preclinical model. Of note, native Asian old-world monkeys, such as the Cynomolgus macaque, do not develop the clinical disease when infected with henipaviruses due to differential immune responses when compared with AGMs [40]. Studies involving challenge with live HeV or NiV can be difficult as they require the use of specialized biosafety level (BSL)-4 facilities to ensure researcher and environmental safety.

2 Preclinical Vaccine Studies

Although no vaccine candidates have been approved for use in humans, various candidate vaccines have been used in animal model preclinical studies including subunit vaccines, lipid nanoparticle (LNP)-encapsulated mRNA vaccines, DNA vaccines, virus-like particles (VLPs), and various vectored vaccine platforms. These vectors include rhabdoviruses (vesicular stomatitis virus [VSV] and rabies virus [RABV]), paramyxoviruses (Newcastle disease virus [NDV] and measles virus [MV]), poxviruses (vaccinia virus and canarypox virus), Venezuelan equine encephalitis virus (VEEV), adeno-associated virus (AAV), chimpanzee adenovirus (ChAd), and bovine herpesvirus (BoHV). Details from all published henipavirus vaccine studies in animal models are shown in Table 1. Henipaviruses have two outer membrane proteins, the glycoprotein (G) and the fusion (F) protein; these proteins have

Table 1
Preclinical henipavirus vaccine studies

Platform	Target antigen	Adjuvant(s)	Vaccination route, dose, and schedule	Challenge route, dose, and virus	Animal model	Ref.
Subunit	HeV-sG	Alhydrogel™	**IM** 100 μg **HeV-sG-V**. primed on day −56 and boosted on day −28; or **IM** 300 μg **HeV-sG-V** given as a single dose on day −56	**IN/IT** 5 × 10^5 PFU **HeV** or **NiV$_B$**[a]	AGM	[45]
	HeV-sG	Alhydrogel™	**IM** 100 μg **HeV-sG-V** given as a single dose on day −7 or − 14; or **IM** 300 μg **HeV-sG-V** given as a single dose on day −14	**IN/IT** 5 × 10^5 PFU **HeV** or **NiV$_B$**[a]	AGM	[45]
	HeV-sG	CpG and Alhydrogel™	**IM** 100 μg **HeV-sG**. Primed on day −42 and boosted on day −21	**IT** 5 × 10^5 PFU **HeV**	AGM	[44]
	HeV-sG	CpG and Alhydrogel™	**IM** 10, 50, or 100 μg **HeV-sG**. Primed on day −42 and boosted on day −21	**IT** 1 × 10^5 $TCID_{50}$ **NiV$_M$**	AGM	[43]
	HeV-sG	Proprietary adjuvant	**IM** 50 or 100 μg **HeV-sG**. Primed on day −49 and boosted on day −28 or primed on day −215 and boosted on day −194	**ON** 2 × 10^6 $TCID_{50}$ **HeV**	Horse	[42]
	HeV-sG	Proprietary adjuvant	**IM** 2 mL of proprietary Zoetis™ vaccine (presumably the same 100 μg/mL dosing of their Equivac® HeV). Primed on day −35 and boosted on day −14	**IN** 5 × 10^5 PFU **HeV** or **NiV$_M$**	Swine	[46]
	HeV-sG	CpG and Alhydrogel™	**SC** 4, 20, or 100 μg **HeV-sG**. Primed on day −40 and boosted on day −20	**ON** 5 × 10^3 $TCID_{50}$ **HeV**	Ferret	[35]
	HeV-sG	CpG and Alhydrogel™	**SC** 4, 20, or 100 μg **HeV-sG**. Primed on day −434 and boosted on day −414 or primed on day −40 and boosted on day −20	**ON** 5 × 10^3 $TCID_{50}$ **NIV$_B$**	Ferret	[34]
	HeV-sG	CSIRO triple adjuvant and Montanide	**SC** 100 μg **HeV-sG**. Primed on day −104 and boosted on days −91 and − 76	**SC** 5 × 10^2 $TCID_{50}$ **NiV$_M$**	Cat	[41]
	HeV-sG	CpG and Alhydrogel™	**IM** 5, 25, or 50 μg **HeV-sG**. Primed on day −42 and boosted on day −21	**ON** 5 × 10^4 $TCID_{50}$ **NiV$_M$**	Cat	[36]
	NiV-sG	CSIRO triple adjuvant	**SC** 100 μg **NiV$_M$-sG**. Primed on day −104 and boosted on days −91 and − 76	**SC** 5 × 10^2 $TCID_{50}$ **NiV$_M$**	Cat	[41]

(continued)

Table 1 (continued)

Platform	Target antigen	Adjuvant(s)	Vaccination route, dose, and schedule	Challenge route, dose, and virus	Animal model	Ref.
VSV vector	NiV_M G	None	**IM** 1×10^7 PFU **rVSV-NiV_M-G**. single dose on day −29	**IT** 1×10^5 $TCID_{50}$ **NiV_M**	AGM	[32]
	NiV_B F and/ or G	None	**IM** 1×10^7 PFU **rVSV-NiV_B-F, −G, or -F/G**. single dose on day −28	**IT** 2.5 x 10^5 PFU and **IN** 2.5 x 10^5	AGM	[51]
	NiV_B F and/ or G	None	**IM** 1×10^7 PFU **rVSV-NiV_B-F, −G, or -F/G**. single dose on day −28	**IN** 5×10^3 PFU **NiV_M**	Ferret	[50]
	NiV_M F or G	None	**IM** 1×10^6 PFU **rVSV-NiV_M-F or -G**. single dose on day −32	**IP** 1×10^5 $TCID_{50}$ **NiV_M**	Hamster	[48]
	NiV_M F, G, or N	None	**IP** 1×10^5 PFU **rVSV-NiV_M- F, −G or -N**. single dose on day −28	**IP** 6.8×10^4 $TCID_{50}$ **NiV_M**	Hamster	[47]
	NiV_M G	None	**IP** 1×10^5 PFU **rVSV-NiV_M-G**. single dose on day −7, −3, −1, 0, +1, or + 3	**IP** 6.8×10^4 $TCID_{50}$ **NiV_M**	Hamster	[49]
	NiV_M F and/ or G	None	**IM** 1×10^6 PFU **rVSV-NiV_M-F or -G**, or 5×10^5 PFU each of **rVSV-NiV_M-F and -G**. single dose	N/A[b]	BALB/c mice	[55]
	HeV G	None	**IM** 1×10^5 PFU **rVSV-HeV-G**. single dose	N/A[b]	BALB/c mice	[52]
	HeV G	None	**IM** 10 μg of **chemically inactivated rVSV-HeV-G** particles given in three doses each 2 weeks apart	N/A[b]	BALB/c mice	[52]
RABV vector	NiV_M F and/ or G	None	**PO** 1×10^8 FFU **rRABV-ERAG$_{333E}$-NiV_M-F and/or -G** given in two doses 8 weeks apart	N/A[b]	Swine	[53]
	NiV_M F and/ or G	None	**PO** $1 \times 10^{6.5}$ FFU **rRABV-ERAG$_{333E}$-NiV_M-F and/or -G**. single dose	N/A[b]	BALB/c mice	[53]
	HeV G	None	**IM** 1×10^5 FFU **rRABV-HeV-G**. single dose	N/A[b]	BALB/c mice	[52]
	HeV G	None	**IM** 10 μg of **chemically inactivated rRABV-HeV-G** particles given in three doses each 2 weeks apart	N/A[b]	BALB/c mice	[52]
	NiV_B G	None	**IM** 10 μg of **chemically inactivated rRABV-NiV_B-G** particles given in two doses 4 weeks apart	N/A[b]	C57BL/ 6 mice	[54]
	NiV_B G	None	**IM** 1×10^5 FFU of **rRABV-NiV_B-G**. single dose	N/A[b]	C57BL/ 6 mice	[54]

NDV vector	NiV_M F and/ or G	None	**IM** 2×10^9 EID_{50} **rNDV-NiV_M-F and/or -G**. boosted 4 weeks after the first dose	N/A[b]	BALB/c mice	[56]
	NiV_M F and/ or G	None	**IM** 1×10^8 EID_{50} **rNDV-NiV_M-F and/or -G**. boosted 4 weeks after the first dose	N/A[b]	Swine	[56]
MV vector	NiV_M G	None	**IP** 2×10^4 $TCID_{50}$ of **rMV-HL-NiV_M-G** or **rMV-Ed-NiV_M-G**. primed on day −28 and boosted on day −7	**IP** 2×10^3 $TCID_{50}$ **NiV_M**	Hamster	[30]
	NiV_M G	None	**SC** 1×10^5 $TCID_{50}$ **rMV-Ed-NiV_M-G**. primed on day −35 and boosted on day −7	**IP** 1×10^5 $TCID_{50}$ **NiV_M**	AGM	[30]
Vaccinia vector	NiV_M F and/ or G	None	**SC** 1×10^7 PFU of **rVV-NiV_M-F, −G** or 5×10^6 of each **rVV-NiV_M-F and -G**. primed at −4 months and boosted at −3 months	**IP** 1×10^3 PFU **NiV_M**	Hamster	[57]
	NiV_M-sG or G	None	**IM** 1×10^8 PFU of **rMVA-NiV-sG** or **rMVA-NiV-G**. both single dose and prime boost (days −29 and − 8) strategies were used	N/A[b]	$IFNAR^{ko}$ mice	[60]
Canarypox vector	NiV_M G	None	**IM** 1×10^8 PFU **ALVAC-NiV_M-G**. two doses, one each on days 0 and 21	N/A[b]	Swine	[63]
	NiV_M F or G	None	**IM** 1×10^8 PFU **ALVAC-NiV_M-F and/or -G**. primed on day −28 and boosted on day −14	**IN** 2.5×10^5 PFU **NiV_M**	Swine	[58]
	HeV F and G	None	**SC** 7.4 log_{10} $CCID_{50}$ or 5.4 log_{10} $CCID_{50}$ **ALVAC-HeV-G and ALVAC-HeV-F** combination. Primed on day −42 and boosted on day −21	**IP** 1×10^3 LD_{50} HeV	Hamster	[59]
	HeV F and G	None	**SC** 6.0 log_{10} $CCID_{50}$ **ALVAC-HeV-G and ALVAC-HeV-F** combination. Primed on day −42 and boosted on day −21	N/A[b]	Ponies	[59]
VEEV vector	NiV_M G or HeV G	None	**IF** 3.1×10^5 IU **rVEEV-NiV_M-G** or 1.2×10^6 IU **rVEEV-HeV-G**. three doses, one each at weeks 0, 5, and 18	N/A[b]	C3H/he mice	[61]
	NiV_M F or HeV F	None	**IF** 50 μL[c] **rVEEV-NiV_M-F** or **rVEEV-HeV-F**. three doses, one each at weeks 0, 4, and 28	N/A[b]	C3H/he mice	[61]

(continued)

Table 1
(continued)

Platform	Target antigen	Adjuvant(s)	Vaccination route, dose, and schedule	Challenge route, dose, and virus	Animal model	Ref.
AAV vector	NiV_M G	None	**IM** 2.1×10^{10} genome particles or ID 1.1×10^{10} genome particles **rAAV1-NiV_M-G, rAAV8-NiV_M-G,** or **rAAVrh32.33-NiV_M-G**. some boosted after 16 weeks	N/A[b]	BALB/C mice	[33]
	NiV_M G	None	**IM** 6.1×10^{11} genome particles **rAAV8-NiV_M-G**. single dose on day −35	**IP** 1×10^4 PFU **NiV_M** or **HeV**	Hamster	[33]
ChAd vector	NiV_B G	None	**IM** 1×10^8 IU of **ChAdOx1 NiV_B G**. single dose on day −42 or primed on day −70, boosted day −42	**IP** 5.3×10^5 $TCID_{50}$ **NiV_B**	Hamster	[62]
	NiV_B G	None	**IM** 1×10^8 IU of **ChAdOx1 NiV_B G**. single dose on day −28	**IP** 6.8×10^4 $TCID_{50}$ **NiV_M**; 6.0×10^3 $TCID_{50}$ **HeV**	Hamster	[62]
BoHV vector	NiV_M F or G	None	**IM** 1×10^6 $TCID_{50}$ **BoHV-4-NiV_M-G** or **-F**. two doses, one each on days 0 and 21	N/A[b]	Swine	[63]
mRNA vaccine	HeV G	None	**IM** 10 μg or 30 μg of **LNP-encapsulated mRNA HeV-sG**. Single dose on day −30	**IP** 1×10^5 $TCID_{50}$ **NiV_M**	Hamster	[64]
DNA vaccine	NiV_M F and/ or G	None	**IM** 0.2, 0.6, 1.9, 5.6, 16.7, or 50 μg **pSV-NiV-F, and/or -G**. single dose on day −14	**ITh** 4.4×10^6 $TCID_{50}$ HIV pseu dovirus	BALB/c mice	[65]

VLP	NiV F, G, and M	None	**SC** 1.75, 3.5, 7, or 14 μg **NiV_M-VLPs**. Boosted with 6 μg at 2 and 4 weeks	N/A[b]	BALB/c mice	[66]
	NiV F, G, and M	None, MPLA, MPLA + alum, or CpG + alum	**IM** 30 μg **NiV_M-VLPs**. Primed on day −58 and boosted on days −37 and − 16	**IP** 1.6×10^4 PFU **NiV_M**	Hamster	[67]
	NiV F, G, and M	MPLA or CpG + alum	**IM** 30 μg **NiV_M-VLPs**. Single dose on day −28	**IP** 3.3×10^4 PFU **NiV_M**	Hamster	[67]
Attenuated NiV_M	Whole NiV	None	**IN** 5×10^3 PFU **rNiV_M-V^{ko}**. Single dose	N/A[b]	Ferret	[71]
Wild-type NiV_M	Whole NiV	None	**PO** 5×10^4 **NiV_M** single dose on day −28	**IN** 5×10^5 PFU **NiV_M**	Swine	[46]

[a] Dose divided evenly between the intranasal and intratracheal routes
[b] Animals were not challenged, instead neutralizing antibody was measured at various time points
[c] Dose could not be calculated due to the lack of a suitable immunofluorescent assay
AAV Adeno-associated virus, *BoHV* Bovine herpesvirus, *$CCID_{50}$* 50% cell culture infectious dose, *ChAd* Chimpanzee adenovirus, *CSIRO* Commonwealth Scientific and Industrial Research Organisation, *EID_{50}* 50% egg infective doses, *ID* Intradermal, *IF* Intrafootpad, *$IFNAR^{ko}$* Interferon receptor knock out, *IM* Intramuscular, *IN* Intranasal, *IP* Intraperitoneal, *ITh* Intrathoracic, *IU* Infectious units, *LNP* Lipid nanoparticle, *MPLA* Monophosphoryl lipid A, *MV* Measles virus, *NDV* Newcastle disease virus, *PFU* Plaque-forming units, *PO* Per os (oral), *RABV* Rabies virus, *SC* Subcutaneous, *$TCID_{50}$* 50% tissue culture infectious doses, *VEEV* Venezuelan equine encephalitis virus, *VLP* Virus-like particles, *VSV* Vesicular stomatitis virus

been the antigenic targets of almost all experimental vaccine approaches with only a few utilizing the nucleocapsid (N) or matrix (M) proteins as antigenic targets.

When choosing an ideal vaccine candidate for henipaviruses, there are several important factors to consider depending on the situation. In an outbreak scenario, the vaccine candidate would need to provide high levels of protection following a single-dose vaccination and the shorter duration from the time of vaccination to time of protection would be critical. In a standard vaccine program for an endemic nation, the durability of protection and cost would likely be more important than requiring a single-dose platform. The ability of a single vaccine candidate to protect against both HeV and NiV would be an advantage in either situation.

2.1 Subunit Vaccines

The most studied henipavirus vaccine candidate is a subunit vaccine consisting of soluble glycoprotein (sG) from HeV together with one or more adjuvants. The HeV-sG vaccine has been shown to protect 100% of ferrets [34, 35], cats [36, 41], horses [42], and AGMs [43–45] from experimental infection with HeV [35, 44, 45] and with NiV [34, 36, 41, 43, 45]. This is also the basis for the commercially available horse vaccine Equivac® HeV described in more detail below. The protective durability of HeV-sG vaccine is not known, although it is at least 12 months in ferrets that have received a booster after 20 days [34] and at least 6 months in horses boosted after 21 days [42]. In general, the durability of subunit vaccines is typically less than that of live virus vaccines.

Vaccination of swine with HeV-sG was less successful than with other animal models [46], although HeV and NiV are not lethal in swine. Vaccinated swine generated neutralizing antibody against HeV but not against NiV_M. Despite this, subsequent challenge with HeV led to only partial protection with a reduction in RNA load in tissues but no reduction in viral shedding. Challenge with NiV_M was not protective with high levels of viral RNA detected in tissues and no reduction in viral shedding. It was determined that cellular immunity was needed in swine and that neutralizing antibody was not sufficient to provide protection. Further studies elucidating the cellular immune responses have been performed using canarypox and BoHV vectors described below.

A NiV-sG vaccine was also shown to be 100% protective against experimental infection with NiV in cats [41], although further studies with this vaccine have not been published as the HeV-sG vaccine was used for all subsequent studies given the cross-protection against both HeV and NiV.

There is currently a version of the HeV-sG vaccine (termed HeV-sG-V) being examined in a phase 1 human clinical trial (NCT04199169) that contains either 10 μg, 30 μg, or 100 μg, with a 1:10 ratio of the adjuvant Alhydrogel™ in a two-dose series at either days 1 and 8 or days 1 and 29. This same formulation (either 100 μg or 300 μg of HeV-sG-V with a 1:10 ratio of

Alhydrogel™) was recently used in prime-boost and single-dose formats in AGMs and showed complete protection in as little as 1 week after the single-dose injection against both HeV and NiV_B in AGMs except for a single AGM who succumbed in the 300 μg single-dose group [45].

2.2 Rhabdovirus Vectors

The primary rhabdovirus vector used is VSV [32, 47–52] although RABV vectors have been used in some studies [52–54]. The general strategy involves utilizing recombinant replication-defective vectors that lack the normal glycoprotein and include an henipaviral antigen on the surface (F or G), although in some cases the native viral glycoprotein may be left intact.

VSV vectors expressing NiV F or G have proven to be 100% protective against NiV challenge in hamsters [47–49], ferrets [50], and AGMs [32, 51]. Most studies utilized NiV_M for the antigen and challenge virus, although some studies have utilized NiV_B as the antigen source and/or challenge virus. A VSV vector expressing NiV_M N demonstrated partial protection in hamsters [47].

Although most studies use a traditional method of vaccinating at least several weeks prior to challenge with infectious virus, one study [49] showed complete protection in hamsters when vaccinated as short as 1 day prior to challenge and partial protection when vaccinated 1 h after infection and possibly some minimal protection at 1 day after challenge. It has not yet been seen if this can be replicated in other animal models.

Additionally, multiple studies have shown that VSV and RABV vectors expressing HeV G, NiV_B G, and NiV_M F and/or G lead to the production of neutralizing antibody against HeV or NiV in mice [52–55]. One of these RABV vectors expressing NiV_M F and/or G was also tested in an oral formulation in swine, which subsequently developed neutralizing antibody; however, no viral challenge was performed to demonstrate protection against viral replication or shedding [53].

2.3 Paramyxovirus Vectors

NDV vectors expressing NiV_M F or G produced neutralizing antibody in mice and pigs [56]. This study used VSV-based NiV_M pseudotyped viruses for the neutralizing antibody assays. The neutralizing antibody response in swine lasted for at least 21 weeks but had reduced dramatically by 29 weeks. No challenge with henipaviruses was performed.

MV vectors using either the HL strain or Edmonston B (Ed) strain that expressed NiV_M G protein both demonstrated complete protection in hamsters against challenge with NiV_M in a prime-boost strategy [30]. These were also found to generate neutralizing antibody to MV and NiV_M suggesting that they might be used to vaccinate against both viruses simultaneously. The rMV-Ed-NiV_M-G was subsequently used in a prime-boost strategy in AGMs and protected them from challenge with NiV_M.

2.4 Poxvirus Vectors

Vaccinia virus vectors expressing NiV_M F or G proteins either individually or when mixed together were able to elicit a neutralizing antibody response in hamsters and confer protection from subsequent NiV_M challenge in a prime-boost strategy [57].

A canarypox vector (ALVAC strain) expressing NiV_M F or G proteins either individually, or when mixed together, produced an excellent response in vaccinated swine [58]. When subsequently challenged with NiV_M, none of the swine developed clinical disease or shed the detectable virus. In addition, they produced neutralizing antibody to NiV_M, although only weakly cross-protective for HeV. However, there were low levels of viral genome and antigen detected in some tissues when the animals were necropsied at the end of the study. While this was not a lethal model in the swine, control animals did shed high levels of virus, and they developed significant clinical disease, including neurologic disease, with significant viral levels and antigen detected in many tissues.

A subsequent study using a combination of two ALVAC vectors expressing HeV F and G evaluated different doses in hamsters and demonstrated significant protection against HeV challenge (89% or 8/9 hamsters with the high dose and 63% or 5/8 with the low dose) while producing the neutralizing antibody, decreasing viral shedding, and decreasing replication in tissues [59]. Challenge with NiV was not tested. The same combination was then used to vaccinate ponies, which demonstrated high levels of neutralizing antibody. Although the ponies were not subsequently challenged with either HeV or NiV, the level of neutralizing antibody was sufficiently high to be considered protective based on prior studies, albeit with the HeV-sG subunit vaccine.

Another vaccinia virus termed modified vaccinia Ankara (MVA) expressing either NiV_M G or sG was used to study immune responses in interferon receptor α and β knockout ($IFNAR^{ko}$) mice [60] using either single-dose regimens or a prime-boost regimen. These mice developed antibody, CD4 T-cell, and CD8 T-cell responses. Of note, using sG as the antigen target elicited stronger T-cell responses than the full-length G antigen.

2.5 VEEV Vector

VEEV vectors expressing NiV_M F, NiV_M G, HeV F, or HeV G were able to produce neutralizing antibody in vaccinated mice as determined utilizing an HIV pseudotype virus assay that was cross-reactive against both NiV_M and HeV regardless of which antigen was used [61]. Again, no henipavirus challenge was performed as immunocompetent mice are not susceptible.

2.6 AAV Vector

Prime-boost vaccination with AAV1, AAV8, and AAVrh32.33 vectors expressing NiV_M G was able to elicit comparable neutralizing antibody production in mice [33]. The AAV8-NiV_M-G vector was subsequently used to vaccinate hamsters in a single-dose strategy conferring complete protection from subsequent challenge with NiV_M, but only 50% protection from challenge with HeV.

2.7 ChAd Vector

A ChAd vector expressing NiV_B G protein conferred complete protection for vaccinated hamsters against lethal challenge with NiV_B with either a prime-boost or single-dose strategy. The same vaccine also conferred complete protection against lethal challenge with NiV_M and partial protection (33% or 2/6 hamsters surviving) against lethal challenge with HeV after a single-dose vaccination [62].

2.8 BoHV Vector

Innate and adaptive immune responses to vaccination in swine were examined using BoHV vectors expressing either NiV_M F or G, or with the canarypox ALVAC vector expressing NiV_M G [63]. The swine were not challenged with NiV or HeV, but potent neutralizing antibody against NiV_M and NiV_B pseudoviruses, CD4 T-cell, and CD8 T-cell responses was observed with both BoHV vectors and the ALVAC vector.

2.9 Nucleic Acid-Based Vaccines

The use of an LNP-encapsulated mRNA vaccine encoding HeV-sG was found to be partially protective against NiV_M in hamsters when given as a single dose of either 10 μg (3/10 hamsters survived) or 30 μg (7/10 hamsters survived) [64]. There was a poor antibody response found in hamsters 25 days after vaccination, which may account for the vaccine being only partially protective.

DNA vaccines utilizing plasmids expressing NiV_M F and/or G were subsequently challenged with an HIV-based NiV_M pseudovirus to test the vaccine in mice under BSL-2 conditions [65]. This demonstrated that the mice produced neutralizing antibody against the pseudovirus. It is not yet clear if this translates to protection against henipaviruses in a susceptible host.

2.10 VLP

NiV_M-VLPs produced using NiV_M F, G, and M were shown to induce a neutralizing antibody response in mice [66]. No challenge could be performed as mice are not susceptible to henipavirus infection; therefore, a subsequent study demonstrated that NiV_M-VLPs induced neutralizing antibody and also conferred protection in hamsters given a subsequent lethal challenge with NiV_M [67]. This occurred with either a three-dose series or a single-dose series with adjuvant administration.

2.11 Attenuated Live Virus

Various $rNiV_M$ mutants have been produced that are attenuated in animal models. NiV_M mutants lacking expression of either the C protein or V protein were attenuated in the hamster model [68] although these animals were not subsequently challenged with wild-type virus, nor was the presence of any neutralizing antibody assessed making it unclear if this could function as a vaccine at the doses used. In contrast, in the ferret model, a NiV_M mutant lacking C protein expression [69] or a functional STAT1 binding domain [70] was not attenuated. A NiV_M mutant lacking V protein expression was attenuated, and all infected ferrets survived without significant clinical disease while also generating neutralizing antibody

[71]; however, these ferrets were not subsequently challenged with wild-type virus. A NiV_M mutant lacking expression of both the C and W proteins was partially attenuated in ferrets [69]; the surviving ferrets demonstrated significant disease, and they were not subsequently challenged with wild-type virus.

2.12 Wild-Type Live Virus

As swine were associated with the initial NiV_M outbreak, but they do not develop the lethal disease, one study has demonstrated that infection with wild-type NiV_M leads to natural immunity that prevents subsequent experimental infection 4 weeks later [46].

2.13 Summary of Henipavirus Vaccine Candidates

Numerous platforms have been used to examine candidate henipavirus vaccines. Most of these have used NiV_M challenge to prove effectiveness, although a few have also been tested against HeV and/or NiV_B. The most studied vaccine is the subunit HeV-sG vaccine, which is protective against HeV, NiV_M, and NiV_B in multiple animal models including AGMs; one formulation is licensed for use in horses, and a similar formulation is currently in a phase 1 human clinical trial. The second most studied platform is the VSV vector, although it is important to note that there are slight variations in the VSV vectors used in the various studies; taken together, these studies demonstrate that the VSV vector is a robust vaccine platform that is protective against NiV_M and NiV_B in multiple animal models including AGMs. It is not clear if these would offer cross-protection against HeV infection, although several of the various vaccine studies suggest that NiV antigens do not completely cross-protect against HeV. Although there are numerous other platforms, these have not been as robustly studied; often, they have been examined only in single studies and in single animal models. Some of these have only been examined in mice without subsequent henipavirus challenge. With the recent implantation of two highly successful LNP-encapsulated mRNA vaccines in humans against SARS-CoV-2 during the COVID-19 pandemic [72], there is likely to be considerably more emphasis on this as a vaccine platform in the near future for other diseases, including for henipaviruses.

3 Domesticated Animal Vaccines

All human cases of HeV have been tied to outbreaks in horses in Australia. These outbreaks have also affected the lucrative racehorse industry in Australia. This has led to the pursuit of equine vaccines to protect against HeV [73, 74]. Additionally, the initial outbreak of NiV was linked to a massive swine outbreak in Malaysia that led to the culling of 1.1 million swine (45% of all swine in Malaysia) with an enormous economic impact [75]. Therefore, significant interest has led to attempts to develop a swine vaccine to protect the swine industry in Southeast Asia and to prevent subsequent transmission to humans. These animal vaccines fit in with the "One Health" concept [42].

3.1 Horse Vaccines

Due to the success of the HeV-sG vaccine studies described above in multiple animal models, including horses [42, 73], this same vaccine approach was used to produce a commercially available equine vaccine, Equivac® HeV by Zoetis™, which became available in November 2012 in Australia as the first commercially available vaccine against a BSL-4 agent. Equivac® HeV is formulated using 100 μg of HeV-sG prepared in cell culture with a proprietary adjuvant. It is administered to horses as two intramuscular injections 3–6 weeks apart followed by boosting at six-month intervals [29]. Subsequently, a post-marketing microchip database was created for all vaccinated horses (>120,000) and no significant side effects were reported; however, injection site reactions were reported in <0.25% of horses [73]. No vaccinated horses have become infected in subsequent outbreaks, while at least 22 laboratory-confirmed cases of HeV in horses have occurred in nonvaccinated horses in Australia since Equivac® HeV became available. Also notable is that no human cases have been reported since horses began being vaccinated, lending support to the "One Health" concept.

3.2 Swine Vaccines

Despite the success of HeV-sG subunit vaccines in multiple animal models as discussed above, this has failed to protect swine against NiV challenge and was only partially protective against HeV challenge [46]. As discussed above, a canarypox virus vector expressing NiV_M G or F has been reported to protect swine against developing the disease with NiV_M challenge [58]. Both recombinant NDV [56] and RABV [53] vectors expressing NiV G and/or F demonstrated the ability to induce durable NiV-specific neutralizing antibodies in swine; however, no challenge was performed in these studies; therefore, it is unclear if this translates into true protection against henipavirus infection. Interestingly, the RABV vector was trialed as an oral vaccine, which would decrease the cost of administration to mass livestock populations. The unique technical and economic challenges to developing a swine vaccine for henipaviruses, as well as a detailed discussion on the current state of vaccine candidates and future directions, were recently reviewed [75].

4 Experimental Therapeutics

Given the sporadic nature of henipavirus outbreaks, vaccinating entire populations may not be a feasible option. In these cases, having access to effective antiviral therapies would be of tremendous benefit. Various established and novel therapeutics have been trialed to determine antiviral activity against henipaviruses. Although numerous compounds have been examined in vitro for anti-henipaviral activity, here we will only discuss those that have been examined in at least on the animal model.

4.1 Ribavirin

Ribavirin is known to have broad-spectrum antiviral activity and is effective against many RNA and DNA viruses. During the initial NiV outbreak in 1998, ribavirin was empirically used and was initially reported in nonrandomized trials to have a 36% reduction in mortality [76], although there were other confounding factors that might have contributed. Subsequent animal studies showed no mortality benefit with the use of ribavirin in hamsters or AGMs infected with NiV or HeV [77–79].

4.2 Chloroquine

Chloroquine is an antimalarial drug and was found to be effective against henipaviruses in vitro by itself or when combined with ribavirin; however, it was ineffective in protecting hamsters [79] and ferrets [80].

4.3 Antibodies

Passive immunization using antibodies directed against the surface glycoproteins of HeV has proven effective against HeV and NiV in both pre- and post-exposure therapeutic approaches in hamsters, ferrets, and AGMs [57, 81–88]. This was also demonstrated using an HIV-based NiV pseudovirus in mice [65]. The most studied passive immunization therapeutic is m102.4, which is a human monoclonal antibody specific for the HeV G protein [81, 89] and blocks the receptor-binding site. This has protected AGMs when given as late as 5 and 7 days after infection with a lethal dose of NiV_M [27, 83]; however, it is notable that this is still before any clinical signs of disease develop, although all AGMs were positive for NiV_M RNA in blood beginning at day 5. This antibody was shown to be safe in a human phase 1 clinical trial [90] and has been given to at least 11 humans under compassionate use who had significant exposure risk with henipaviruses [29, 74, 91]. Recently, the humanized antibody h5B3.1 against the F protein of HeV and NiV has been shown to be protective in ferrets infected with either HeV or NiV_M when given as late as 3 and 5 days after infection [88]. It is reasonable to consider that cocktail containing antibodies targeting both the G and F proteins (such as m102.4 and h5B3.1) could prove to be a potent post-exposure therapeutic combination.

4.4 Purine Analogs

A purine analog with broad-spectrum antiviral activity, favipiravir (T-705; 6-fluoro-3-hydroxy-2-pyrazinecarboxamide), which has been approved for use in Japan against emerging influenza strains and is currently being evaluated in multiple clinical trials in the United States and Europe, demonstrated the ability to protect hamsters from experimental infection with NiV_M [92]. This medication works as a viral RNA-dependent RNA polymerase inhibitor.

When hamsters were administered favipiravir either twice daily orally or once daily subcutaneously for 14 days, beginning on the day of infection with a lethal dose of NiV_M, 100% were protected from disease. In both cases, a loading dose of 600 mg/kg/day was used on day 0 and 300 mg/kg/day on all subsequent days. It is not yet clear how long after henipavirus infection this could be administered and still be effective, or if the duration could be shortened.

The purine analog prodrug remdesivir (GS-5734) is a 1′-cyano-substituted adenosine nucleotide analog with broad-spectrum antiviral activity including against coronaviruses (including SARS-CoV-2), filoviruses, and paramyxoviruses that were shown to confer complete protection against lethal NiV_B challenge in AGMs when given as an IV infusion (10 mg/kg) beginning 24 hours after infection and repeated daily for 12 days [93]. Of note, all treated animals seroconverted within 15 days of infection. Half (two of four AGMs) developed mild, self-resolving signs of respiratory disease, and only one AGM had a transient viremia detected. All AGMs were observed until 92 days post-infection to monitor for signs of late-onset encephalitis, but no neurologic signs were detected. Additional studies will be needed to determine if the treatment duration could be decreased or started later than 24 hours post-infection and still be protective.

4.5 Fusion Inhibitors

Cholesterol-tagged peptides derived from C-terminal heptad repeat regions of paramyxovirus F proteins are able to potently inhibit the fusion of NiV with infected target cells in vitro [94] and were partially effective in hamsters [95]. This was most effective when given prior to infection, with less protective effect the further out from the time of infection it was administered.

4.6 Interferon Inducers

Interferon antagonism is known to be important in the pathogenesis of many paramyxoviruses, and henipaviruses have developed multiple mechanisms to evade the interferon response [28, 69, 71, 96–102]. The interferon inducer poly(I)-poly(C_{12}U) was found to be partially protective against NiV infection in the hamster model when given as daily injections for 10 consecutive days after NiV_M infection [78]. This molecule has a well-established safety profile in humans [103].

4.7 Inhibitors of Pyrimidine Nucleotides

Examined at the same time as poly(I)-poly(C_{12}U) and ribavirin mentioned above, the orotidine 5′-phosphate (OMP) decarboxylase inhibitor 6-azauridine was found to not be effective in treating hamsters infected with NiV_M [78].

4.8 Summary of Therapeutics

Of the various experimental therapeutics tested in animals, only monoclonal antibodies, especially m102.4, have had multiple robust preclinical studies showing complete effectiveness in multiple animal models against both HeV and NiV, and m102.4 has been safely given to humans under compassionate use and in a phase 1 clinical trial. This antibody is effective even when given several days after exposure to lethal doses, which makes it a useful therapeutic option with the caveat that it does not appear to be effective when given after symptoms of henipavirus infection have arisen. It may prove to be even more effective when combined in a cocktail with antibodies targeting additional henipavirus proteins such as h5B3.1.

Favipiravir and remdesivir have each only been used in a single study in a single animal model; however, these therapeutics have the advantage of not requiring a cold chain and the ability to easily stockpile. They are also further along in the pipeline for approval for use in humans for other viral diseases than the other therapeutics described; remdesivir particularly has the advantage that it has been used extensively in humans to treat SARS-CoV-2 infection and has robust and excellent safety data [104]. Favipiravir and remdesivir also have the potential for broad-spectrum antiviral therapy making them attractive options. Further studies in additional animal models and against other henipavirus strains will be helpful to understand the potential benefits of these therapies.

Fusion inhibitors and interferon inducers have both shown partial efficacy in single studies in hamsters without any additional follow-up studies being performed in other animal models making it hard to draw too firm of conclusions about their potential use. Ribavirin, despite initial hope of efficacy in humans, does not appear to be effective when examined under more controlled in vivo models.

5 Concluding Remarks

Significant progress has been made in the development of potential vaccines and therapeutics against henipavirus infection. There are multiple platforms that have undergone robust preclinical studies. One vaccine, HeV-sG-V, is currently in a human phase 1 clinical trial and one therapeutic, monoclonal antibody m102.4, was shown to be safe in a completed human phase 1 clinical trial, while remdesivir has extensive safety data from use against SARS-CoV-2. Additional vaccine and therapeutic candidates discussed here are likely to proceed into human clinical trials in the future as well. With the unfortunate realization of the current COVID-19 pandemic, the need for urgent preparation of vaccines and therapeutics against other viral illnesses with significant pandemic potential, such as henipaviruses, has become even more clear.

References

1. Mathieu C, Horvat B (2015) Henipavirus pathogenesis and antiviral approaches. Expert Rev Anti-Infect Ther 13(3):343–354. https://doi.org/10.1586/14787210.2015.1001838
2. Weatherman S, Feldmann H, de Wit E (2018) Transmission of henipaviruses. Curr Opin Virol 28:7–11. https://doi.org/10.1016/j.coviro.2017.09.004
3. Clayton BA, Wang LF, Marsh GA (2013) Henipaviruses: an updated review focusing on the pteropid reservoir and features of transmission. Zoonoses Public Health 60(1): 69–83. https://doi.org/10.1111/j.1863-2378.2012.01501.x
4. Halpin K, Young PL, Field HE, Mackenzie JS (2000) Isolation of Hendra virus from pteropid bats: a natural reservoir of Hendra virus. J Gen Virol 81(Pt 8):1927–1932
5. Field H, Schaaf K, Kung N, Simon C, Waltisbuhl D, Hobert H, Moore F, Middleton D, Crook A, Smith G, Daniels P, Glanville R, Lovell D (2010) Hendra virus outbreak with novel clinical features, Australia. Emerg Infect Dis 16(2):338–340. https://doi.org/10.3201/eid1602.090780
6. Playford EG, McCall B, Smith G, Slinko V, Allen G, Smith I, Moore F, Taylor C, Kung YH, Field H (2010) Human Hendra virus encephalitis associated with equine outbreak, Australia, 2008. Emerg Infect Dis 16(2): 219–223. https://doi.org/10.3201/eid1602.090552
7. McCormack JG, Allworth AM, Selvey LA, Selleck PW (1999) Transmissibility from horses to humans of a novel paramyxovirus, equine morbillivirus (EMV). J Infect 38(1): 22–23
8. Selvey LA, Wells RM, McCormack JG, Ansford AJ, Murray K, Rogers RJ, Lavercombe PS, Selleck P, Sheridan JW (1995) Infection of humans and horses by a newly described morbillivirus. Med J Aust 162(12): 642–645
9. Westbury HA (2000) Hendra virus disease in horses. Rev Sci Tech 19(1):151–159
10. Chua KB, Goh KJ, Wong KT, Kamarulzaman A, Tan PS, Ksiazek TG, Zaki SR, Paul G, Lam SK, Tan CT (1999) Fatal encephalitis due to Nipah virus among pig-farmers in Malaysia. Lancet 354(9186): 1257–1259. https://doi.org/10.1016/S0140-6736(99)04299-3
11. Chua KB, Bellini WJ, Rota PA, Harcourt BH, Tamin A, Lam SK, Ksiazek TG, Rollin PE, Zaki SR, Shieh W, Goldsmith CS, Gubler DJ, Roehrig JT, Eaton B, Gould AR, Olson J, Field H, Daniels P, Ling AE, Peters CJ, Anderson LJ, Mahy BW (2000) Nipah virus: a recently emergent deadly paramyxovirus. Science 288(5470):1432–1435
12. Gurley ES, Montgomery JM, Hossain MJ, Bell M, Azad AK, Islam MR, Molla MA, Carroll DS, Ksiazek TG, Rota PA, Lowe L, Comer JA, Rollin P, Czub M, Grolla A, Feldmann H, Luby SP, Woodward JL, Breiman RF (2007) Person-to-person transmission of Nipah virus in a Bangladeshi community. Emerg Infect Dis 13(7): 1031–1037. https://doi.org/10.3201/eid1307.061128
13. Harcourt BH, Lowe L, Tamin A, Liu X, Bankamp B, Bowden N, Rollin PE, Comer JA, Ksiazek TG, Hossain MJ, Gurley ES, Breiman RF, Bellini WJ, Rota PA (2005) Genetic characterization of Nipah virus, Bangladesh, 2004. Emerg Infect Dis 11(10):1594–1597
14. Homaira N, Rahman M, Hossain MJ, Epstein JH, Sultana R, Khan MS, Podder G, Nahar K, Ahmed B, Gurley ES, Daszak P, Lipkin WI, Rollin PE, Comer JA, Ksiazek TG, Luby SP (2010) Nipah virus outbreak with person-to-person transmission in a district of Bangladesh, 2007. Epidemiol Infect 138(11):1630–1636. https://doi.org/10.1017/S0950268810000695
15. Hossain MJ, Gurley ES, Montgomery JM, Bell M, Carroll DS, Hsu VP, Formenty P, Croisier A, Bertherat E, Faiz MA, Azad AK, Islam R, Molla MA, Ksiazek TG, Rota PA, Comer JA, Rollin PE, Luby SP, Breiman RF (2008) Clinical presentation of Nipah virus infection in Bangladesh. Clin Infect Dis 46(7):977–984. https://doi.org/10.1086/529147
16. Hsu VP, Hossain MJ, Parashar UD, Ali MM, Ksiazek TG, Kuzmin I, Niezgoda M, Rupprecht C, Bresee J, Breiman RF (2004) Nipah virus encephalitis reemergence, Bangladesh. Emerg Infect Dis 10(12): 2082–2087
17. Luby SP, Rahman M, Hossain MJ, Blum LS, Husain MM, Gurley E, Khan R, Ahmed BN, Rahman S, Nahar N, Kenah E, Comer JA, Ksiazek TG (2006) Foodborne transmission of Nipah virus, Bangladesh. Emerg Infect Dis 12(12):1888–1894. https://doi.org/10.3201/eid1212.060732
18. Quddus R, Alam S, Majumdar MA, Anwar S, Khan MR, Zahid Mahmud Khan AKS, Arif SM, Alam R, Siddique FM, Tan CT (2004)

A report of 4 patients with Nipah encephalitis from Rajbari district, Bangladesh in the January 2004 outbreak. Neurol Asia 9:33–37
19. Rahman MA, Hossain MJ, Sultana S, Homaira N, Khan SU, Rahman M, Gurley ES, Rollin PE, Lo MK, Comer JA, Lowe L, Rota PA, Ksiazek TG, Kenah E, Sharker Y, Luby SP (2012) Date palm sap linked to Nipah virus outbreak in Bangladesh, 2008. Vector Borne Zoonotic Dis 12(1):65–72. https://doi.org/10.1089/vbz.2011.0656
20. Arankalle VA, Bandyopadhyay BT, Ramdasi AY, Jadi R, Patil DR, Rahman M, Majumdar M, Banerjee PS, Hati AK, Goswami RP, Neogi DK, Mishra AC (2011) Genomic characterization of Nipah virus, West Bengal, India. Emerg Infect Dis 17(5): 907–909. https://doi.org/10.3201/eid1705.100968
21. Chadha MS, Comer JA, Lowe L, Rota PA, Rollin PE, Bellini WJ, Ksiazek TG, Mishra A (2006) Nipah virus-associated encephalitis outbreak, Siliguri, India. Emerg Infect Dis 12(2):235–240
22. Chatterjee P (2018) Nipah virus outbreak in India. Lancet 391(10136):2200
23. Ching PKG, de los Reyes VC, Sucaldito MN, Tayag E, Columna-Vingno AB, Malbas FF, Bolo GC, Sejvar JJ, Eagles D, Payford G, Dueger E, Kaku Y, Marikawa S, Kuroda M, Marsh GA, McCullough S, Foxwell AR (2015) Outbreak of Henipavirus infection, Philippines, 2014. Emerg Infect Dis 21:328
24. Goh KJ, Tan CT, Chew NK, Tan PS, Kamarulzaman A, Sarji SA, Wong KT, Abdullah BJ, Chua KB, Lam SK (2000) Clinical features of Nipah virus encephalitis among pig farmers in Malaysia. N Engl J Med 342(17):1229–1235. https://doi.org/10.1056/NEJM200004273421701
25. Islam MS, Sazzad HMS, Satter SM, Sultana S, Hossain MJ, Hasan M, Rahman M, Campbell S, Cannon DL, Ströher U (2016) Nipah virus transmission from bats to humans associated with drinking traditional liquor made from date palm sap, Bangladesh, 2011–2014. Emerg Infect Dis 22(4):664
26. Chong HT, Hossain MJ, Tan CT (2008) Differences in epidemiologic and clinical features of Nipah virus encephalitis between the Malaysian and Bangladesh outbreaks. Neurology Asia 13:23–26
27. Mire CE, Satterfield BA, Geisbert JB, Agans KN, Borisevich V, Yan L, Chan Y-P, Cross RW, Fenton KA, Broder CC, Geisbert TW (2016) Pathogenic differences between Nipah virus Bangladesh and Malaysia strains in primates: implications for antibody therapy. Sci Rep 6:30916
28. Satterfield BA, Geisbert TW, Mire CE (2016) Inhibition of the host antiviral response by Nipah virus: current understanding and future perspectives. Futur Virol 11(5): 331–344
29. Satterfield BA, Dawes BE, Milligan GN (2016) Status of vaccine research and development of vaccines for Nipah virus. Vaccine 34(26):2971–2975. https://doi.org/10.1016/j.vaccine.2015.12.075
30. Yoneda M, Georges-Courbot M-C, Ikeda F, Ishii M, Nagata N, Jacquot F, Raoul H, Sato H, Kai C (2013) Recombinant measles virus vaccine expressing the Nipah virus glycoprotein protects against lethal Nipah virus challenge. PLoS One 8(3):e58414
31. Vigant F, Lee B (2011) Hendra and Nipah infection: pathology, models and potential therapies. Infect Disord Drug Targets 11(3): 315–336. BSP/ID-DT/E-Pub/000178-11-3 [pii]
32. Prescott J, DeBuysscher BL, Feldmann F, Gardner DJ, Haddock E, Martellaro C, Scott D, Feldmann H (2015) Single-dose live-attenuated vesicular stomatitis virus-based vaccine protects African green monkeys from Nipah virus disease. Vaccine 33(24): 2823–2829
33. Ploquin A, Szecsi J, Mathieu C, Guillaume V, Barateau V, Ong KC, Wong KT, Cosset FL, Horvat B, Salvetti A (2013) Protection against henipavirus infection by use of recombinant adeno-associated virus-vector vaccines. J Infect Dis 207(3):469–478. https://doi.org/10.1093/infdis/jis699
34. Pallister JA, Klein R, Arkinstall R, Haining J, Long F, White JR, Payne J, Feng YR, Wang LF, Broder CC, Middleton D (2013) Vaccination of ferrets with a recombinant G glycoprotein subunit vaccine provides protection against Nipah virus disease for over 12 months. Virol J 10:237. https://doi.org/10.1186/1743-422X-10-237
35. Pallister J, Middleton D, Wang LF, Klein R, Haining J, Robinson R, Yamada M, White J, Payne J, Feng YR, Chan YP, Broder CC (2011) A recombinant Hendra virus G glycoprotein-based subunit vaccine protects ferrets from lethal Hendra virus challenge. Vaccine 29(34):5623–5630. https://doi.org/10.1016/j.vaccine.2011.06.015
36. McEachern JA, Bingham J, Crameri G, Green DJ, Hancock TJ, Middleton D, Feng YR, Broder CC, Wang LF, Bossart KN (2008) A recombinant subunit vaccine formulation protects against lethal Nipah virus challenge in cats. Vaccine 26(31):3842–3852. https://doi.org/10.1016/j.vaccine.2008.05.016

37. Meganck RM, Baric RS (2021) Developing therapeutic approaches for twenty-first-century emerging infectious viral diseases. Nat Med 27(3):401–410
38. Plotkin SA (2017) Vaccines for epidemic infections and the role of CEPI. Hum Vaccin Immunother 13(12):2755–2762. https://doi.org/10.1080/21645515.2017.1306615
39. Satterfield BA (2017) The future of preventing and treating Nipah virus infection, vol 3. Future Sci
40. Prasad AN, Woolsey C, Geisbert JB, Agans KN, Borisevich V, Deer DJ, Mire CE, Cross RW, Fenton KA, Broder CC (2020) Resistance of Cynomolgus monkeys to Nipah and Hendra virus disease is associated with cell-mediated and humoral immunity. J Infect Dis 221(Suppl 4):S436–S447
41. Mungall BA, Middleton D, Crameri G, Bingham J, Halpin K, Russell G, Green D, McEachern J, Pritchard LI, Eaton BT, Wang LF, Bossart KN, Broder CC (2006) Feline model of acute Nipah virus infection and protection with a soluble glycoprotein-based subunit vaccine. J Virol 80(24):12293–12302. https://doi.org/10.1128/JVI.01619-06
42. Middleton D, Pallister J, Klein R, Feng Y-R, Haining J, Arkinstall R, Frazer L, Huang J-A, Edwards N, Wareing M (2014) Hendra virus vaccine, a one health approach to protecting horse, human, and environmental health. Emerg Infect Dis 20(3):372
43. Bossart KN, Rockx B, Feldmann F, Brining D, Scott D, LaCasse R, Geisbert JB, Feng YR, Chan YP, Hickey AC (2012) A Hendra virus G glycoprotein subunit vaccine protects African Green monkeys from Nipah virus challenge. Sci Transl Med 4(146):146ra107-146ra107
44. Mire CE, Geisbert JB, Agans KN, Feng YR, Fenton KA, Bossart KN, Yan L, Chan YP, Broder CC, Geisbert TW (2014) A recombinant Hendra virus G glycoprotein subunit vaccine protects nonhuman primates against Hendra virus challenge. J Virol 88(9):4624–4631. https://doi.org/10.1128/JVI.00005-14
45. Geisbert TW, Bobb K, Borisevich V, Geisbert JB, Agans KN, Cross RW, Prasad AN, Fenton KA, Yu H, Fouts TR (2021) A single dose investigational subunit vaccine for human use against Nipah virus and Hendra virus. NPJ Vaccines 6(1):1–12
46. Pickering BS, Hardham JM, Smith G, Weingartl ET, Dominowski PJ, Foss DL, Mwangi D, Broder CC, Roth JA, Weingartl HM (2016) Protection against henipaviruses in swine requires both, cell-mediated and humoral immune response. Vaccine 34(40):4777–4786. https://doi.org/10.1016/j.vaccine.2016.08.028
47. DeBuysscher BL, Scott D, Marzi A, Prescott J, Feldmann H (2014) Single-dose live-attenuated Nipah virus vaccines confer complete protection by eliciting antibodies directed against surface glycoproteins. Vaccine 32(22):2637–2644
48. Lo MK, Bird BH, Chattopadhyay A, Drew CP, Martin BE, Coleman JD, Rose JK, Nichol ST, Spiropoulou CF (2014) Single-dose replication-defective VSV-based Nipah virus vaccines provide protection from lethal challenge in Syrian hamsters. Antivir Res 101:26–29
49. DeBuysscher BL, Scott D, Thomas T, Feldmann H, Prescott J (2016) Peri-exposure protection against Nipah virus disease using a single-dose recombinant vesicular stomatitis virus-based vaccine. NPJ Vaccines 1:16002
50. Mire CE, Versteeg KM, Cross RW, Agans KN, Fenton KA, Whitt MA, Geisbert TW (2013) Single injection recombinant vesicular stomatitis virus vaccines protect ferrets against lethal Nipah virus disease. Virol J 10:353. https://doi.org/10.1186/1743-422X-10-353
51. Mire CE, Geisbert JB, Agans KN, Versteeg KM, Deer DJ, Satterfield BA, Fenton KA, Geisbert TW (2019) Use of single-injection recombinant vesicular stomatitis virus vaccine to protect nonhuman primates against lethal Nipah virus disease. Emerg Infect Dis 25(6):1144–1152. https://doi.org/10.3201/eid2506.181620
52. Kurup D, Wirblich C, Feldmann H, Marzi A, Schnell MJ (2015) Rhabdovirus-based vaccine platforms against henipaviruses. J Virol 89(1):144–154. https://doi.org/10.1128/JVI.02308-14
53. Shuai L, Ge J, Wen Z, Wang J, Wang X, Bu Z (2020) Immune responses in mice and pigs after oral vaccination with rabies virus vectored Nipah disease vaccines. Vet Microbiol 241:108549
54. Keshwara R, Shiels T, Postnikova E, Kurup D, Wirblich C, Johnson RF, Schnell MJ (2019) Rabies-based vaccine induces potent immune responses against Nipah virus. NPJ Vaccines 4:15. https://doi.org/10.1038/s41541-019-0109-5
55. Chattopadhyay A, Rose JK (2011) Complementing defective viruses that express separate paramyxovirus glycoproteins provide a new vaccine vector approach. J Virol 85(5):2004–2011
56. Kong D, Wen Z, Su H, Ge J, Chen W, Wang X, Wu C, Yang C, Chen H, Bu Z

(2012) Newcastle disease virus-vectored Nipah encephalitis vaccines induce B and T cell responses in mice and long-lasting neutralizing antibodies in pigs. Virology 432(2): 327–335

57. Guillaume V, Contamin H, Loth P, Georges-Courbot MC, Lefeuvre A, Marianneau P, Chua KB, Lam SK, Buckland R, Deubel V (2004) Nipah virus: vaccination and passive protection studies in a hamster model. J Virol 78(2):834–840
58. Weingartl HM, Berhane Y, Caswell JL, Loosmore S, Audonnet J-C, Roth JA, Czub M (2006) Recombinant Nipah virus vaccines protect pigs against challenge. J Virol 80(16): 7929–7938
59. Guillaume-Vasselin V, Lemaitre L, Dhondt KP, Tedeschi L, Poulard A, Charreyre C, Horvat B (2016) Protection from Hendra virus infection with canarypox recombinant vaccine. NPJ Vaccines 1(1):1–8
60. Kalodimou G, Veit S, Jany S, Kalinke U, Broder CC, Sutter G, Volz A (2020) A soluble version of Nipah virus glycoprotein G delivered by vaccinia virus MVA activates specific CD8 and CD4 T cells in mice. Viruses 12(1): 26
61. Defang GN, Khetawat D, Broder CC, Quinnan GV (2010) Induction of neutralizing antibodies to Hendra and Nipah glycoproteins using a Venezuelan equine encephalitis virus in vivo expression system. Vaccine 29(2): 212–220
62. van Doremalen N, Lambe T, Sebastian S, Bushmaker T, Fischer R, Feldmann F, Haddock E, Letko M, Avanzato VA, Rissanen I, LaCasse R, Scott D, Bowden TA, Gilbert S, Munster V (2019) A single-dose ChAdOx1-vectored vaccine provides complete protection against Nipah Bangladesh and Malaysia in Syrian golden hamsters. PLoS Negl Trop Dis 13(6):e0007462. https://doi.org/10.1371/journal.pntd.0007462
63. Pedrera M, Macchi F, McLean RK, Franceschi V, Thakur N, Russo L, Medfai L, Todd S, Tchilian EZ, Audonnet J-C (2020) Bovine herpesvirus-4-vectored delivery of Nipah virus glycoproteins enhances T cell immunogenicity in pigs. Vaccine 8(1):115
64. Lo MK, Spengler JR, Welch SR, Harmon JR, Coleman-McCray JD, Scholte FE, Shrivastava-Ranjan P, Montgomery JM, Nichol ST, Weissman D (2020) Evaluation of a single-dose nucleoside-modified messenger RNA vaccine encoding Hendra virus-soluble glycoprotein against lethal Nipah virus challenge in Syrian hamsters. J Infect Dis 221(Suppl 4):S493–S498
65. Nie J, Liu L, Wang Q, Chen R, Ning T, Liu Q, Huang W, Wang Y (2019) Nipah pseudovirus system enables evaluation of vaccines in vitro and in vivo using non-BSL-4 facilities. Emerg Microbes Infect 8(1):272–281. https://doi.org/10.1080/22221751.2019.1571871
66. Walpita P, Barr J, Sherman M, Basler CF, Wang L (2011) Vaccine potential of Nipah virus-like particles. PLoS One 6(4):e18437. https://doi.org/10.1371/journal.pone.0018437
67. Walpita P, Cong Y, Jahrling PB, Rojas O, Postnikova E, Yu S, Johns L, Holbrook MR (2017) A VLP-based vaccine provides complete protection against Nipah virus challenge following multiple-dose or single-dose vaccination schedules in a hamster model. NPJ Vaccines 2:21. https://doi.org/10.1038/s41541-017-0023-7
68. Yoneda M, Guillaume V, Sato H, Fujita K, Georges-Courbot MC, Ikeda F, Omi M, Muto-Terao Y, Wild TF, Kai C (2010) The nonstructural proteins of Nipah virus play a key role in pathogenicity in experimentally infected animals. PLoS One 5(9):e12709. https://doi.org/10.1371/journal.pone.0012709
69. Satterfield BA, Cross RW, Fenton KA, Borisevich V, Agans KN, Deer DJ, Graber J, Basler CF, Geisbert TW, Mire CE (2016) Nipah virus C and W proteins contribute to respiratory disease in ferrets. J Virol 90(14): 6326–6343. https://doi.org/10.1128/JVI.00215-16
70. Satterfield BA, Borisevich V, Foster SL, Rodriguez SE, Cross RW, Fenton KA, Agans KN, Basler CF, Geisbert TW, Mire CE (2019) Antagonism of STAT1 by Nipah virus P gene products modulates disease course but not lethal outcome in the ferret model. Sci Rep 9(1):1–18
71. Satterfield BA, Cross RW, Fenton KA, Agans KN, Basler CF, Geisbert TW, Mire CE (2015) The immunomodulating V and W proteins of Nipah virus determine disease course. Nat Commun 6:7483
72. Huang Q, Zeng J, Yan J (2021) COVID-19 mRNA vaccines. J Genet Genomics 48:107
73. Broder CC, Weir DL, Reid PA (2016) Hendra virus and Nipah virus animal vaccines. Vaccine 34(30):3525–3534. https://doi.org/10.1016/j.vaccine.2016.03.075
74. Broder CC, Xu K, Nikolov DB, Zhu Z, Dimitrov DS, Middleton D, Pallister J, Geisbert

TW, Bossart KN, Wang LF (2013) A treatment for and vaccine against the deadly Hendra and Nipah viruses. Antivir Res 100(1): 8–13. https://doi.org/10.1016/j.antiviral.2013.06.012

75. McLean RK, Graham SP (2019) Vaccine development for Nipah virus infection in pigs. Front Vet Sci 6:16. https://doi.org/10.3389/fvets.2019.00016

76. Chong HT, Kamarulzaman A, Tan CT, Goh KJ, Thayaparan T, Kunjapan SR, Chew NK, Chua KB, Lam SK (2001) Treatment of acute Nipah encephalitis with ribavirin. Annal Neurol 49(6):810–813

77. Rockx B, Bossart KN, Feldmann F, Geisbert JB, Hickey AC, Brining D, Callison J, Safronetz D, Marzi A, Kercher L, Long D, Broder CC, Feldmann H, Geisbert TW (2010) A novel model of lethal Hendra virus infection in African green monkeys and the effectiveness of ribavirin treatment. J Virol 84(19):9831–9839. https://doi.org/10.1128/JVI.01163-10

78. Georges-Courbot MC, Contamin H, Faure C, Loth P, Baize S, Leyssen P, Neyts J, Deubel V (2006) Poly(I)-poly(C12U) but not ribavirin prevents death in a hamster model of Nipah virus infection. Antimicrob Agents Chemother 50(5):1768–1772. https://doi.org/10.1128/AAC.50.5.1768-1772.2006

79. Freiberg AN, Worthy MN, Lee B, Holbrook MR (2010) Combined chloroquine and ribavirin treatment does not prevent death in a hamster model of Nipah and Hendra virus infection. J Gen Virol 91(Pt 3):765–772. https://doi.org/10.1099/vir.0.017269-0

80. Pallister J, Middleton D, Crameri G, Yamada M, Klein R, Hancock TJ, Foord A, Shiell B, Michalski W, Broder CC (2009) Chloroquine administration does not prevent Nipah virus infection and disease in ferrets. J Virol 83(22):11979–11982

81. Zhu Z, Bossart KN, Bishop KA, Crameri G, Dimitrov AS, McEachern JA, Feng Y, Middleton D, Wang LF, Broder CC, Dimitrov DS (2008) Exceptionally potent cross-reactive neutralization of Nipah and Hendra viruses by a human monoclonal antibody. J Infect Dis 197(6):846–853. https://doi.org/10.1086/528801

82. Mire CE, Satterfield BA, Geisbert JB, Agans KN, Borisevich V, Yan L, Chan YP, Cross RW, Fenton KA, Broder CC, Geisbert TW (2016) Pathogenic differences between Nipah virus Bangladesh and Malaysia strains in primates: implications for antibody therapy. Sci Rep 6: 30916. https://doi.org/10.1038/srep30916

83. Geisbert TW, Mire CE, Geisbert JB, Chan YP, Agans KN, Feldmann F, Fenton KA, Zhu Z, Dimitrov DS, Scott DP, Bossart KN, Feldmann H, Broder CC (2014) Therapeutic treatment of Nipah virus infection in nonhuman primates with a neutralizing human monoclonal antibody. Sci Transl Med 6(242):242ra282. https://doi.org/10.1126/scitranslmed.3008929

84. Bossart KN, Geisbert TW, Feldmann H, Zhu Z, Feldmann F, Geisbert JB, Yan L, Feng YR, Brining D, Scott D, Wang Y, Dimitrov AS, Callison J, Chan YP, Hickey AC, Dimitrov DS, Broder CC, Rockx B (2011) A neutralizing human monoclonal antibody protects African green monkeys from Hendra virus challenge. Sci Transl Med 3 (105): 105ra103:105ra103. https://doi.org/10.1126/scitranslmed.3002901

85. Bossart KN, Zhu Z, Middleton D, Klippel J, Crameri G, Bingham J, McEachern JA, Green D, Hancock TJ, Chan YP, Hickey AC, Dimitrov DS, Wang LF, Broder CC (2009) A neutralizing human monoclonal antibody protects against lethal disease in a new ferret model of acute Nipah virus infection. PLoS Pathog 5(10):e1000642. https://doi.org/10.1371/journal.ppat.1000642

86. Guillaume V, Contamin H, Loth P, Grosjean I, Courbot MCG, Deubel V, Buckland R, Wild TF (2006) Antibody prophylaxis and therapy against Nipah virus infection in hamsters. J Virol 80(4):1972–1978

87. Mire CE, Chan YP, Borisevich V, Cross RW, Yan L, Agans KN, Dang HV, Veesler D, Fenton KA, Geisbert TW, Broder CC (2019) A Cross-reactive humanized monoclonal antibody targeting fusion glycoprotein function protects ferrets against lethal Nipah virus and Hendra virus infection. J Infect Dis. https://doi.org/10.1093/infdis/jiz515

88. Mire CE, Chan Y-P, Borisevich V, Cross RW, Yan L, Agans KN, Dang HV, Veesler D, Fenton KA, Geisbert TW (2020) A cross-reactive humanized monoclonal antibody targeting fusion glycoprotein function protects ferrets against lethal Nipah virus and Hendra virus infection. J Infect Dis 221(Suppl 4):S471–S479

89. Broder CC (2013) Passive immunization and active vaccination against Hendra and Nipah viruses. Dev Biol 135:125–138

90. Playford EG, Munro T, Mahler SM, Elliott S, Gerometta M, Hoger KL, Jones ML, Griffin P, Lynch KD, Carroll H (2020) Safety, tolerability, pharmacokinetics, and immunogenicity of a human monoclonal antibody targeting the G glycoprotein of henipaviruses in healthy adults: a first-in-human, randomised,

controlled, phase 1 study. Lancet Infect Dis 20(4):445–454

91. Thakur N, Bailey D (2019) Advances in diagnostics, vaccines and therapeutics for Nipah virus. Microbes Infect. https://doi.org/10.1016/j.micinf.2019.02.002

92. Dawes BE, Kalveram B, Ikegami T, Juelich T, Smith JK, Zhang L, Park A, Lee B, Komeno T, Furuta Y, Freiberg AN (2018) Favipiravir (T-705) protects against Nipah virus infection in the hamster model. Sci Rep 8(1):7604. https://doi.org/10.1038/s41598-018-25780-3

93. Lo MK, Feldmann F, Gary JM, Jordan R, Bannister R, Cronin J, Patel NR, Klena JD, Nichol ST, Cihlar T, Zaki SR, Feldmann H, Spiropoulou CF, de Wit E (2019) Remdesivir (GS-5734) protects African green monkeys from Nipah virus challenge. Sci Transl Med 11(494). https://doi.org/10.1126/scitranslmed.aau9242

94. Steffen DL, Xu K, Nikolov DB, Broder CC (2012) Henipavirus mediated membrane fusion, virus entry and targeted therapeutics. Viruses 4(2):280–308. https://doi.org/10.3390/v4020280

95. Porotto M, Rockx B, Yokoyama CC, Talekar A, Devito I, Palermo LM, Liu J, Cortese R, Lu M, Feldmann H, Pessi A, Moscona A (2010) Inhibition of Nipah virus infection in vivo: targeting an early stage of paramyxovirus fusion activation during viral entry. PLoS Pathog 6(10):e1001168. https://doi.org/10.1371/journal.ppat.1001168

96. Uchida S, Horie R, Sato H, Kai C, Yoneda M (2018) Possible role of the Nipah virus V protein in the regulation of the interferon beta induction by interacting with UBX domain-containing protein 1. Sci Rep 8(1):7682. https://doi.org/10.1038/s41598-018-25815-9

97. Mire CE, Satterfield BA, Geisbert TW (2015) Pathogenesis of Hendra virus in humans. Human Emerging and Re-emerging Infections Set:207

98. Shaw ML, Garcia-Sastre A, Palese P, Basler CF (2004) Nipah virus V and W proteins have a common STAT1-binding domain yet inhibit STAT1 activation from the cytoplasmic and nuclear compartments, respectively. J Virol 78(11):5633–5641. https://doi.org/10.1128/JVI.78.11.5633-5641.2004

99. Rodriguez JJ, Cruz CD, Horvath CM (2004) Identification of the nuclear export signal and STAT-binding domains of the Nipah virus V protein reveals mechanisms underlying interferon evasion. J Virol 78(10):5358–5367

100. Rodriguez JJ, Horvath CM (2004) Host evasion by emerging paramyxoviruses: Hendra virus and Nipah virus v proteins inhibit interferon signaling. Viral Immunol 17(2):210–219. https://doi.org/10.1089/0882824041310568

101. Rodriguez JJ, Wang LF, Horvath CM (2003) Hendra virus V protein inhibits interferon signaling by preventing STAT1 and STAT2 nuclear accumulation. J Virol 77(21):11842–11845

102. Rodriguez JJ, Parisien JP, Horvath CM (2002) Nipah virus V protein evades alpha and gamma interferons by preventing STAT1 and STAT2 activation and nuclear accumulation. J Virol 76(22):11476–11483

103. Thompson KA, Strayer DR, Salvato PD, Thompson CE, Klimas N, Molavi A, Hamill AK, Zheng Z, Ventura D, Carter WA (1996) Results of a double-blind placebo-controlled study of the double-stranded RNA drug polyI:polyC12U in the treatment of HIV infection. Eur J Clin Microbiol Infect Dis 15(7):580–587

104. Jiang Y, Chen D, Cai D, Yi Y, Jiang S (2021) Effectiveness of remdesivir for the treatment of hospitalized COVID-19 persons: a network meta-analysis. J Med Virol 93(2):1171–1174

Part I

Studying Henipaviruses Under Biosafety Level 2 Conditions

Chapter 2

A Revised Diagnostic Quantitative RT-PCR for the Detection of Nipah Virus Infection

Ketan Patel, John Klena, and Michael K. Lo

Abstract

From its discovery in Malaysia in the late 1990s, the spillover of the Nipah virus from its pteropid reservoir into the human population has resulted in sporadic outbreaks of fatal encephalitis and respiratory disease. In this chapter, we revise a previously described quantitative reverse transcription polymerase chain reaction method, which now utilizes degenerate nucleotides at certain positions in the probe and the reverse primer to accommodate the sequence heterogeneity observed within the Nipah henipavirus species.

Key words Nipah virus, Quantitative RT-PCR, Primer, Probe, Nucleoprotein gene

1 Introduction

Since its initial emergence in Malaysia in 1998–1999, the Nipah virus (NiV) has caused near-annual outbreaks of fatal encephalitis and respiratory disease in humans in Bangladesh and India, with an overall mortality rate of greater than 75% [1, 2]. Since there is currently no approved therapeutics for NiV infection, early diagnosis is crucial to implement infection control measures to curb potential secondary chains of transmission among healthcare workers and family caregivers [3]. Although virus isolation in cell culture remains the gold standard for diagnosing a NiV-positive patient specimen, it is time- and resource-intensive, requiring up to 2 weeks under biosafety level 4 (BSL-4) containment for a determination. Quantitative real-time reverse transcription polymerase chain reaction (qRT-PCR) is a sensitive method to detect the presence of NiV infection. Although several nested RT-PCR protocols have been developed for NiV surveillance and diagnosis [4, 5], one particular primer/probe set has been used to diagnose the majority of human NiV cases in Bangladesh, in which spillover from pteropid bat reservoirs has been documented for over a decade [6]. Given the sporadic but continual spillovers of NiV in

Alexander N. Freiberg and Barry Rockx (eds.), *Nipah Virus: Methods and Protocols*, Methods in Molecular Biology, vol. 2682, https://doi.org/10.1007/978-1-0716-3283-3_2, © Springer Science+Business Media, LLC, part of Springer Nature 2023

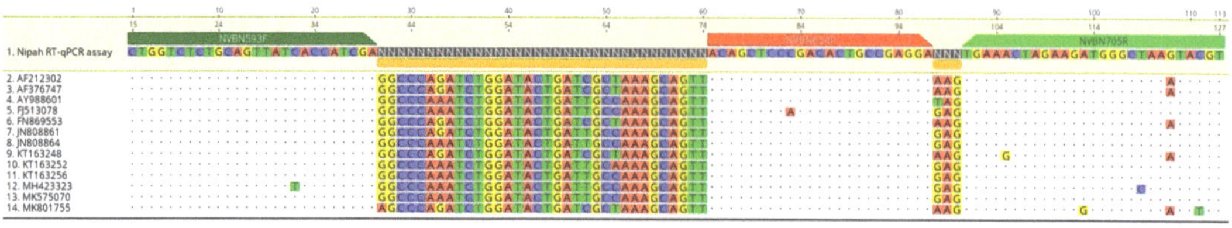

Fig. 1 Partial alignments of oligonucleotide binding regions, Nipah virus
Alignment of the nucleoprotein gene sequence window targeted by the primer/probe set across 13 available Nipah virus sequences (accession numbers from National Center for Biotechnology Information (NCBI)) displaying the heterogeneity observed in samples collected across both humans and bats (*see* **Note 1** for sequence information). Dots represent identical nucleotides compared with the Nipah qRT-PCR assay primer/probe sequences. Nucleotide substitutions are specified. Green (primers) and red (probe) arrows: oligonucleotides as specified in Table 1

Bangladesh and more recently in the southern part of India, here we update our previously described protocol with minor modifications to the reverse primer and probe to account for some sequence heterogeneity observed across Malaysian and Bangladesh genotypes of NiV (Fig. 1). In addition, a shorter synthetic positive control RNA sequence was designed to replace the previously described positive control in vitro transcribed RNA, which encoded the entire nucleoprotein (N) gene coding sequence.

2 Samples, Materials, Reagents, and Equipment

2.1 Patient Sample Handling

1. Patient samples from nasopharyngeal swabs are collected in viral transport medium (VTM) (BD Diagnostic Systems, USA) and are stored at temperatures ≤ −80 °C until the time of use. Undiluted patient cerebrospinal fluid and urine are collected and stored at temperatures ≤ −80 °C until the time of use.

2.2 RNA Extraction

1. 2× MagMAX Lysis buffer (Thermo Fisher, USA).
2. 100% isopropanol, molecular grade.
3. 100% ethanol, molecular grade.
4. MagMAX Pathogen RNA/DNA Kit (Life Technologies #4462359)—includes lysis/binding buffer and magnetic beads for nucleic acid capture.
5. Sterile nuclease-free water.
6. MagMAX Express-96 Standard Plates (Thermo Fisher #4388475).
7. MagMAX Express-96 Deep Well Plates (Thermo Fisher #4388476).

Table 1
Primers, probes, and synthetic RNA control for NiV-specific qRT-PCR

Oligonucleotide ID	Sequence[a]	Concentration[b]
NVBN593F (forward)	5′-CTGGTCTCTGCAGTTATCACCATCGA-3′	Use 750 nM per reaction
NVBN705R (reverse)	5′-ACGTAYTTAGCCCATCTTCTAGTTTCA-3′	Use 600 nM per reaction
NVBN654P (probe)	5′-/FAM/-AC AGC TCC M/ZEN/G ACA CTG CCG AGG A-/IBFQ/−3′	Use 400 nM per reaction
Synthetic RNA control[c]	5′-CAC CCU GGU CUC UGC AGU UAU CAC CAU CGA GGC CCG UAA CAG AUG AAA GAG CAA GCU ACU AGU UAC AGC UCC CGA CAC UGC CGA GGA AAG UGA AAC UAG AAG AUG GGC UAA AUA CGU CCA-3′	Dilutions of synthetic RNA control ranging from ~10^1 to 10^7 copies per μL of sterile nuclease-free water

[a] Y is C, T; M is A, C. ZEN Double-Quenched Probes: ZEN Double-Quenched Probes contain a 5′ fluorophore FAM-6-carboxyfluorescein (FAM); 3′ Iowa Black FQ (IBFQ) quencher; and proprietary, internal ZEN quencher

[b] Optimized concentrations are given in nanomole per liter (nM) based on the final reaction mix (e.g., 1.0 μL of a 10 μM primer stock solution per 25 μL total reaction volume yields a final concentration of 400 nM as indicated in the table

[c] For synthetic RNA control: green = forward primer binding region; red = probe binding region; blue = NVBN705R reverse primer binding region

8. MicroAmp Optical Adhesive Covers (Thermo Fisher #4311971).
9. MagMAX Express-96 Deep Well Magnetic Particle Retriever (Thermo Fisher #4456933).

2.3 qRT-PCR

1. SuperScript™ III Platinum™ One-Step qRT-PCR Kit (Thermo Fisher #11732020).
2. Primers and synthetic RNA control: forward primer NVBN593F, probe NVBN654P, and reverse primer NVBN705R. The primers are prepared in a stock solution of nuclease-free Tris borate EDTA (TBE) buffer at a concentration of 10 μM. Primer and probe sequences, along with that of the synthetic RNA-positive control, are shown in Table 1. All oligonucleotides were synthesized and provided by Integrated DNA Technologies, Inc.
3. CFX Connect Real-Time PCR Detection System (Bio-Rad Laboratories, Inc.).
4. MicroSeal "C" PCR Plate Sealing Film, adhesive, optical (Bio-Rad Laboratories, Inc. #MSC1001).

5. Hard-shell 96-Well PCR Plates, low profile, thin wall, skirted, white/white (Bio-Rad Laboratories, Inc., #HSP9655).
6. CFX Manager™ Software (Bio-Rad Laboratories, Inc.).

2.4 Reagent Preparation and Stability

1. MagMAX Kit: Store the wash solutions, the elution buffer, and the lysis buffer solution at room temperature. Store the RNA-binding beads at 4 °C and the lysis enhancer and carrier RNA at −20 °C until use.
   (a) Add an appropriate volume of 100% isopropanol to the Wash Solution 1 concentrate. Mix well by shaking and mark the bottle to indicate that this has been done.
   (b) Add an appropriate volume of 100% ethanol to the Wash Solution 2 concentrate. Mix well by shaking and mark on the bottle to indicate that this has been done.
   (c) Dilute 2× MagMAX lysis buffer 1:1 with 100% isopropanol to reach a working concentration.
2. SuperScript™ III Platinum™ One-Step qRT-PCR Kit: Store contents at −20 °C until use. When in use, keep kit contents on ice after briefly thawing appropriate components to prepare master mixes. Primer and probe sequences, as well as optimized concentrations, are shown in Table 1. All oligonucleotides were synthesized and provided by Integrated DNA Technologies, Inc. (Iowa, USA).
3. Synthetic RNA control: On the day of use, prepare tenfold serial dilutions (in duplicate) of the synthetic RNA control ranging from 10^1 to 10^7 copies per μL in order to generate a standard curve to quantitate NiV N gene copy numbers from RNA extracted from patient samples.

3 Methods

3.1 Sample Inactivation

1. Since NiV is classified as a BSL-4 pathogen, suspected NiV patient samples stored in VTM require appropriate inactivation, which is performed within a class II biosafety cabinet within a BSL-4 laboratory containment facility.
2. Inactivate 100 μL of the patient sample in 400 μL of MagMAX lysis buffer. To ensure inactivation, thoroughly mix the sample by vortexing or pipetting up and down.

3.2 RNA Extraction

1. Using the MagMAX Express™-96 bead retriever, perform the RNA extraction according to the manufacturer's instructions by transferring 500 μL of inactivated sample into a deep well plate containing 20 μL bead/lysis binding solution mix. Once the extraction is complete, carefully remove the RNA (elution)

plate from the machine. Add an adhesive cover to the plate, and either use RNA immediately for qRT-PCR or store RNA at −80 °C (*see* **Note 2** for general procedures regarding the handling of RNA).

3.3 NiV-Specific One-Step qRT-PCR

1. Evaluating a sample for the presence of NiV is conducted by amplification of a 113-bp fragment of the NiV nucleoprotein (N) gene using the primer/probe set: NVBN593F, NVBN705R, and NVBN654P (*see* Table 1 for sequence information).
2. Prepare the master mix for qRT-PCR based on the number of samples to be tested, including that for nontemplate controls and standard curve-positive controls. Each reaction should consist of 12.5 μL of 2× reaction buffer provided with the SuperScript™ III Platinum™ One-Step qRT-PCR Kit, 0.5 μL of reverse transcriptase/Taq mixture from the kit, 750 nM of NVBN593F, 600 nM of NVBN507R, 400 nM of NVBN654P, and nuclease-free water up to 20 uL.
3. Add 5 μL of extracted sample RNA, positive control, or negative control (nuclease-free water) to a well containing 20 μL of the master mix, for a total reaction volume of 25 μL.
4. Perform thermal cycling at 50 °C for 15 minutes for reverse transcription, followed by 95 °C for 2 min and then 45 cycles of 95 °C for 15 s and 60 °C for 30 s on a CFX Connect Real-Time PCR Detection System.
5. Analyze amplification curves and quantitate sample NiV N gene RNA copy numbers using CFX Manager software (Fig. 2).

4 Notes

1. The alignment of 13 NiV N gene fragments utilized the following accession numbers for NiV sequences collected from Malaysia (AF212302—human, AF376747—bat, FN869553—bat), Bangladesh (AY988601—human, JN808861—human, JN808864—human, MK575070—bat), Thailand (KT163248—bat, KT163252—bat, KT163256—bat), India (MH432323—human, FJ513078—human), and Cambodia (MK801755—bat).
2. Avoid both RNA and RNase contamination when conducting qRT-PCR. Such precautionary measures include wearing gloves and gowns and opening tubes using the tissue to avoid forming aerosols, which could lead to sample cross-contamination.

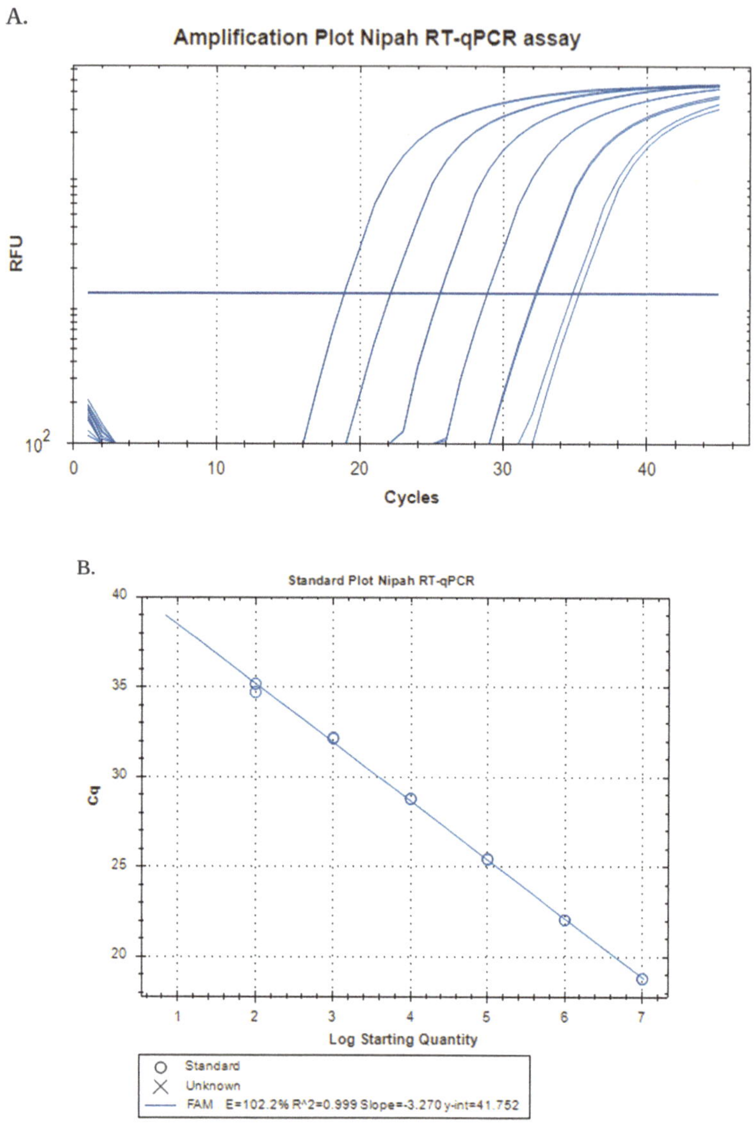

Fig. 2 Determination of efficiency of amplification based on the reference Nipah virus genome sequence-specific synthetic RNA
(**a**) Amplification plot of serial dilutions of a synthetic RNA control using the optimized primer probe concentrations in Table 1. (**b**) Standard plot efficiency of Nipah qRT-PCR amplification of synthetic synthetic RNA control containing the NiV N gene-specific amplicon region (NC_002728). Cq on Y-axis signifies the cycle threshold of detection. X-axis denotes starting quantity of synthetic RNA control present

References

1. Lo MK, Rota PA (2008) The emergence of Nipah virus, a highly pathogenic paramyxovirus. J Clin Virol 43(4):396–400
2. Arunkumar G et al (2019) Outbreak investigation of Nipah virus disease in Kerala, India, 2018. J Infect Dis 219(12):1867–1878
3. Nikolay B et al (2019) Transmission of Nipah virus – 14 years of investigations in Bangladesh. N Engl J Med 380(19):1804–1814
4. Yadav PD et al (2019) Nipah virus sequences from humans and bats during Nipah outbreak, Kerala, India, 2018. Emerg Infect Dis 25(5): 1003–1006
5. Wacharapluesadee S et al (2005) Bat Nipah virus, Thailand. Emerg Infect Dis 11(12): 1949–1951
6. Lo MK et al (2012) Characterization of Nipah virus from outbreaks in Bangladesh, 2008-2010. Emerg Infect Dis 18(2):248–255

Chapter 3

Recombinant Soluble Henipavirus Glycoprotein Preparation

Lianying Yan, Spencer L. Sterling, Deborah L. Fusco, Yee-Peng Chan, Kai Xu, Eric D. Laing, and Christopher C. Broder

Abstract

Henipaviruses possess two envelope glycoproteins, the attachment (G) and the fusion (F) proteins that mediate cellular entry and are the major targets of virus-neutralizing antibody responses. Recombinant expression technologies have been used to produce soluble G and F proteins (sG and sF) that retain native-like oligomeric conformations and epitopes, which are advantageous for the development and characterization of vaccines and antiviral antibody therapeutics. In addition to Hendra virus and Nipah virus tetrameric sG and trimeric sF production, we also describe the expression and purification of Cedar virus tetrameric sG and Ghana virus trimeric sF glycoproteins. These henipavirus glycoproteins were also used as immunizing antigens to generate monoclonal antibodies, and binding was demonstrated with a pan-henipavirus multiplex microsphere immunoassay.

Key words Henipaviruses, Hendra virus, Nipah virus, Cedar virus, Ghana virus, Mòjiāng virus, F glycoprotein, G glycoprotein, Expression, Purification, Cross-linking, Multiplex microsphere immunoassay

1 Introduction

Hendra virus (HeV) and Nipah virus (NiV) are pathogenic, zoonotic viruses and the prototypical henipaviruses [1]. HeV and NiV first emerged in the mid and late 1990s in Australia [2] and Malaysia [3], respectively, and are the causative agents of fatal respiratory and neurologic diseases in livestock and humans [2, 4, 5]. *Pteropus* spp. of bats have been shown to be the natural hosts of HeV and NiV [6] and are responsible for the zoonotic transmission of these viruses. Biosurveillance efforts have uncovered an additional diversity of henipaviruses in African fruit bats, including Ghana virus (GhV), which is known only from sequence data [7, 8] and a nonpathogenic henipavirus, Cedar virus (CedV) isolated from Australian *Pteropus* spp. [9]. Within the African continent, *Eidolon helvum*, a panmictic population, is suspected to be a key animal host of African henipaviruses [10, 11] and human exposure to African

Alexander N. Freiberg and Barry Rockx (eds.), *Nipah Virus: Methods and Protocols*, Methods in Molecular Biology, vol. 2682, https://doi.org/10.1007/978-1-0716-3283-3_3,

henipaviruses was detected in a human population in Cameroon [12]. A fifth henipavirus, Mòjiāng virus (MojV), was discovered from rodents sampled in China and is also known only from sequence data [13].

The henipaviruses encode two envelope glycoproteins, the receptor-binding protein (RBP) for attachment known as the G glycoprotein and the fusion (F) glycoprotein, which together mediate receptor engagement and membrane fusion allowing cellular entry of the virus nucleocapsid and the initiation of infection. Unlike many other paramyxoviruses, the G glycoprotein lacks hemagglutinin or neuraminidase activities and does not recognize sialic acid moieties. The virus entry receptors of HeV and NiV are the B-class ephrin ligands, ephrin-B2 and ephrin-B3 [14–16]. Receptor-mediated fusion and virus entry occur through the sequential engagement of the G glycoprotein with ephrin-B2 or ephrin-B3 ligands followed by the triggering of a conformational change in the F glycoprotein that facilitates membrane fusion between the virion and host cell (reviewed in [17]). Structural analysis has demonstrated that G is a tetramer (a dimer of dimers) [18, 19] and that F is a trimer [20]. Henipavirus entry can be neutralized by antibodies reactive to either the G or F glycoproteins (reviewed in [21]).

Neutralizing antibody (NAb) induction is considered a correlate of protection for many viral vaccines [22]. Antibody-mediated neutralization occurs in large part through engagement with virus envelope glycoproteins, interference with receptor-binding domains, and inhibition of virus entry into the cell. HeV and NiV G glycoproteins possess conserved receptor-binding pocket that is the target of NAbs [23–25]. Recombinant expressed and soluble versions of the G and F henipavirus glycoproteins (sG and sF) retain native-like, oligomeric, and quaternary structures and are able to generate neutralizing humoral responses [26] and have been used to identify monoclonal antibodies for passive immunization [27–30], and the HeV-sG protein has been extensively tested as a subunit vaccine against HeV and NiV in multiple animal models including nonhuman primates [31] and has been commercialized, and fully licensed, as a vaccine against HeV for horses in Australia (Equivac® HeV) [32]. The HeV-sG immunogen has also proven effective as a single-dose immunogen in nonhuman primates and is currently being evaluated in a phase I clinical trial sponsored by the Coalition for Epidemic Preparedness Innovations (CEPI) [33].

Here, we describe updated methodology [34] for the production of recombinant oligomeric, soluble G (sG), and F (sF) proteins including detailed steps in the design and expression, purification, and analysis of sG and sF. These sG and sF proteins are expressed in a mammalian FreeStyle™ 293F suspension cell culture system, retain post-translational modifications, and are purified as native-like tetrameric or trimeric proteins, respectively. The CedV sG and

GhV sF glycoproteins are also described here, while the CedV sF and GhV sG along with MojV sF and sG have been recently detailed elsewhere [35]. All of these soluble henipavirus glycoproteins have been used to generate murine monoclonal antibodies (mAbs).

2 Materials

2.1 Cell Culture

1. The FreeStyle™ 293 Expression System and FreeStyle™ 293 Expression Medium were purchased from Thermo Fisher Scientific (Waltham, MA, USA). Additional cell culture media: Dulbecco's Modified Eagle's Medium (DMEM) (Quality Biological, Gaithersburg, MD, USA) supplemented with 2 mM L-Glutamine (Quality Biological) and 5% Cosmic Calf serum (GE Healthcare, Chicago, IL, USA) (referred henceforth as DMEM-5). 0.25% trypsin/0.02% EDTA (Quality Biological). Sterile 1X PBS for cell culture (Quality Biological).
2. Hygromycin B, 50 mg/mL (Invitrogen, Carlsbad, CA, USA).
3. Plastic ware: 75 cm^2 and 150 cm^2 tissue culture flasks (Corning Inc., Corning, NY, USA). Polypropylene 15 mL and 50 mL conical centrifuge tubes (Corning Inc.). 6-, 24-, and 96-well flat-bottom tissue culture plates (Corning Inc.). Nonpyrogenic polycarbonate 500 mL Erlenmeyer flasks (Corning Inc.). 250 mL conical bottom centrifuge tubes (Corning Inc.). Sterilizing filter units, low protein-binding membrane, 0.22 μm PES (Corning Inc.).

2.2 DNA Transfection

1. The plasmids (pUC57) bearing codon-optimized open reading frame (ORF) sequences of henipavirus envelope glycoproteins (HeV, NiV CedV, and GhV F or G) were generated in part by GenScript Biotech (Piscataway, NJ, USA). The ORFs were cloned into pcDNA3.1 Hygro-CMV expression plasmids.
2. 0.1 mg/mL Poly-D-Lysine hydrobromide (Sigma-Aldrich, St. Louis, MO, USA).
3. DMEM (no additives) and DMEM-5.
4. X-tremeGENE 9 DNA Transfection Reagent (Roche Holding AG, Basel, SUI).

2.3 Affinity Precipitations

1. Lysis buffer: Pierce RIPA Buffer (Thermo Fisher Scientific) supplemented with EDTA-free Complete Mini Protease Inhibitor (Roche).
2. 1.7 mL centrifuge tubes (Thomas Scientific, Swedesboro, NJ, USA).
3. 50% slurry S-protein Agarose beads (MilliporeSigma, Burlington, MA, USA, MA).

4. XCell II™ Blot Module (Invitrogen).
5. NuPAGE 4–12% Bis–Tris Gel (Invitrogen).
6. NuPAGE LDS Sample Buffer (4X) (Life Technologies, Carlsbad, CA, USA).
7. 2-Mercaptoethanol (Sigma-Aldrich).
8. 20X SDS MOPS Running Buffer (Invitrogen).
9. 20X Transfer Buffer (Invitrogen).
10. Tween 20 (Sigma-Aldrich, MO).
11. Blocking buffer: 5% skim milk blocker, 1X PBS, 0.1% Tween 20.
12. Mouse anti-S-tag antibody, HRP-conjugated (Southern Biotech, Birmingham, AL, USA).
13. SuperSignal West Pico Chemiluminescent Substrate (Thermo Fisher Scientific).

2.4 Henipavirus Soluble G (sG)

1. S-Protein Agarose (MilliporeSigma).
2. XK26 column (GE Healthcare).
3. Centriprep® molecular weight cutoff centrifugal filter units, YM 30 (MilliporeSigma).
4. Acrodisc® Syringe Filter 0.2 μm HT Tuffryn Low Protein-Binding Membrane (MilliporeSigma).
5. Wash Buffer I: PBS, 0.1% Triton® X-100, 0.3 M NaCl.
6. Wash Buffer II: PBS, 0.1% Triton® X-100.
7. 20% Ethanol.
8. Elution buffer: 0.2 M citrate, pH 2.
9. Neutralization buffer: 1 M Tris–HCl pH 8.0 or 1 M HEPES buffer pH 9.0.
10. Protein buffer: PBS, pH 7.4.

2.5 Henipavirus Soluble F (sF)

1. S-Protein Agarose (MilliporeSigma).
2. XK26 column (GE Healthcare).
3. Centriprep® molecular weight cutoff centrifugal filter units, YM 30 (MilliporeSigma).
4. Acrodisc® Syringe Filter 0.2 μm HT Tuffryn Low Protein-Binding Membrane (MilliporeSigma).
5. XCell II™ Blot Module (Invitrogen).
6. Wash buffer I: PBS, 0.5% Triton® X-100, 0.5 M NaCl, 0.1 M L-Arginine, 0.02 M Tris–HCl, pH 7.5.
7. Wash buffer II: PBS, 0.1% Triton® X-100, 0.1 M L-Arginine.
8. 20% ethanol.

9. Elution buffer: 0.2 M citrate, 0.2 M L-Arginine, pH 2.
10. Neutralization buffer: 1 M HEPES buffer pH 9.0.
11. Protein buffer: PBS, 0.01% Triton® X-100, 0.1 M L-Arginine.

2.6 Size Exclusion Chromatography

All buffers should be sterile-filtered and degassed.

1. A Fast Protein Liquid Chromatography (FPLC) system such as a P-500 pump (GE Healthcare) or similar, UA-6 UV detector (ISCO) and fraction collector (ISCO).
2. Analytic column: Superdex 200 10/300 GL gel filtration column (GE Healthcare).
3. Preparative column: HiLoad 16/60 Superdex 200 prep grade XK 16 gel filtration column (GE Healthcare).
4. Centriprep® molecular weight cutoff centrifugal filter units (MilliporeSigma).
5. Reagents: PBS; 20% ethanol; PBS 0.01% Triton® X-100.

2.7 Polyacrylamide Gel Electrophoresis (PAGE) and Western Blotting

2.7.1 Blue Native Polyacrylamide Gel Electrophoresis (BN-PAGE) (Invitrogen)

1. XCell SureLock® Mini-Cell.
2. NativePAGE™ Novex® 3–12% Bis–Tris Gels 1.0 mm, 15 well.
3. NativePAGE™ Running Buffer (20X).
4. NativePAGE™ Cathode Buffer Additive (20X).
5. NativePAGE™ 5% G-250 Sample Additive.
6. NativePAGE™ Sample Buffer (4X).
7. NativeMark™ Unstained Protein Standard.
8. Fixing solution (40% methanol, 10% acetic acid).
9. Destain solution (8% acetic acid).

2.7.2 Western Blotting and Immunodetection

1. Polyvinylidene difluoride (PVDF) membrane for native gel analysis and nitrocellulose membrane (0.45 μm) for denatured gel analysis (Bio-Rad Laboratories, Hercules, CA, USA).
2. NuPAGE® Transfer Buffer (20X).
3. Blocking buffer: 5% skim milk blocker (Bio-Rad Laboratories), 1X PBS, 0.1% Tween 20.
4. Wash buffer: 1X PBS, 0.1% Tween 20.

2.8 Cross-Linking

1. BS^3 (bis(sulfosuccinimidyl)suberate), No-Weigh™ Format cross-linking agent (Thermo Fisher Scientific).
2. XCell II™ Blot Module (Invitrogen).
3. NuPAGE 4–12% Bis–Tris Gel (Invitrogen).
4. NuPAGE LDS Sample Buffer (4X) (Thermo Fisher Scientific).
5. 2-Mercaptoethanol (Sigma-Aldrich).

6. 20X SDS MOPS Running Buffer (Invitrogen).
7. 20X Transfer Buffer (Invitrogen).
8. Blocking buffer: 5% skim milk blocker, 1X PBS, 0.1% Tween 20.

2.9 Removing S-Tag for Soluble F (sF)

1. Factor Xa Cleavage Capture Kit (MilliporeSigma).
2. Xarrest™ Agarose (MilliporeSigma).
3. Spin Filter 0.2 mL (included with the kit).
4. XCell SureLock® Mini-Cell.
5. XCell II™ Blot Module (Invitrogen).
6. NuPAGE 4–12% Bis–Tris Gel (Invitrogen).
7. NuPAGE LDS Sample Buffer (4X) (Thermo Fisher Scientific).
8. 2-Mercaptoethanol (Sigma-Aldrich, MO).
9. 20X SDS MOPS Running Buffer (Invitrogen).
10. 20X Transfer Buffer (Invitrogen).
11. SimplyBlue™ SafeStain (Thermo Fisher Scientific).
12. Blocking buffer: 5% skim milk blocker, 1X PBS, 0.1% Tween 20.

2.10 Multiplex Microsphere Immunoassay

1. Bio-Plex Pro™ magnetic COOH beads 36, 26, 55, 63.46, 43, 53, 35, and 62 (Bio- Rad Laboratories).
2. Standard clear flat-bottom 96-well plates to set serial dilutions.
3. Black flat-bottom 96- well plates to run the experiment and take Bio-Plex 200 reads.
4. 96-well plate micro-seal film.
5. Magnetic separator.
6. Orbit P2 Labnet Shaker.
7. Ca^2/Mg^{2+} free PBS (PBSA).
8. PBSA-Tween (0.05%. PBSA-T).
9. Bead activation buffer (10% PBS, pH 6.2).
10. 1-Ethyl-3 (3-dimethylaminopropyl) carbodiimide HCI (EDC) (Thermo Fisher Scientific).
11. N-Hydroxysulfosuccinimide (Sulfo-NHS) (Thermo Fisher Scientific).
12. Bead storage buffer (1% BSA/PBSA/0.05 sodium azide) (Sigma-Aldrich) with protease inhibitor tablet (1 tablet. 10 ml of 1x storage buffer).
13. 2 mL sterile screw top cap tube (Sarstedt Inc., Newton, NC, USA).

14. mAb: mouse α-Hendra (HeV) and Nipah (NiV) sF 5G7 (IgG2b); mouse α-Cedar sF 19E7 (IgG1); mouse α-GhV sF 5B7 (IgG2b); mouse α-Hendra (HeV), Nipah (NiV) sG 7B7 (IgG1); mouse α-Cedar-sG 14F3 (IgG2b); mouse α-Ghana (GhV) sG 10D5 (IgG2b); and mouse α-D61 (IgG1) linear gp41 [36] as a negative control.
15. Human: hu102.4 ((HeV), Nipah (NiV) sG; hu5B3 (HeV), Nipah (NiV) sF, and hu 150.8 IgG ephrin B2 negative control.
16. Goat Anti-Mouse IgG-Biotin conjugates (Thermo Fisher Scientific) and Goat Anti-Human IgG-Biotin conjugates (Thermo Fisher Scientific). Secondary antibodies.
17. Streptavidin-PE (Qiagen, Hilden, DEU).

3 Methods

3.1 Constructions of the Plasmids That Express Henipaviruses Surface Proteins (HeV, NiV CedV, and GhV sF or sG)

Here, we describe the technique used to design and express the attachment (G) and fusion (F) glycoproteins of HeV (GenBank NC 001906.3), NiV (GenBank NC 002728.1), CedV (GenBank KP271122.1), and GhV (GenBank NC 025256.1) as native-like oligomeric, soluble proteins (sF, sG).

1. Cloning of trimeric soluble F (sF): The human codon-optimized HeV, NiV, CedV, and GhV F ORFs were modified by replacing the predicted C-terminal transmembrane anchor domain with a GCN_t trimeric folding motif [26]. (MKQIED KIEEILSKIYHIENEIARIKKLIGE) in heptad repeat phase with HR2 (*see* **Note 1**) followed by a factor Xa protease cleavage site (IEGR) and a 15 amino acid S-tag (KETAAAKFERQHMDS) appended to the C-terminus of the constructs. The genes were cloned into a promoter-modified mammalian expression vector pcDNA 3.1.
2. Hygro(+) (Invitrogen) as described in [34]. The correct constructs were confirmed by DNA sequencing. Figure 1A shows a schematic diagram of the construction.
3. Cloning of tetrameric soluble G (sG): The human codon-optimized HeV, NiV, CedV, and GhV G ORFs were modified by replacing the predicted transmembrane anchor domain with an Igκ leader sequence (METDTLLLWVLLLWVPGSTGD) followed by an N-terminal S-tag (KETAAAKFERQHMDS), a factor Xa protease cleavage site (IEGR), and a GCN_4 tetrameric folding motif, GCN_{tet} (MKQIEDKLEEIESKLKKIENELARIKK) [37]. The genes were cloned into a modified pcDNA 3.1 as described above. The correct constructs were confirmed by DNA sequencing. Figure 1B shows a schematic diagram of the constructs.

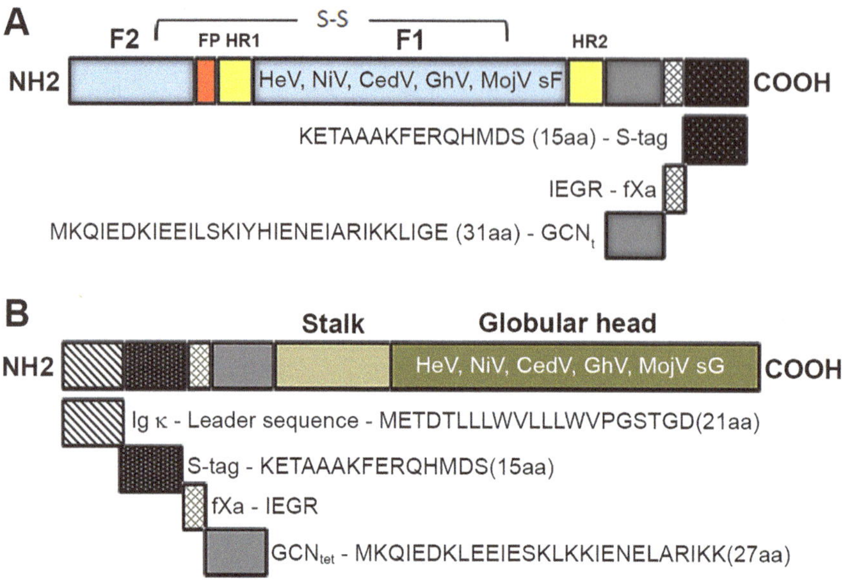

Fig. 1 Schematic representations of HeV, NiV, CedV, GhV, and MojV virus sF or sG expression plasmids. (**a**) To generate the recombinant, sF construct, the transmembrane, and cytoplasmic tail domains were replaced by the trimeric coil-coiled motif GCN_t (trimeric) and S-peptide sequence was appended to the C-terminus of the construct. A factor Xa protease cleavage site was engineered upstream to the S-tag allowing the removal of S-tag by enzymatic digestion. (**b**) To construct sG, the predicted transmembrane anchor domain was replaced with an Igκ leader sequence, S-peptide sequence, and a factor Xa protease cleavage site followed by GCN_{tet} (tetrameric) motif. The correct constructs were confirmed by DNA sequencing

3.2 Transient Transfection of FreeStyle™ 293F Cells

1. One day prior to transfection, incubate a 6-well tissue culture plate with coating buffer (0.1 mg/mL poly-D-lysine hydrobromide). Add 2 mL of coating buffer to each well of a 6-well plate in a biosafety cabinet and incubate at room temperature for 15 min. Aspirate the buffer and let the plate dry for 1–2 h. Wash twice with 1X PBS and then seed with 0.5×10^6 FreeStyle™ 293F cells per well in 3 mL DMEM-5.
2. Allow the cells to adhere and grow at 37 °C, 5–8% CO_2 overnight. Cells should be 70–90% confluent the next day.
3. Transfect one well with the vector pcDNA 3.1 without the gene of interest as a negative control.
4. Setup duplicate wells for each transfection, one for expression assessment and the other for stable cell line generation.
5. Prepare the transfection mixture as follows (per well): Add 6 μL of X-tremeGENE 9 DNA Transfection Reagent (Roche) to 0.5 mL of serum-free DMEM. Gently mix the solution. Add 2 μg of plasmid DNA to the mixture and vortex briefly. Incubate the transfection mixture at room temperature for 30 min.
6. Aspirate the medium from the 6-well plate and replace it with 0.5 mL of fresh DMEM-5 per well. Add the transfection mixture to the cell at the side of the well without disturbing the monolayer. Gently rock the plate to mix.

7. Incubate the cells at 37 °C, 5–8% CO_2 for at least 4 hours (h) before adding an additional 0.5 mL of DMEM-5.
8. Continue to incubate the cells at 37 °C, 5–8% CO_2 for 48 h to allow protein expression and secretion to occur.

3.3 Supernatant Harvest and Affinity Precipitation

1. Collect the supernatant from the negative control, expression assessment, and stable cell line generation wells into 1.7 mL centrifuge tubes. Centrifuge at 18,000 × g for 1 min to pellet cells.
2. Transfer the supernatant to fresh 1.7 mL tubes and add 30 μL of 50% slurry S-protein agarose beads to each tube. Rotate at room temperature for 1 h or at 4 °C for 2 h.
3. Add 1 tablet of complete protease inhibitor cocktail tablets to 50 mL of lysis buffer. Add 0.7 mL of this lysis buffer to the wells designated as negative control and expression assessment. Do not lyse the duplicate well meant for stable cell line generation. Allow lysis on ice for 10 min (*see* **Note 2**).
4. Transfer the lysate to 1.7 mL centrifuge tubes and rotate at 4 °C for 10–30 min to allow complete lysis.
5. Centrifuge the lysate at 18,000 × g for at least 10 min to pellet cell debris.
6. Transfer the cleared lysate to fresh tubes and add 30 μL of 50% slurry S-agarose beads to each tube. Rotate at room temperature for 1 h or at 4 °C 2 h.
7. After the affinity binding, centrifuge the samples at 3000 × g for 1 min to pellet the agarose beads. Aspirate the unbound lysate or supernatant without disturbing the agarose beads.
8. Wash the agarose beads by adding 1 mL of lysis buffer and mix by inverting the tubes several times.
9. Repeat steps 7 and 8 twice.
10. Aspirate the lysis buffer after the last wash, and add 50 μL of 2X NuPAGE LDS sample loading buffer with 2.5 μL of 5% 2-mercaptoethanol to the agarose beads.
11. Boil the samples for 10 min. Centrifuge the samples at 3000 × g for 1 min. Load 25 μL of each sample into a NuPAGE 4–12% Bis–Tris Gel followed by Western blotting procedures.
12. For immunodetection, incubate the blot with a 1:20,000 dilution of mouse anti-S-tag antibody and HRP-conjugate in blocking buffer for 1 h at room temperature. Apply the SuperSignal West Pico Chemiluminescent Substrate as the HRP substrate to the blot. See Fig. 2 for the Western blot.

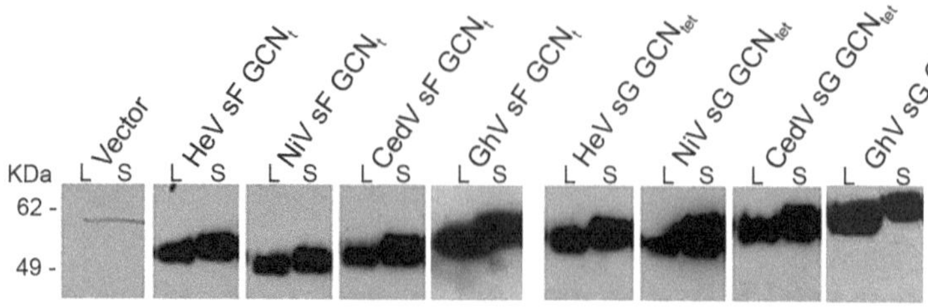

Fig. 2 Transient expression of various HeV, NiV, CedV, and GhV sF and sG proteins. FreeStyle™-293F cells were transfected with sF and sG constructs under the CMV-driven promoter in pcDNA3.1. The cell lysate and supernatant were precipitated with S-protein agarose. The Western blot was probed with HRP-conjugated rabbit α-S-peptide antibody. *L* lysate, *S* supernatant. Vector: empty vector (negative control)

3.4 Stable Cell Line Production

3.4.1 Transfected Cell Selection

1. At 48 h post-transfection, replace the culture medium with the selection medium daily to ensure complete selection (*see* **Note 3**).
2. Once new colonies form and become 90% confluent, aspirate medium from the 6-well plate and add 2 mL of PBS. Gently rock the plate before aspirating the PBS.
3. Add 0.5 mL of trypsin-EDTA and leave for 5 s. Aspirate the trypsin and add 1 mL of fresh selection medium to resuspend the cells, and then transfer the cells into a T-75 cm^2 tissue culture flask.
4. Add 17 mL of selection medium to the flask allowing the cells to grow and form a monolayer at 37 °C, 5–8% CO_2.
5. Once the cells have reached 80–90% confluence, split the cells 1:5 in the selection medium. Repeat this for a total of three passages. Keep 1 mL of the supernatant at each passage for affinity precipitation to monitor the protein secretion level.
6. When cells reach confluency at the third passage, proceed to the next step.

3.4.2 Single Cell Isolation

1. Aspirate the medium from the 75 cm^2 flask and add 8 mL PBS. Gently rock the flask before aspirating the PBS.
2. Add 4 mL of trypsin-EDTA and leave for 5 s. Aspirate the trypsin and use 10 mL of fresh selection medium to resuspend the cells and transfer the cells into a 50 mL conical centrifuge tube.
3. Pellet the cells at 800 × g for 10 min. Remove the supernatant and resuspend the pellet in 20 mL selection medium.
4. Count the cells using trypan blue to determine cell density.
5. In three 96-well plates, add 200 μL PBS to the outer-most wells (rows A and H, columns 1 and 12) to prevent evaporation. Add 100 μL selection media to the remaining wells.

6. Dilute cells of interest in the selection media to 8 cells/mL, and add 100 μL of this dilution to each of the selection media-containing wells. Each well now should have an average of 0.8 cell/well (*see* **Note 4**).
7. Incubate the cells at 37 °C, 5–8% CO_2 for 10 to 14 days, permitting colonies to form and until single colonies of cells are observable under a light microscope.
8. When the color of the medium begins to change, transfer all single colonies individually by pipetting up and down to 24-well plates with 1 mL selection medium added to each well.
9. Incubate single colonies in 24-well plates at 37 °C, 5–8% CO_2 for 4 to 6 days, at which time a monolayer should form. When cells reach 70–90% confluence, take 0.9 mL of supernatant from each well for immuno-precipitation and Western blotting to identify clonal lines that express the most amount of secreted protein. Replace the selection medium. Once the best clone has been determined via immunoblot, then expand this clonal line into a larger tissue culture flask.
10. To expand the clonal line, aspirate the medium from the well of the selected clone. Add 1 mL PBS to wash cells and then aspirate. Add 0.3 mL trypsin-EDTA for 3 s. Remove trypsin and resuspend cells in 1 mL selection medium.
11. Transfer the resuspended cells into a T-75-cm^2 tissue culture flask added with 19 mL of selection medium. Incubate the cells until confluent at 37 °C, 5–8% CO_2.
12. Repeat steps 1 to 11 with selected clone(s) one to two more times to further select a stable clonal line with the maximal expression of the targeted soluble protein.
13. Once a desirable clone has been obtained, expand the selected cell line to larger flasks for storage and expression.

3.5 Expression and Collection of Protein in Suspension

3.5.1 Expression of Soluble Proteins

1. Once a good candidate has been selected for protein expression, move cells into two T-150-cm^2 tissue culture flasks with 30 mL of selection medium. Allow the cells to adhere and incubate at 37 °C, 5–8% CO_2 for a few days.
2. When the cells are 70–80% confluent, wash twice with 20 mL PBS, and then add 30 mL of FreeStyle™ 293 Expression Medium. Incubate the cells at 37 °C, 5–8% CO_2 overnight.
3. Next day, two T-150 cm^2 flasks of FreeStyle™ 293 cells are transferred into one 500 mL Erlenmeyer flask with FreeStyle™ 293 Expression Medium. To facilitate the transfer and select for less adherent cells, tap the flasks with your hands until most cells are nonadherent. Transfer the supernatant and FreeStyle™ 293 cells in suspension from the two T-150 cm^2 flasks

to the one 500 mL Erlenmeyer flask, add media to a final volume of 100 mL, and allow the cells to grow in suspension, shaking at 125 rpm in the 37 °C, 5–8% CO_2 incubator. Monitor the cell density and viability daily using a Trypan blue stain. When cells reach a density greater than $1.5x10^6$ / mL, the cells are split into multiple 500-mL Erlenmeyer flasks (e.g., 25 mL cell per flask; final volume 100 mL expression medium). When the split cells again reach a density greater than $1.5x10^6$ / mL, add expression medium to a final volume of 250 mL. Continually monitor the cells daily for 4 to 5 days until cell viability falls below 80%. The supernatant is then collected for protein purification procedures (*see* **Note 5**).

3.5.2 Harvesting Supernatant from Erlenmeyer Flasks

1. Collect the medium from each Erlenmeyer flask into 250 mL conical bottom centrifuge tubes. Spin at 2500 × g for 1 h to pellet the cells.
2. Collect the supernatant by decantation with a 0.2 μm low protein-binding filter membrane unit. Add three protease inhibitor tablets per 1 L of supernatant and Triton X-100 to a final concentration of 0.1%.
3. Filter the supernatant through the vacuum filter apparatus. Store the supernatant at 4 °C for affinity purification.

3.6 Affinity Purification of S-Tag Proteins

The steps for purifying S-tagged sF or sG protein through S-agarose affinity column are almost the same. The procedure for soluble F purification has been previously described [34], in which arginine was added during the course of purification to prevent protein aggregation and promote proper protein folding. In this part, we focus on soluble G, which because of its stability, the addition of arginine is not necessary.

1. Load 10 mL bed volume of S-protein Agarose into a XK 26 column. Always maintain at least 2–3 cm of buffer above the surface of the agarose.
2. Allow the column inlet adaptor to be 3–5 cm above the buffer level, allowing the input buffer to enter the column dropwise. Use a peristaltic pump to apply buffer through the inlet tubing. The solution passing through the column outlet depends on gravity.
3. Wash the column with 6-bed volumes of Wash Buffer I.
4. Apply the prepared supernatant to the column. Maintain a flow rate of 3 to 4 mL per minute by adjusting the peristaltic pump and a stopcock connected at the outlet tubing of the column.
5. Wash the column with 3x bed volumes of Wash Buffer I followed by 6x bed volumes of Wash Buffer II to remove triton.

6. To elute the bound protein, stop the pump and allow the Wash buffer II to drain until it reaches the surface of the beads. Add 12 mL of elution buffer. Incubate the elution buffer with the beads for 10 min (after collecting the first 4 mL of flow through; this should still be the Wash Buffer II).
7. Collect 12 mL of the elution into a 50 mL sterile conical centrifuge tube containing 20 mL of neutralization buffer. Check the pH with pH strips and add more neutralization buffer if needed to obtain neutral pH.
8. Repeat the elution and incubation 2 to 3 times.
9. Wash the column with 6X bed volume of wash buffer II follow by 6X bed volume of storage buffer. Store the beads in the storage buffer at 2 °C to 8 °C. Do not freeze the washed beads! The beads can be reused up to five times.
10. Combine all neutralized elution with the first 4 mL flow through from step 7.
11. Concentrate the elution by Amicon Ultra Centrifuge Filters 30 K to ~1 mL.
12. Exchange the elution into PBS.
13. Pre-wet an Acrodisc® Syringe Filter 0.2 μm HT Tuffryn Membrane, Low Protein-Binding filtration unit with PBS. Filter the purified protein, determine the concentration, and then store at 4 °C.

3.7 Size Exclusion Chromatography

1. Wash the analytic column: Superdex 200 10/300 GL gel filtration (GE Healthcare) with at least 3x column volume with sterile deionized water.
2. Equilibrate the column with at least three column volumes of the appropriate protein buffer (PBS for sG, PBS with 0.01% Triton X-100 for sF), keeping track of UV measurements. The column is ready for use when UV measurements are stable.
3. Inject protein into the machine at the entry port.
4. Use 3 mL syringe and tubing for sample injection. The column flow rate should be 60 mL/h
5. Start fractions collector.
6. Stop collection when the last UV peak has been observed.
7. Wash the column with at least 2x column volume of sterile deionized water followed by 3x column volume of 20% ethanol. Store the column in 20% ethanol.
8. Take 1 to 10 μl from each fraction of all peaks from the soluble glycoprotein for native gel analysis to observe the oligomeric species. The Coomassie blue and Western blot of Native PAGE gels for the peak-producing fractions.

3.8 Analysis of Proteins by Native PAGE System

3.8.1 Electrophoresis

1. Prepare running buffers: Dilute 20X Native PAGE™ running buffer to 1X solution in deionized water. Dilute 20X Native PAGE™ Cathode Buffer Additive to 1X solution for Coomassie detection and 0.1X solution for Western blotting in 1X Native PAGE™ running buffer.
2. Prepare samples: For 20 μL, add 5 μL of 4X NativePAGE™ Sample Buffer and 0.5 μL of NativePAGE™ 5% G-250 to 14.5 μL protein sample.
3. Set up the electrophoresis system using the NativePAGE™ Novex® 3–12% Bis–Tris Gels 1.0 mm, 15 well, and the XCell SureLock™ Mini-Cell as described by the manufacturer.
4. Rinse the wells with 1X running buffer and load the samples before adding the cathode buffer.
5. Load 5 μL of NativeMark™ Unstained Protein Standard for Coomassie stain and 10 μL added with 1 μL of 5% G-250 for Western blotting.
6. Perform the electrophoresis at 150 V for 2 h at room temperature.

3.8.2 Coomassie Stain

The G-250 reagent in the Cathode buffer stains the proteins during electrophoresis. Therefore, further staining is not required. However, a more sensitive staining protocol is available as described by the manufacturer.

1. After electrophoresis, place the gel in a container with enough fixing solution to cover the gel. Microwave the gel to near boiling and cool for 1 min on an orbital shaker at room temperature.
2. Repeat step 1 for two to three times and allow the gel to cool at room temperature for 15 min on an orbital shaker with gentle shaking.
3. Replace the fix solution with destain solution and microwave to near boiling two to three times as described in steps 1 and 2.
4. Shake the gel on an orbital shaker at room temperature until the desired background is obtained. See Fig. 3 for examples of Coomassie-stained gels.

3.8.3 Western Blotting

1. Use only 0.1X cathode buffer in 1X NativePAGE™ running buffer for Western blot.
2. Prepare 1X transfer buffer from 20X NuPAGE® Transfer Buffer in 20% methanol.
3. Activate the PVDF membrane in methanol for 1 min and rinse with deionized water.
4. Equilibrate PVDF membrane and filter paper in 1X transfer buffer for at least 5 min at room temperature.

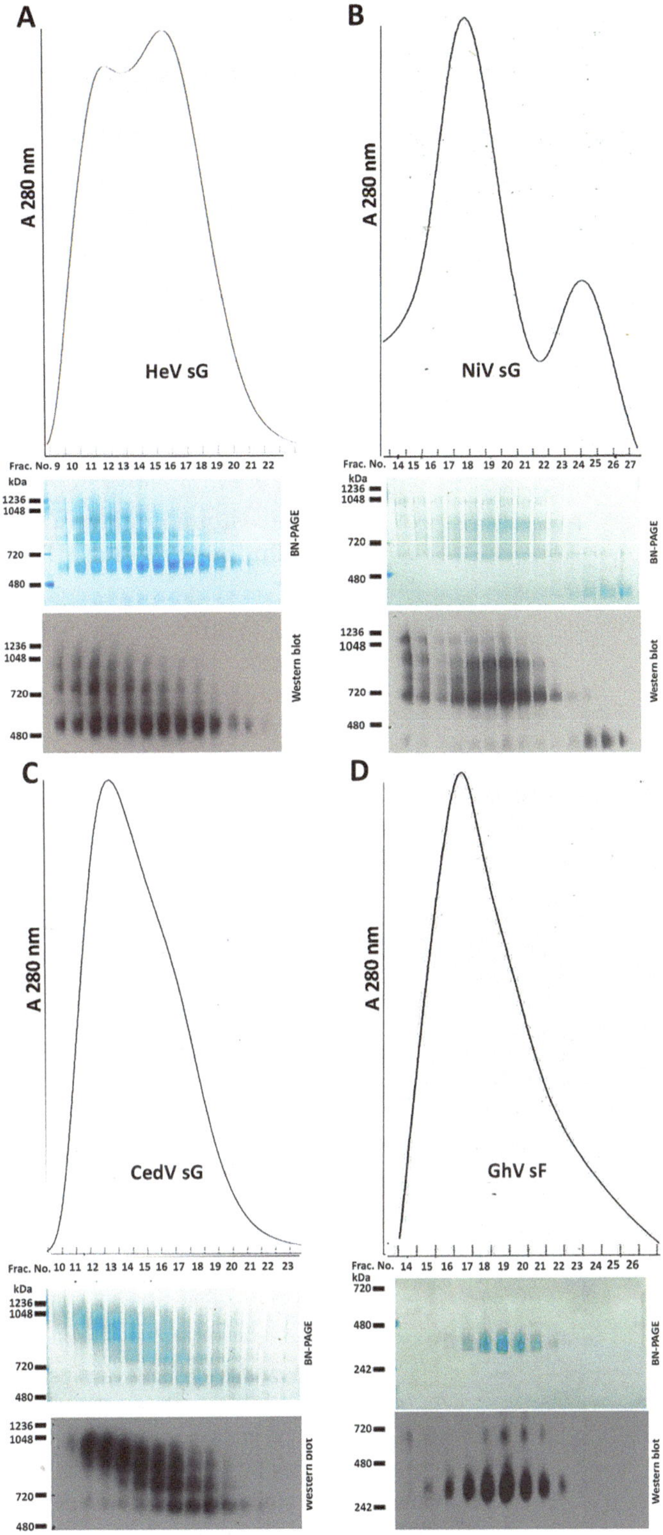

Fig. 3 Size exclusion chromatography analysis of various oligomeric envelope glycoproteins. Proteins were purified from FreeStyle™ 293F stable cell line supernatants. (**a**) HeV sG GCN_{tet} S-tag. (**b**) NiV sG GCN_{tet} S-tag. (**c**) CedV sG GCN_{tet} S-tag. (**d**) GhV sF-GCN_{t} S-tag. Supernatant protein (2 mg) was applied to a calibrated Superdex 200 10/300 gel filtration column, 400 μL of each fraction

5. After electrophoresis, place the gel in a transfer buffer with 0.1% SDS. Let this incubate while setting up the transfer apparatus using the XCell II™ Blot Module as described by the manufacturer.
6. Transfer at 42 V constant for 2 h at 4 °C.
7. After transfer, incubate the membrane in 20 mL of 8% acetic acid for 15 min at room temperature. Rinse with deionized water and air dry the membrane.
8. Rewet the membrane with methanol, and then rinse it with deionized water.
9. Place the membrane in blocking buffer and incubate at room temperature for at least 1 h or 4 °C overnight.
10. Proceed to immunodetection. To detect S-tagged, use 1: 20,000 dilution of α-S-tag HRP-conjugated antibody in blocking buffer.
11. Wash the membrane for 5 min in wash buffer and repeat washing three times. Add SuperSignal West Pico Chemiluminescent Substrate and incubate for 5 min at room temperature. Proceed to film exposure. See Fig. 3 for the results.

3.9 Determination of Glycoprotein Oligomerization Status by Cross-Linking

Surface glycoproteins of henipaviruses mediate successful entry of host cell. To validate the oligomeric formation of soluble forms of surface glycoproteins, we used a water-soluble, non-cleaveable bis-sulfosuccinimidyl suberate (BS^3) as a cross-linker. Here, we have optimized the conditions and confirmed the oligomeric status of those proteins.

1. Add 140 μL water to a 2 mg-size BS^3 tube to make a 25 mM stock solution. Use immediately and discard leftover.
2. For each protein, set up six different concentrations of BS^3 from 0.02, 0.04, 0.08, 0.12, 0.5, and 1.0 mM in a 50 μL reaction.
3. Add 1 μg protein at the last and incubate at 4 °C overnight. On the next day, add 2 μL Tris–HCL (1 M) to quench each reaction and incubate at room temperature for 15 min. Split

Fig. 3 (continued) was collected, and gel filtration elution profiles are presented in the top panels. Blue native polyacrylamide gel electrophoresis (BN-PAGE) analysis of elution profiles are presented in the middle panels. Fractions (10 μL) were analyzed by BN-PAGE and stained with Coomassie Brilliant Blue. Western blots of elution profile fractions (1 μL) probed with rabbit anti-S-tag antibody and HRP conjugate are presented on the bottom panels. Elution fractions with a profile corresponding to predicted native-like molecular weight, (**a**) fractions 14–21, (**b**) fractions 17–22, (**c**) fractions 16–21, and (**d**) fractions 16–22 were combined for concentration, S-tag removal, and further characterization

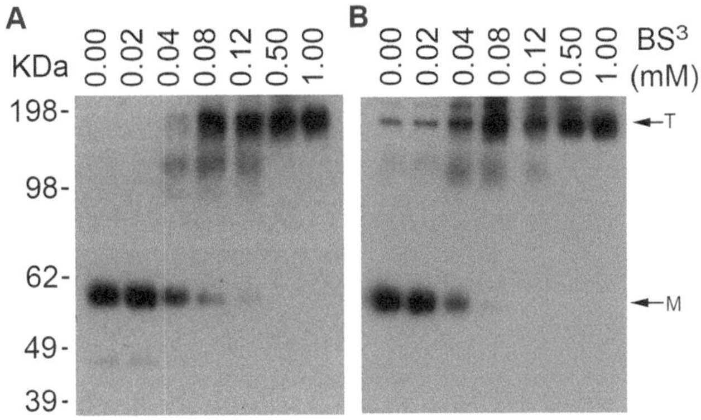

Fig. 4 Predicted sizes of purified oligomeric CedV sF-GCN$_t$. (**a**) Western blot, reduced conditions; (**b**) Western blot, nonreduced conditions. Purified CedV sF-GCN$_t$ protein (1.0 μg) was split into two equal volumes and cross-linked with a series of BS^3 cross-linker reagents at indicated concentrations. The purified protein (0.1 μg) from each reaction was electrophoresed on denaturing NuPAGE (4–12% polyacrylamide) gels and probed with α-S-tag HRP conjugate. Arrowheads from bottom to top indicate the positions of monomer (M) (~58 kDa) and trimer (T) (~174 kDa) of CedV sF-GCN$_t$ protein, respectively

each reaction into two tubes of equal volume (25 μL/ each) and then add 25 μL each to the reducing and nonreducing sample loading buffer. Load 0.1 μg (10 μL) of each reaction separately onto a 4–12% NuPAGE gel. Probe the blot with α-S-tag HRP-conjugated antibody. See Fig. 4. Cross-linking results shown for CedV sF-GCN$_t$ (*see* **Note 6**).

3.10 Removal of S-Tag for Soluble F Proteins

To generate monoclonal antibodies and reduce the chance of producing anti-S-tag antibodies, the S-tags were removed from each purified soluble protein by enzymatic digestion with Factor Xa (Millipore-Sigma) before being used to immunize mice. Protease digestion was carried out following the manufacturer's recommended protocol.

3.10.1 Factor Xa Cleavage of Recombinant Protein

1. Use 15 U enzyme to digest 1 mg protein in 1X Factor Xa Cleavage/Capture Buffer.
2. Incubate the reactions at 4 °C overnight.
3. Determine the extent of cleavage of the samples by SDS-PAGE analysis followed by Western blotting using α-S-tag Ab and Coomassie stain.

3.10.2 Removal of Factor Xa Enzyme

1. Prepare 1X Factor Xa Cleavage/Capture Buffer by diluting the supplied 10X stock with sterile deionized water.
2. Mix the Xarrest Agarose (supplied as a 50% slurry) by inversion until fully resuspended.

3. Centrifuge at 1000 × g for 1 min and carefully remove and discard the supernatant.
4. Resuspend the agarose in ten-bed volumes of 1X Factor Xa Cleavage/Capture Buffer, centrifuge again, and remove and discard the supernatant. Repeat three times.
5. Add one-bed volume of 1x Factor Xa Cleavage/Capture Buffer and fully resuspend. The Xarrest Agarose is now equilibrated and ready to use.
6. Transfer the prepared Xarrest Agarose from step 5 to the sample cup of a 2 mL spin filter. Add the entire volume of the cleavage reaction (1 mL from Sect. 1) to the prepared Xarrest Agarose. Mix gently to resuspend the agarose. Do not vortex.
7. Incubate and rotate at room temperature for 30 min.
8. Centrifuge the reaction at 1000 × g for 1 min to remove the Xarrest agarose. Bound Factor Xa is retained in the sample cup, and the cleaved target protein flows into the filtrate tube during centrifugation. Save the filtrated protein for the removal of residual S-tag.

3.10.3 Removal of Residual S-Tag

1. Wash S-Beads with 1x binding/washing buffer three times.
2. Transfer the cleaved protein from above into a tube with S-beads.
3. Incubate and rotate at room temperature for 45 min.
4. Centrifuge at 1000 × g for 1 min to remove the S-beads.
5. Save the filtrated fraction (the protein without S-tag).
6. Buffer exchange with PBS 0.01% Triton and determine concentration.
7. Determine the extent of cleavage of the samples by 4–12% NuPAGE gel analysis and stained with Coomassie Simply-BlueTM SafeStain or Western blot probed with anti-S-tag HRP-conjugated antibody. See Fig. 5, shown for HeV, NiV, and CedV sF-GCN$_t$ (*see* **Note 7**).

3.11 Henipavirus Multiplex Microsphere Immunoassay

Multiplex microsphere immunoassays based on Luminex xMAP technology that facilitate the measurements of multiple analytes in a single microplate well requiring very small sample volumes are a powerful approach compared to traditional ELISAs. A multiplex microsphere immunoassay (MMIA) using a Bio-Rad Bio-Plex platform was established to differentiate between HeV and NiV sera immunoglobulins [38]. Here, we incorporate CedV and GhV sF and sG along with HeV and NiV sF and sG in a single MMIA and demonstrate that monoclonal antibodies raised against the sF and sG are specific to the immunizing virus proteins. Manufacturer guidelines for activation of Bio-Plex Pro magnetic COOH beads and antigen coupling were followed (*see* **Note 8**). Antibody

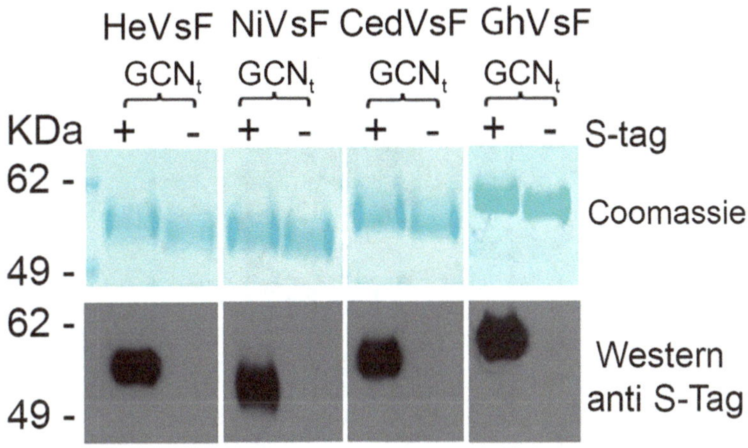

Fig. 5 Removal of peptide S-tag after oligomeric glycoprotein purification. Proteins from fractions corresponding with trimeric sizes were combined after size exclusion chromatography. The proteins marked with (–) were treated with Factor Xa Cleavage Capture Kit. The uncleaved and cleaved proteins were analyzed by 4–12% SDS-PAGE, stained with Coomassie blue (top panel), and confirmed by Western blotting detected with α--S-tag HRP conjugate (bottom panel). The + / – indicates with or without S-tag

dilutions were made to the final concentrations of 0.25 μg/mL. For washing steps, either automated or handheld magnetic plate washers are suitable following manufacturer guidelines or optimization.

1. Vortex each sF- or sG-coupled bead for 1 min and then sonicate all the beads for 1 min (*see* **Note 9**).
2. Prepare a master mix containing all the sF- or sG-coupled beads based on 1 μL of each sF- or sG-coupled bead per well in 100 μl PBSA (*see* **Note 10**).
3. Add 100 μL of sF/sG-bead master mix beads to each well, 96-well flat-bottom plates (*see* **Note 11**).
4. Wash the plate wells twice to remove the bead storage buffer.
5. Take 100 μl of all diluted antibodies and add them to designated wells.
6. Cover the 96-well plate with aluminum foil, and shake (900 rpm) at room temperature for 45 min.
7. Wash the plate three times to remove excess primary antibodies that have not bound to the sF- or sG-coupled beads.
8. Add 100 μL of biotinylated anti-mouse or anti-human IgG diluted 1:500 to each well. Cover the 96-well plate with aluminum foil and shake (900 rpm) at room temperature for 30 min.
9. Wash the plate to remove unbound secondary antibodies.

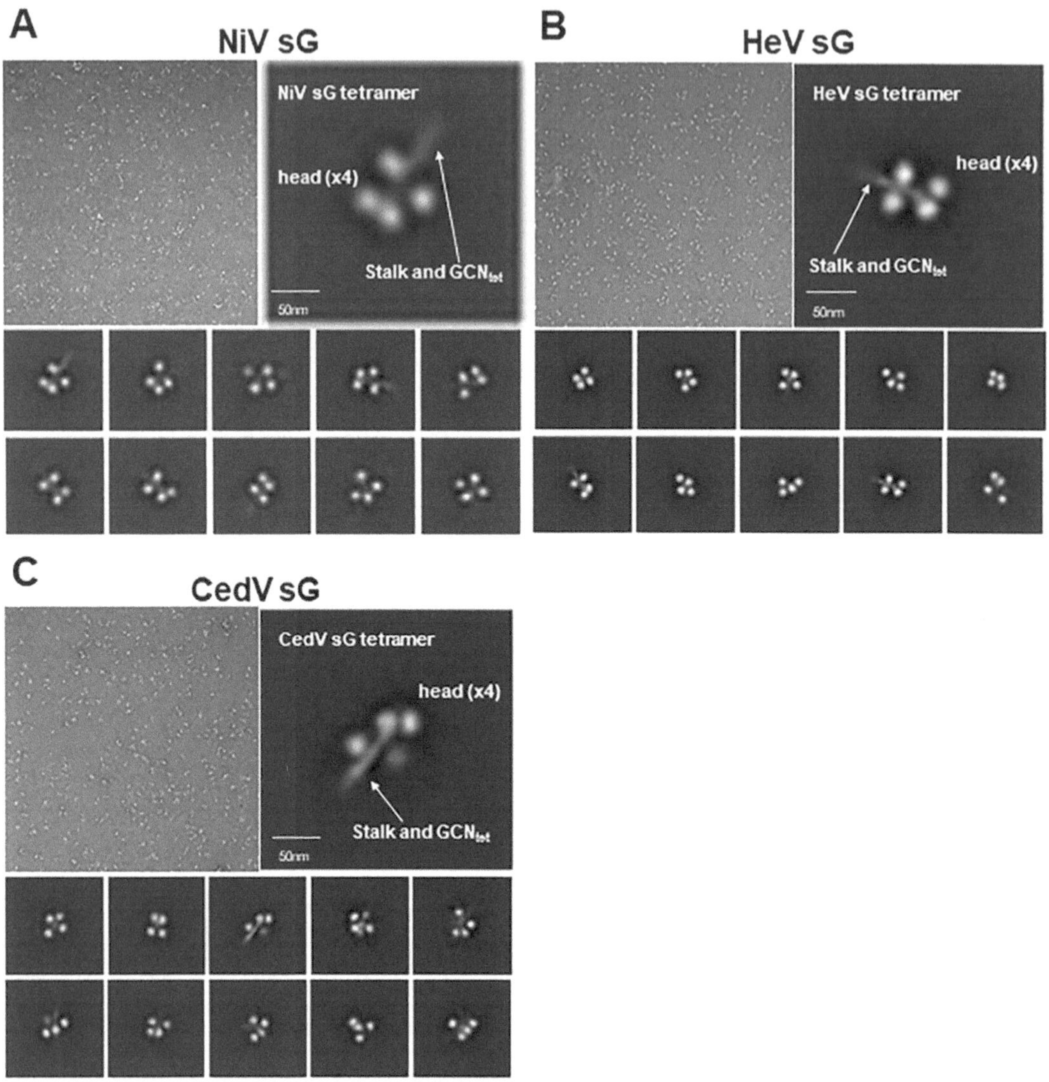

Fig. 6 Electron microscopy analysis of henipavirus sG glycoproteins. (**a**) NiV sG: A raw negative stain electron microscopy (nsEM) micrograph, select 2D classification and a representative class showing tetramer, including head, stalk, and GCN$_{tet}$ regions. (**b**) HeV sG: A raw nsEM micrograph, select 2D classification and a representative class showing tetramer, including head, stalk, and GCN$_{tet}$ regions. (**c**) CedV sG: A raw nsEM micrograph, select 2D classification and a representative class showing tetramer, including head, stalk, and GCN$_{tet}$ regions

10. Add 100 μL of Streptavidin-PE master mix (1:1000 in PBSA), cover the 96-well black plate with aluminum foil, and shake (900 rpm) at room temperature for 30 min.
11. Wash the plate to remove unbound Streptavidin-PE.
12. Resuspend each well with 120 μL PBSA-T to each well, and shake (900 rpm) for at least 15 min. Plates were then analyzed with a Bio-Rad Bio-Plex 200 machine with a High RP1 target setting. See Figs. 6, 7, and 8.

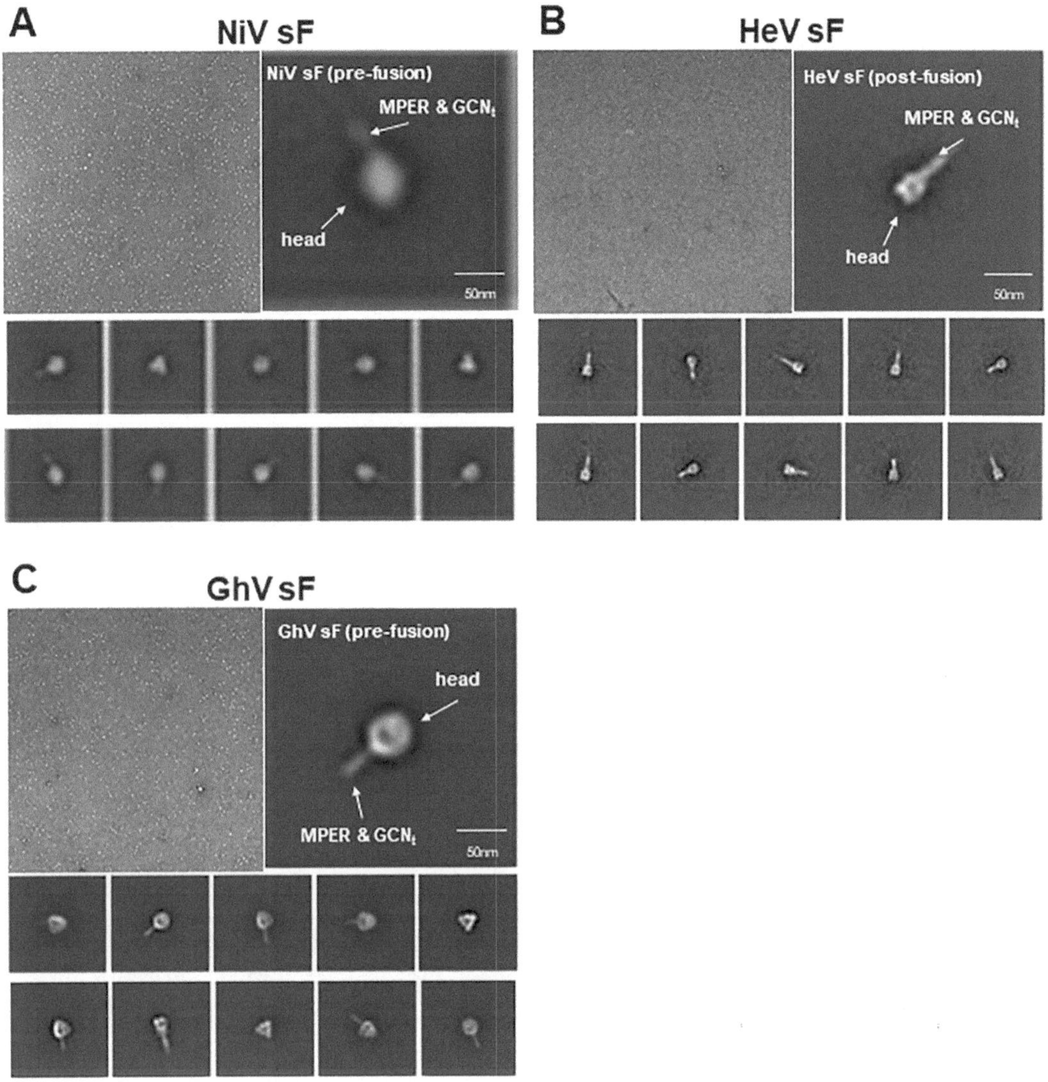

Fig. 7 Electron microscopy analysis of henipavirus sF glycoproteins. (**a**) NiV sF: A raw nsEM micrograph, 2D classification (pre-fusion form), and a representative pre-fusion class showing the globular head, membrane-proximal external region (MPER), and GCN$_t$ regions. (**b**) HeV sF: A raw nsEM micrograph, 2D classification (post-fusion form), and a representative post-fusion class showing head, membrane-proximal external region (MPER), and GCN$_t$ regions. (**c**) GhV sF: A raw nsEM micrograph, 2D classification (both pre-fusion and post-fusion forms), and a representative pre-fusion class showing the globular head, membrane-proximal external region (MPER), and GCN$_t$ regions

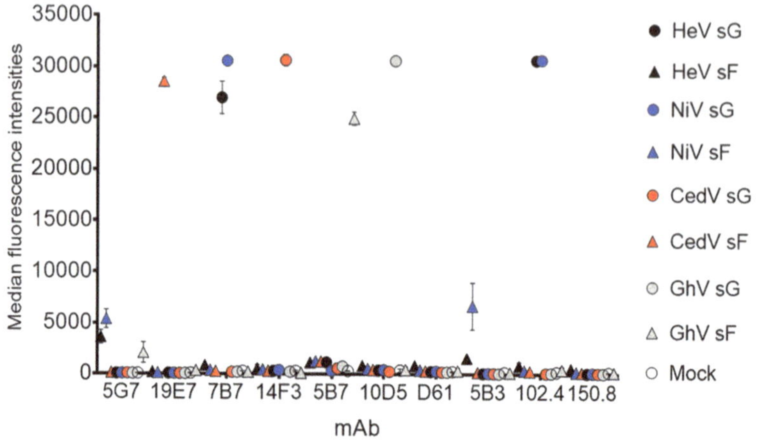

Fig. 8 Monoclonal antibodies react specifically with henipavirus glycoproteins. Purified sF and sG from HeV, NiV, CedV, and GhV were coupled to magnetic microspheres (Bio-Plex Pro™) and incubated with primary mouse monoclonal antibodies (0.125 μg/mL) followed by a secondary biotinylated anti-mouse IgG and detection with streptavidin–phycoerythrin. Glycoprotein-coupled microspheres and fluorescent signals were detected with a Bio-Rad Bio-Plex 200

4 Notes

1. To ensure proper folding and the stability of trimeric recombinant sF proteins, the GCN_t motif must be in heptad repeat phase with HR2 of F. HR2 and GCN_t both have a characteristic seven residues repeat, $(a,b,c,d,e,f,g)_n$ with hydrophobic residues at positions a and d. Therefore, when replacing the TM and CT domains of F with GCN_t, truncation of F must be downstream of position g of the C-terminal heptad repeat if position a of the GCN_t N-terminal heptad repeat follows.
2. Do not add lysis buffer to cell line generation well. Instead, replace supernatant with DMEM-5 supplemented with 300 μg/mL hygromycin B, henceforth discussed as selection media.
3. The nonexpressing cells should be dying within several days, and expressing colonies will start to form. For FreeStyle™ 293F cells, this may take 7 to 10 days depending on the transfection efficiency. When all dead cells have been removed and resistant colonies are growing well, the cells should be transferred into a 75 cm^2 tissue culture flask.
4. We also prepare one 96-well plate as described above, but with cells diluted to 1.6 cells/mL in order to ensure that enough single colonies could grow.

5. This procedure is scalable depending on the production efficiency of the cell lines, as well as the amount of protein needed.
6. HeV sF or NiV sF cross-linking procedures and results mirrored CedV sF results.
7. It was noticed that the N-terminally S-tag fused upstream of GCN_{tet} of sG was not cleavable. If the S-tag has to be cleaved from the protein for any purpose, we suggest adding a small linker (GGGGG) between fXa and GCN_{tet}, in which the fXa site can be accessible to Factor Xa protease and S-tag can be cleaved off.
8. Use extra caution to ensure beads do not get mixed, and also remember that beads are fluorescent so minimize exposure to light at all times.
9. For the sonication, place each tube containing virus sF- or sG-coupled beads into an Eppendorf tube foam floater. Place this foam floater into the ultrasound cleanser water bath. Put on ear protection, then turn the ON dial, and sonicate for 1 min.
10. Use 15 mL conical tube to make a master mix containing all the sF or sG-couples beads. For 96-well plates, make a 10 mL master mix. Add 100 μL of each sG- or sF-coupled bead stock, and bring the final volume to 10 mL PBSA. Gently vortex for 1 min.
11. Make sure all the tips are equally engaged, and when you go back and forth into the liquid reservoir containing the master mix, gently mix the solution to ensure that all sF- or sG-coupled beads are evenly distributed. Do not go past the first stop on the pipet when mixing.

Acknowledgments

The views expressed in the manuscript are solely those of the authors and do not represent official views or opinions of the Department of Defense or the Uniformed Services University of the Health Sciences.

Funding

Research support was provided by National Institutes of Health grants AI054715, AI077995, and AI142764 to C.C.B.

References

1. Wang LF, Yu M, Hansson E, Pritchard LI, Shiell B, Michalski WP, Eaton BT (2000) The exceptionally large genome of Hendra virus: support for creation of a new genus within the family Paramyxoviridae. J Virol 74(21): 9972–9979
2. Selvey LA, Wells RM, McCormack JG, Ansford AJ, Murray K, Rogers RJ, Lavercombe PS, Selleck P, Sheridan JW (1995) Infection of humans and horses by a newly described morbillivirus. Med J Aust 162(12):642–645
3. Centers for Disease C, Prevention (1999) Outbreak of Hendra-like virus – Malaysia and Singapore, 1998–1999. MMWR Morb Mortal Wkly Rep 48(13):265–269
4. Mohd Nor MN, Gan CH, Ong BL (2000) Nipah virus infection of pigs in peninsular Malaysia. Rev Sci Tech 19(1):160–165
5. Chua KB, Goh KJ, Wong KT, Kamarulzaman A, Tan PS, Ksiazek TG, Zaki SR, Paul G, Lam SK, Tan CT (1999) Fatal encephalitis due to Nipah virus among pig-farmers in Malaysia. Lancet 354(9186): 1257–1259. https://doi.org/10.1016/S0140-6736(99)04299-3
6. Halpin K, Hyatt AD, Fogarty R, Middleton D, Bingham J, Epstein JH, Rahman SA, Hughes T, Smith C, Field HE, Daszak P (2011) Pteropid bats are confirmed as the reservoir hosts of henipaviruses: a comprehensive experimental study of virus transmission. Am J Trop Med Hyg 85(5):946–951. https://doi.org/10.4269/ajtmh.2011.10-0567
7. Drexler JF, Corman VM, Gloza-Rausch F, Seebens A, Annan A, Ipsen A, Kruppa T, Muller MA, Kalko EK, Adu-Sarkodie Y, Oppong S, Drosten C (2009) Henipavirus RNA in African bats. PLoS One 4(7):e6367. https://doi.org/10.1371/journal.pone.0006367
8. Drexler JF, Corman VM, Muller MA, Maganga GD, Vallo P, Binger T, Gloza-Rausch F, Cottontail VM, Rasche A, Yordanov S, Seebens A, Knornschild M, Oppong S, Adu Sarkodie Y, Pongombo C, Lukashev AN, Schmidt-Chanasit J, Stocker A, Carneiro AJ, Erbar S, Maisner A, Fronhoffs F, Buettner R, Kalko EK, Kruppa T, Franke CR, Kallies R, Yandoko ER, Herrler G, Reusken C, Hassanin A, Kruger DH, Matthee S, Ulrich RG, Leroy EM, Drosten C (2012) Bats host major mammalian paramyxoviruses. Nat Commun 3:796. https://doi.org/10.1038/ncomms1796
9. Marsh GA, de Jong C, Barr JA, Tachedjian M, Smith C, Middleton D, Yu M, Todd S, Foord AJ, Haring V, Payne J, Robinson R, Broz I, Crameri G, Field HE, Wang LF (2012) Cedar virus: a novel Henipavirus isolated from Australian bats. PLoS Pathog 8(8):e1002836. https://doi.org/10.1371/journal.ppat.1002836
10. Hayman DT, Suu-Ire R, Breed AC, McEachern JA, Wang L, Wood JL, Cunningham AA (2008) Evidence of henipavirus infection in west African fruit bats. PLoS One 3(7): e2739. https://doi.org/10.1371/journal.pone.0002739
11. Peel AJ, Sargan DR, Baker KS, Hayman DT, Barr JA, Crameri G, Suu-Ire R, Broder CC, Lembo T, Wang LF, Fooks AR, Rossiter SJ, Wood JL, Cunningham AA (2013) Continent-wide panmixia of an African fruit bat facilitates transmission of potentially zoonotic viruses. Nat Commun 4:2770. https://doi.org/10.1038/ncomms3770
12. Pernet O, Schneider BS, Beaty SM, LeBreton M, Yun TE, Park A, Zachariah TT, Bowden TA, Hitchens P, Ramirez CM, Daszak P, Mazet J, Freiberg AN, Wolfe ND, Lee B (2014) Evidence for henipavirus spillover into human populations in Africa. Nat Commun 5:5342. https://doi.org/10.1038/ncomms6342
13. Wu Z, Yang L, Yang F, Ren X, Jiang J, Dong J, Sun L, Zhu Y, Zhou H, Jin Q (2014) Novel Henipa-like virus, Mojiang Paramyxovirus, in rats, China, 2012. Emerg Infect Dis 20(6): 1064–1066. https://doi.org/10.3201/eid2006.131022
14. Negrete OA, Levroney EL, Aguilar HC, Bertolotti-Ciarlet A, Nazarian R, Tajyar S, Lee B (2005) EphrinB2 is the entry receptor for Nipah virus, an emergent deadly paramyxovirus. Nature 436(7049):401–405. https://doi.org/10.1038/nature03838
15. Bonaparte MI, Dimitrov AS, Bossart KN, Crameri G, Mungall BA, Bishop KA, Choudhry V, Dimitrov DS, Wang LF, Eaton BT, Broder CC (2005) Ephrin-B2 ligand is a functional receptor for Hendra virus and Nipah virus. Proc Natl Acad Sci U S A 102(30): 10652–10657. https://doi.org/10.1073/pnas.0504887102
16. Xu K, Broder CC, Nikolov DB (2012) Ephrin-B2 and ephrin-B3 as functional henipavirus receptors. Semin Cell Dev Biol 23(1): 116–123. https://doi.org/10.1016/j.semcdb.2011.12.005
17. Bossart KN, Fusco DL, Broder CC (2013) Paramyxovirus entry. Adv Exp Med Biol 790:

95–127. https://doi.org/10.1007/978-1-4614-7651-1_6

18. Bowden TA, Crispin M, Harvey DJ, Jones EY, Stuart DI (2010) Dimeric architecture of the Hendra virus attachment glycoprotein: evidence for a conserved mode of assembly. J Virol 84(12):6208–6217. https://doi.org/10.1128/JVI.00317-10
19. Xu K, Chan YP, Rajashankar KR, Khetawat D, Yan L, Kolev MV, Broder CC, Nikolov DB (2012) New insights into the Hendra virus attachment and entry process from structures of the virus G glycoprotein and its complex with Ephrin-B2. PLoS One 7(11):e48742. https://doi.org/10.1371/journal.pone.0048742
20. Xu K, Chan YP, Bradel-Tretheway B, Akyol-Ataman Z, Zhu Y, Dutta S, Yan L, Feng Y, Wang LF, Skiniotis G, Lee B, Zhou ZH, Broder CC, Aguilar HC, Nikolov DB (2015) Crystal structure of the pre-fusion Nipah virus fusion glycoprotein reveals a novel hexamer-of-trimers assembly. PLoS Pathog 11(12):e1005322. https://doi.org/10.1371/journal.ppat.1005322
21. Broder CC (2012) Henipavirus outbreaks to antivirals: the current status of potential therapeutics. Curr Opin Virol 2(2):176–187. https://doi.org/10.1016/j.coviro.2012.02.016
22. VanBlargan LA, Goo L, Pierson TC (2016) Deconstructing the antiviral neutralizing-antibody response: implications for vaccine development and immunity. Microbiol Mol Biol Rev 80(4):989–1010. https://doi.org/10.1128/mmbr.00024-15
23. Bossart KN, Crameri G, Dimitrov AS, Mungall BA, Feng YR, Patch JR, Choudhary A, Wang LF, Eaton BT, Broder CC (2005) Receptor binding, fusion inhibition, and induction of cross-reactive neutralizing antibodies by a soluble G glycoprotein of Hendra virus. J Virol 79(11):6690–6702. https://doi.org/10.1128/jvi.79.11.6690-6702.2005
24. Xu K, Rajashankar KR, Chan YP, Himanen JP, Broder CC, Nikolov DB (2008) Host cell recognition by the henipaviruses: crystal structures of the Nipah G attachment glycoprotein and its complex with ephrin-B3. Proc Natl Acad Sci U S A 105(29):9953–9958. https://doi.org/10.1073/pnas.0804797105
25. Xu K, Rockx B, Xie Y, DeBuysscher BL, Fusco DL, Zhu Z, Chan Y-P, Xu Y, Luu T, Cer RZ, Feldmann H, Mokashi V, Dimitrov DS, Bishop-Lilly KA, Broder CC, Nikolov DB (2013) Crystal structure of the Hendra virus attachment G glycoprotein bound to a potent cross-reactive neutralizing human monoclonal antibody. PLoS Pathog 9(10):e1003684. https://doi.org/10.1371/journal.ppat.1003684
26. Chan YP, Lu M, Dutta S, Yan L, Barr J, Flora M, Feng YR, Xu K, Nikolov DB, Wang LF, Skiniotis G, Broder CC (2012) Biochemical, conformational, and immunogenic analysis of soluble trimeric forms of henipavirus fusion glycoproteins. J Virol 86(21):11457–11471. https://doi.org/10.1128/jvi.01318-12
27. Zhu Z, Bossart KN, Bishop KA, Crameri G, Dimitrov AS, McEachern JA, Feng Y, Middleton D, Wang L-F, Broder CC, Dimitrov DS (2008) Exceptionally potent cross-reactive neutralization of Nipah and Hendra viruses by a human monoclonal antibody. J Infect Dis 197(6):846–853. https://doi.org/10.1086/528801
28. Bossart KN, Zhu Z, Middleton D, Klippel J, Crameri G, Bingham J, McEachern JA, Green D, Hancock TJ, Chan Y-P, Hickey AC, Dimitrov DS, Wang L-F, Broder CC (2009) A neutralizing human monoclonal antibody protects against lethal disease in a new ferret model of acute Nipah virus infection. PLoS Pathog 5(10):e1000642. https://doi.org/10.1371/journal.ppat.1000642
29. Bossart KN, Geisbert TW, Feldmann H, Zhu Z, Feldmann F, Geisbert JB, Yan L, Feng YR, Brining D, Scott D, Wang Y, Dimitrov AS, Callison J, Chan YP, Hickey AC, Dimitrov DS, Broder CC, Rockx B (2011) A neutralizing human monoclonal antibody protects African green monkeys from Hendra virus challenge. Sci Transl Med 3(105):105ra103. https://doi.org/10.1126/scitranslmed.3002901
30. Geisbert TW, Mire CE, Geisbert JB, Chan Y-P, Agans KN, Feldmann F, Fenton KA, Zhu Z, Dimitrov DS, Scott DP, Bossart KN, Feldmann H, Broder CC (2014) Therapeutic treatment of Nipah virus infection in nonhuman primates with a neutralizing human monoclonal antibody. Sci Transl Med 6(242):242ra282. https://doi.org/10.1126/scitranslmed.3008929
31. Broder CC, Weir DL, Reid PA (2016) Hendra virus and Nipah virus animal vaccines. Vaccine 34(30):3525–3534. https://doi.org/10.1016/j.vaccine.2016.03.075
32. Middleton D, Pallister J, Klein R, Feng YR, Haining J, Arkinstall R, Frazer L, Huang JA, Edwards N, Wareing M, Elhay M, Hashmi Z, Bingham J, Yamada M, Johnson D, White J, Foord A, Heine HG, Marsh GA, Broder CC, Wang LF (2014) Hendra virus vaccine, a one health approach to protecting horse, human, and environmental health. Emerg Infect Dis

20(3):372–379. https://doi.org/10.3201/eid2003.131159

33. Geisbert TW, Bobb K, Borisevich V, Geisbert JB, Agans KN, Cross RW, Prasad AN, Fenton KA, Yu H, Fouts TR, Broder CC, Dimitrov AS (2021) A single dose investigational subunit vaccine for human use against Nipah virus and Hendra virus. NPJ Vaccines 6(1):23. https://doi.org/10.1038/s41541-021-00284-w
34. Chan YP, Yan L, Feng YR, Broder CC (2009) Preparation of recombinant viral glycoproteins for novel and therapeutic antibody discovery. Methods Mol Biol 525:31–58, xiii. https://doi.org/10.1007/978-1-59745-554-1_2
35. Cheliout Da Silva S, Yan L, Dang HV, Xu K, Epstein JH, Veesler D, Broder CC (2021) Functional analysis of the fusion and attachment glycoproteins of Mojiang Henipavirus. Viruses 13(3):517. https://doi.org/10.3390/v13030517
36. Earl PL, Broder CC, Doms RW, Moss B (1997) Epitope map of human immunodeficiency virus type 1 gp41 derived from 47 monoclonal antibodies produced by immunization with oligomeric envelope protein. J Virol 71(4):2674–2684. https://doi.org/10.1128/jvi.71.4.2674-2684.1997
37. Harbury PB, Zhang T, Kim PS, Alber T (1993) A switch between two-, three-, and four-stranded coiled coils in GCN4 leucine zipper mutants. Science 262(5138):1401–1407
38. Bossart KN, McEachern JA, Hickey AC, Choudhry V, Dimitrov DS, Eaton BT, Wang LF (2007) Neutralization assays for differential henipavirus serology using bio-Plex protein array systems. J Virol Methods 142(1–2):29–40. https://doi.org/10.1016/j.jviromet.2007.01.003

Chapter 4

Cell–Cell Fusion Assays to Study Henipavirus Entry and Evaluate Therapeutics

I. Abrrey Monreal and Hector C. Aguilar

Abstract

Henipaviruses include the deadly zoonotic Nipah (NiV) and Hendra (HeV) paramyxoviruses, which have caused recurring outbreaks in human populations. A hallmark of henipavirus infection is the induction of cell–cell fusion (syncytia), caused by the expression of the attachment (G) and fusion (F) glycoproteins on the surface of infected cells. The interactions of G and F with each other and with receptors on cellular plasma membranes drive both viral entry and syncytia formation and are thus of great interest. While F shares structural and functional homologies with class I fusion proteins of other viruses such as influenza and human immunodeficiency viruses, the intricate interactions between the G and F glycoproteins allow for unique approaches to studying the class I membrane fusion process. This allows us to study cell–cell fusion and viral entry kinetics for BSL-4 pathogens such as NiV and HeV under BSL-2 conditions using recombinant DNA techniques. Here, we present approaches to studying henipavirus-induced membrane fusion for currently identified and emerging henipaviruses, including more traditional syncytia counting-based cell–cell fusion assay and a new heterologous fluorescent dye exchange cell–cell fusion assay.

Key words Membrane fusion, Henipavirus, Class I fusion protein, Heptad repeat, Entry kinetics, Luciferase reporter assay, Split GFP, Split protein, F-triggering, Syncytia

1 Introduction

The membrane fusion process utilized by henipaviruses is of high interest as this is not only the means of viral entry but also the cause of pathognomonic features of henipavirus infection: syncytia formation. The latter is the generation of multinucleated cells (syncytia) that can be found in the lungs, CNS, and various other receptor-expressing tissues. The World Health Organization (WHO) has identified NiV and related viruses on the list of Blueprint priority diseases [1]. This, coupled with the discovery of new species of henipaviruses and increasing spillover events to new territories [2], urges the formulation of assays to measure viral entry kinetics and cell–cell fusion in various host cell types and species. These assays will in turn facilitate screens that assess the

Alexander N. Freiberg and Barry Rockx (eds.), *Nipah Virus: Methods and Protocols*, Methods in Molecular Biology, vol. 2682, https://doi.org/10.1007/978-1-0716-3283-3_4,

inhibition of membrane fusion in vitro. Dealing with BSL-4 pathogens is costly, cumbersome, and time-consuming. While some research requires the use of a live virus, the ability to study the membrane fusion process and test potential therapeutics at BSL-2 conditions greatly increases the speed of henipavirus research and discovery. Since viral infection depends on membrane fusion, in vitro inhibitors of this process could also yield therapeutic candidates for in vivo use.

Membrane fusion for the henipaviruses is carried out in a pH-independent manner and is mediated by the viral attachment (G) and fusion (F) glycoproteins. This has been described extensively in the literature [1c, 3]. Briefly, G first binds a protein receptor (ephrin-B2 or ephrin-B3 for NiV and HeV), which then causes a series of conformational changes in G that in turn trigger F to drive the fusion of viral–cell and cell–cell membranes. Traditionally, membrane fusion assays are carried out using recombinant versions of the attachment and fusion glycoproteins transfected into permissive cell lines, followed by quantification of fusion via syncytia counting [4a]. This approach can also be used to screen fusion inhibitors, such as the previously described heptad repeat region peptides, including HR2 [5]. Cell–cell fusion assays may also be used to identify permissive cell lines and virus receptors by generating recombinant versions of the F and G glycoproteins of newly identified henipaviral species and assessing the induction of cell–cell fusion [4a]. Additionally, we recently developed a related cell–cell fusion assay described in detail using fluorescent markers to track the fusion process. This heterologous cell fusion assay uses a nonpermissive cell line, incapable of undergoing fusion, to express the attachment and fusion glycoproteins, which are then overlaid with receptor-containing cells fluorescently labeled with lipid, cytoplasmic, and DNA stains. Hemifusion and full membrane fusion can then be tracked over time by monitoring the amount of lipid and cytoplasmic dye exchanged, respectively. Hemifusion is an intermediate state of the membrane fusion process in which the juxtaposed outer membranes have been mixed, but the inner membranes and cytoplasmic contents have not.

The steps from receptor binding to full membrane fusion are an active area of research, and determining all the membrane fusion intermediates remains important. One of the tools used to study intermediate steps in fusion utilizes a peptide that traps the fusion glycoprotein in the pre-hairpin intermediate (PHI) [6]. At this stage, the fusion process has gone from receptor binding to F-triggering by G, a process that exposes the heptad repeat regions of F. This intermediate is trapped in this PHI confirmation by the HR2 peptide, ultimately blocking fusion. This peptide-based approach was the basis of an antiviral for HIV [7] and has been developed as an important tool for studying the viral–cell membrane fusion process for class I fusion proteins. This allows probing of hyper- and hypofusogenic mutants to determine what aspect of the F/G interactions is affected to generate various fusion phenotypes.

While not covered in detail here, entry kinetics from a viral standpoint can also be studied outside of BSL-4 settings via a pseudotyped virus reporter assay, using vesicular stomatitis virus (VSV) with a luciferase reporter gene, pseudotyped with henipaviruses G and F, which is extensively described in the literature [8].

Additionally, we have recently adapted to the study of henipaviruses a described approach to study the kinetics of fusion pore formation, using a dual-split protein assay adapted from Nakane and Matsuda [9] This assay can be used to complement syncytia counting and specifically can differentiate between F and G mutants that may be deficient in full fusion but capable of undergoing fusion pore formation. Since this assay depends on the exchange of cytoplasmic contents, where a split GFP–luciferase complex combines to make an active luciferase or GFP protein, it is possible to identify mutants that form pores but may not be able to undergo complete membrane fusion as observed through syncytia counting.

Here, we present quantitative approaches to assess cell–cell fusion via traditional syncytia counting, as well as the newly adapted quantitative heterologous cell–cell fusion assay, which assesses fusion pore formation and hemifusion.

2 Materials

The amount of fusion observed can be affected by the level of proteins expressed on the cell surface, proper F processing (proper proteolytic cleavage), the ratio of F to G, and time. We have included the general protocol followed in our laboratory for Nipah (NiV) and Hendra (HeV), but conditions should be adapted to other henipaviruses and F/G mutants to ensure that comparisons within experimental designs are valid. In addition, flow cytometry and Western blot analysis should be carried out to assess glycoprotein expression at the cell surface, as well as F processing, respectively, as these parameters can severely affect cell–cell fusion quantification. While this assay can be readily adapted to other permissive cell lines, we describe it using HEK-293 T and Vero cells.

2.1 Syncytia Counting and Cell–Cell Fusion Inhibition Assays

2.1.1 Cell Culture and Transfection

1. Permissive cell line culture and reagents: HEK-293 T cells or Vero cells, grown in complete media. DMEM supplemented with 10% fetal bovine serum and 100 u/mL penicillin 0.1 mg/mL streptomycin (from 100× solution).
2. Recombinant proteins: Appropriate recombinant DNA expression plasmids encoding for F and G *henipavirus* proteins in vectors suitable for mammalian expression in the cells of choice (*see* **Note 1**).

3. Transfection reagents: 6-well plates, 25 kD linear polyethyleneimine (PEI) prepared at 1 mg/mL pH 7.0 and sterile-filtered, or lipofectamine 2000/3000, or TurboFect, depending on the cell of choice, Opti-MEM, or serum-free DMEM.

2.1.2 Counting

1. Giemsa stain (optional).
2. Light microscope with phase contrast or suitable setup to visualize unstained cells.
3. Counter/clicker.

2.1.3 Inhibition

1. Potential inhibitors at desired concentrations.

2.2 Heterologous Fusion Assay

This assay can be done using various cell types. In the case below, we present the use of PK13 (a nonpermissive cell line herein termed effector cells) overlaid with Vero cells (target cells) containing the receptor and which undergo fusion only when mixed with the effector cells. Depending on the need, this assay can be adapted in the case of NiV and HeV using BSRT7 cells, HEK-293 T, or other cell lines as target cells. For initial trials and optimization, it is suitable to observe fusion events at 200X using standard clear bottom 6-well plates. For higher magnification, we recommend the use of coverslips or suitable plates amenable to higher-power microscopy.

2.2.1 Transfection and Seeding

1. Vero cells in 10 cm dishes.
2. 6-well plates for PK13 cells.
3. Plasmids of interest including GFP, RFP, or similar protein.
4. Complete media as above.
5. Lipofectamine 2000.

2.2.2 Labeling and Overlaying Veros

1. CellTracker Green CMFDA.
2. DiI stain (1,1′-dioctadecyl-3,3,3′,3′-tetramethylindocarbocyanine perchlorate (‘DiI’; DiIC18 (3))).
3. Hoechst 33342.
4. Pre-warmed (37 °C) complete media and Opti-MEM.

2.2.3 Microscopy

1. 6-well clear bottom plates or u-slide of choice (*see* **Note 2**).
2. Poly-lysine-coated coverslips #1½.
3. Glass slides.
4. Mounting media, 20 mM Tris pH 8.0, 50% glycerol, 0.5% N-propyl gallate (*see* **Note 3**).
5. Coverslip sealant (clear fast-drying nail polish).
6. Microscope with proper filter sets and inverted microscope for observing 6-well plates.

3 Methods

3.1 Syncytia Counting and Cell–Cell Fusion Inhibition Assays

Standard biosafety measures and cell line-specific incubation procedures must be followed unless specified otherwise. Cell numbers and procedures outlined below are for use with HEK-293 T cells. Other cell types may require further optimization, i.e., seeding densities, transfection procedure, and requirement of Giemsa staining.

3.1.1 Transfection

1. Day 0: Split cells to be transfected 1 day before inappropriate complete media. 6-well dish: Seed ~0.3–0.5 × 10^6 cells/well and aim for 80–95% confluency on the day of transfection (*see* **Note 4**).
2. Day 1: Prior to transfection, bring all reagents to room temperature. Continue to step 3 if using cell lines amenable to PEI transfection. If using a commercially available transfection reagent, follow the manufacturer's protocol using 2–3 μg total DNA and then proceed to step 8.
3. In a sterile tube, add plasmid DNA (2 μg total) to 1 mL of serum-free DMEM or Opti-MEM per well (*see* **Note 5**).
4. Add 6 μL PEI (1 μg/μL) to the diluted DNA. Mix immediately by gentle vortexing or pipetting (*see* **Note 6**).
5. Incubate for 15 min at room temperature.
6. Add DNA/PEI mixture to cells after aspirating incubation media, and rinse gently with pre-warmed PBS before adding DNA/PEI mixture, if desired.
7. Add 2 mL of pre-warmed complete media to transfected cells 4 h after transfection, and it is not necessary to remove/rinse transfection media (*see* **Note 7**).
8. Observe cells for syncytia formation and fix cells in 0.5% PFA solution at the appropriate time (~16 h depending on the viral glycoproteins), and syncytia should be countable and distinguishable between mutants or conditions.
9. Optional Giemsa staining: If cell type makes it difficult to distinguish between fused and unfused cells, staining with Giemsa is recommended to help visualize nuclei inside syncytia. To fixed cells, add Giemsa Stain diluted 1:20 with deionized water for 15–60 min before rinsing with deionized water and air-drying before counting.

3.1.2 Syncytia Counting

1. Using a handheld counter or similar device count, the total number of nuclei within syncytia found in each field, counting five fields per well at 200X magnification. Nuclei are counted when there are ≥4 nuclei to avoid counting cell division events

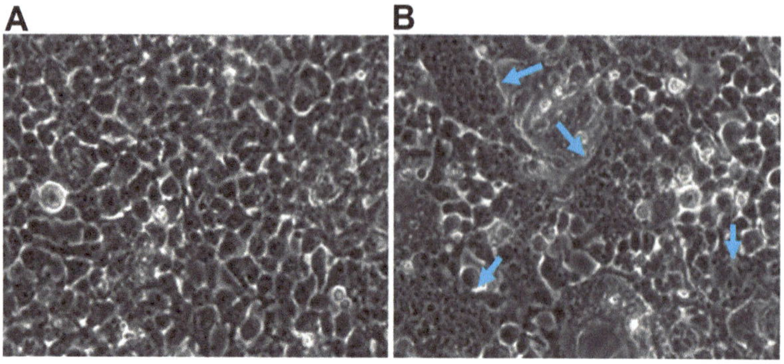

Fig. 1 Syncytia formation obtained by glycoprotein expression plasmid transfection. (**a**) HEK-293 T cells mock-transfected with pCDNA3.1+ showing no syncytia formation. (**b**) Representative image of HEK-293 T cells undergoing fusion after transfection of NiV F and G DNA expression plasmids. Blue arrows point to formed syncytia

(*see* **Note 8**). Optionally, nuclei outside of syncytia may also be counted per field, to calculate a percentage of fused cells per field (Fig. 1).

3.1.3 Inhibition Assays

1. The addition of the desired inhibitor can be done as early as 0–4 h post-transfection in the media of choice depending on the stability of the inhibitor but should be added prior to the beginning of fusion events. Make sure that the inhibitor does not affect transfection efficiency, for example, using a GFP or luciferase DNA expression vector as a marker of transfection efficiency.

3.2 Heterologous Fusion Assay

3.2.1 Cell Seeding and Coverslip Preparation

1. Day 0: If observing cells under high magnification, prepare coverslip using poly-lysine before placing them in individual wells. Alternatively, use commercially available vessels suitable for higher magnification, as mentioned in *see* **Note 2**.
2. Seed 6-well plate with 0.3–0.5 × 10^6, or plate of choice, of PK13s to be transfected. Aim for 80–90% confluency at the time of transfection. If observing fusion under high power, add the poly-lysine-coated coverslips prior to seeding.
3. Seed Vero cells in a 10-cm dish using ~2.2 × 10^6 cells aiming for 70–85% confluency upon completion of transfection. On average, a single 10-cm dish of Vero cells is suitable to overlay a 6-well plate of PK13s when using 250,000 Vero cells per well.

3.2.2 Transfection and Labeling

1. Day 1: Transfect PK13s using 2 μg of total DNA and a 1:1–3:1 (or other desired) ratio of F/G using Lipofectamine 2000 following the manufacturer's protocol. It is recommended to transfect a control-well with a fluorescent marker protein to monitor transfection efficiency.

2. Day 2: Stain receptor-positive cells using 2 μM CellTracker (CT) and 0.25 μM DiI (*see* **Note 9**).
3. Add DiI and CellTracker to 5 mL pre-warmed complete media/10-cm culture dish from 10 mM working stocks in DMSO. Ensure that dye solutions are completely homogenous prior to adding them to the media. DiI may be diluted 1:1 from 20 mM DMSO stock with EtOH to prevent precipitation and crashing out of dye prior to addition to complete media.
4. Remove media from cells and add the fluorophore solution.
5. Incubate at 37 °C and 5% CO_2 for 30 min.
6. Wash cells 3 × 5 min using 5–10 mL pre-warmed full media.
7. Label Vero nuclei using Hoechst at 2 μM final concentration in 5 mL pre-warmed Opti-MEM for 30 min in the incubator (*see* **Note 10**).
8. Wash cells 3 × 5 min as previously. Cells can sit at this stage for up to 24 h in full media (generally left for 2 h before overlay).

3.2.3 Overlay and Slide Preparation

1. Rinse labeled cells with PBS, then add 5 mL PBS to plate, scrape cells using a cell scraper, and then collect and rinse the plate with an additional 5 mL of PBS.
2. Centrifuge cells at 200 × g for 5 min at 4 °C.
3. Remove supernatant and resuspend in ~250 μL Opti-MEM. Then, count in a hemocytometer to get the desired coverage. The suggested overlay density is ~250,000 cells/well, but this number can be adjusted as necessary (*see* **Note 11**).
4. Add cells evenly and dropwise to PK13 cells. Shake back and forth side to side and ensure even distribution. Do not swirl!
5. Spinoculate if desired at 200 × g for 5 min 4 °C. Cells can be quickly imaged at time zero if needed (be very quick). Leave cells in the incubator for 1 h before fixing for 15 min with 0.5% PFA (*see* **Note 12**).
6. Proceed to imaging if not preparing coverslips for use on slides. If proceeding with mounted slides first ensure slides are clean, and add 8–12 μL of mounting media in the center of the slide.
7. Remove the coverslip from the well and gently dab excess PFA on the kimwipe by touching the thin side of the coverslip before placing it carefully on top of the previously added mounting media.
8. Using a fine brush affix, the coverslip to the slide by adding a small amount of clear fingernail polish to opposite ends before proceeding to the next sample.

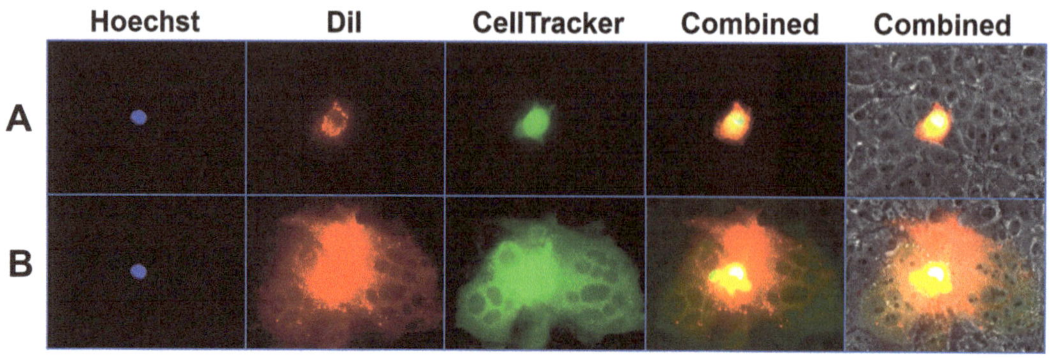

Fig. 2 Heterologous fusion assay. Vero target cells were overlaid on transfected effector PK13 cells at 200X. The target cells are labeled using the nuclear stain Hoechst, lipid dye DiI, and cytoplasmic dye CellTracker green CMFDA. (**a**) No fusion is observed in pCDNA3.1+ mock-transfected effector cells. (**b**) Representative image of dyes diffusing from target to effector cells during cell–cell syncytia formation

9. When done with the last sample, finish sealing the slides and allow them to dry before gently cleaning the exposed side of the coverslip. Then, proceed to imaging.

3.2.4 Microscopy and Imaging

1. Image wells ensuring settings can be maintained between wells with no overexposed regions. If quantification of types of fusion events, i.e., hemifusion vs fusion, will be performed, a lower overlay density of Vero cells is recommended. Then, a full count of events in each well is used to compare between samples (Fig. 2). We routinely use the open-source project software Fiji [10] for image processing and analysis.

4 Notes

1. It is suggested to perform flow cytometry and Western blot analyses, respectively, to determine cell surface expression and F protein processing levels, as these can drastically affect syncytia levels.
2. Traditional 6-well plates are not suitable for use past 200X magnification. There are many commercially available variants and options available depending on need.
3. N-propyl gallate is an optional anti-fade additive. Mounting media can be adjusted from 50% to 90% glycerol. 50% glycerol will give the best brightfield views, and 90% glycerol will give the clearest background during fluorescence imaging. When using the glycerol-based mounting medium, images should be taken within 24 h. For prolonged storage and imaging, other mounting media should be considered.

4. The use of codon-optimized DNA is recommended using vectors that have been designed for high expression in the desired mammalian cell lines, such as pCDNA 3.1^{+}, pCMV, pCAGGS, or other suitable vectors.
5. The order of addition and concentration of DNA will affect transfection efficiency. The DNA solution should be made and mixed prior to adding the 1 μg/μL PEI. Do not add concentrated PEI solutions to DNA.
6. Ratios of PEI/DNA can be varied from 2:1 to 6:1 as determined experimentally.
7. If using Opti-MEM, it is not necessary to add media at 4 h; although protein expression levels may be altered, this must be determined when establishing a set protocol.
8. In HEK-293 T cells, it is not usually necessary to use a stain to aid in seeing syncytia, and the appearance of a "halo" of light can be used to differentiate between fused cells, where fused cells will not allow light to be transmitted. Syncytia will appear as dark, flat patches, and the nuclei within the syncytia will appear as circles within the patches. To assess fusion, the syncytia counted should be averaged across fields and normalized to the wild-type fusion protein of interest. Traditional 6-well plates are not suitable for use past 200X magnification. There are many commercially available variants and options available depending on need.
9. The staining concentration was optimized to be 2 μM Cell Tracker green and 0.25 μM DiI. Modify concentrations depending on individual results.
10. Check labeling of overlay cells before proceeding to the overlay step to ensure adequate dye labeling, and Hoechst dye can "leak" into PK13 cells if not adequately washed from the Vero cells before overlaying.
11. Pipette vigorously to remove clumps for best results. After determining cell concentration, adjust volume as required for desired cell coverage.
12. Incubation can be changed to any desired length of time, and this method is suitable for live cell imaging before fixing. Extended incubation times are also suitable, but will result in large syncytia events.

References

1. (a) Organization, W. H. List of Blueprint priority diseases http://www.who.int/blueprint/priority-diseases/en/; (b) Organization, W. H. Nipah virus outbreaks in the WHO South-East Asia Region. http://www.searo.who.int/entity/emerging_diseases/links/nipah_virus_outbreaks_sear/en/. Accessed 12 Sept 2017; (c) Sharma V, Kaushik S, Kumar R, Yadav JP (2019) Emerging trends of Nipah virus: a review. Rev Med Virol 29(1):6
2. (a) Atherstone C, Diederich S, Weingartl H. M, Fischer K, Balkema-Buschmann A, Grace D, Alonso S, Dhand NK, Ward MP, Mor SM (2019) Evidence of exposure to

henipaviruses in domestic pigs in Uganda. Transbound Emerg Dis 66(2):921–928; (b) Kessler MK, Becker DJ, Peel AJ, Justice NV, Lunn T, Crowley DE, Jones DN, Eby P, Sanchez CA, Plowright RK (2018) Changing resource landscapes and spillover of henipaviruses. Ann N Y Acad Sci 1429(1):78–99; (c) Pernet O, Schneider BS, Beaty SM, LeBreton M, Yun TE, Park A, Zachariah TT, Bowden TA, Hitchens P, Ramirez CM, Daszak P, Mazet J, Freiberg AN, Wolfe ND, Lee B (2014) Evidence for henipavirus spillover into human populations in Africa. Nat Commun 5:10

3. (a) Singh RK, Dhama K, Chakraborty S, Tiwari R, Natesan S, Khandia R, Munjal A, Vora KS, Latheef SK, Karthik K, Malik YS, Singh R, Chaicumpa W, Mourya DT (2019) Nipah virus: epidemiology pathology immunobiology and advances in diagnosis vaccine designing and control strategies – a comprehensive review. Vet Q 39(1):26–55; (b) Satterfield BA, Dawes BE, Milligan GN (2016) Status of vaccine research and development of vaccines for Nipah virus. Vaccine 34(26):2971–2975; (c) Pernet O, Wang YE, Lee B (2012) Henipavirus receptor usage and tropism. In: Lee B, Rota PA (eds) Henipavirus: ecology molecular virology and pathogenesis, vol 359. Springer, Berlin, pp 59–78; (d) Aguilar HC, Iorio RM (2012) Henipavirus membrane fusion and viral entry. In: Lee B, Rota PA (eds) Henipavirus: ecology molecular virology and pathogenesis, vol 359. Springer, Berlin, pp 79–94; (e) Rockx B, Winegar R, Freiberg AN (2012) Recent progress in henipavirus research: molecular biology genetic diversity animal models. Antivir Res 95(2): 135–149; (f) Aguilar HC, Lee B (2011) Emerging paramyxoviruses: molecular mechanisms and antiviral strategies. Expert Rev Mol Med 13:19; (g) Lee B, Ataman ZA (2011) Modes of paramyxovirus fusion: a Henipavirus perspective. Trends Microbiol 19(8):389–399

4. (a) Negrete OA, Levroney EL, Aguilar HC, Bertolotti-Ciarlet A, Nazarian R, Tajyar S, Lee B (2005) EphrinB2 is the entry receptor for Nipah virus an emergent deadly paramyxovirus. Nature 436(7049):401–405; (b) Negrete OA, Chu D, Aguilar HC, Lee B (2007) Single amino acid changes in the Nipah and Hendra virus attachment glycoproteins distinguish EphrinB2 from EphrinB3 usage. J Virol 81(19):10804–10814; (c) Bonaparte MI, Dimitrov AS, Bossart KN, Crameri G, Mungal BA, Bishop KA, Choudhry V, Dimitrov DS, Wang LF, Eaton BT, Broder CC (2005) Ephrin-B2 ligand is a functional receptor for Hendra virus and Nipah virus. Proc Natl Acad Sci U S A 102(30):10652–10657

5. (a) Xu YH, Gao S, Cole DK, Zhu JJ, Su N, Wang H, Gao GF, Rao ZH (2004) Basis for fusion inhibition by peptides: analysis of the heptad repeat regions of the fusion proteins from Nipah and Hendra viruses newly emergent zoonotic paramyxoviruses. Biochem Biophys Res Commun 315(3):664–670; (b) Bossart KN, Mungall BA, Crameri G, Wang LF, Eaton BT, Broder CC (2005) Inhibition of Henipavirus fusion and infection by heptad-derived peptides of the Nipah virus fusion glycoprotein. Virol J 2:15

6. (a) Aguilar HC, Ataman ZA, Aspericueta V, Fang AQ, Stroud M, Negrete OA, Kammerer RA, Lee BA (2009) Novel receptor-induced activation site in the Nipah virus attachment glycoprotein (G) involved in triggering the fusion glycoprotein (F). J Biol Chem 284(3): 1628–1635; (b) Liu Q, Bradel-Tretheway B, Monreal AI, Saludes JP, Lu XN, Nicola AV, Aguilar HC (2015) Nipah virus attachment glycoprotein stalk C-terminal region links receptor binding to fusion triggering. J Virol 89(3):1838–1850; (c) Liu Q, Stone JA, Bradel-Tretheway B, Dabundo J, Montano JAB, Santos-Montanez J, Biering SB, Nicola AV, Iorio RM, Lu XN, Aguilar HC (2013) Unraveling a three-step spatiotemporal mechanism of triggering of receptor-induced Nipah virus fusion and cell entry. PLoS Pathog 9(11): 12; (d) Biering SB, Huang A, Vu AT, Robinson LR, Bradel-Tretheway B, Choi E, Lee B, Aguilar HC (2012) N-Glycans on the Nipah virus attachment glycoprotein modulate fusion and viral entry as they protect against antibody neutralization. J Virol 86(22):11991–12002; (e) Aguilar HC, Aspericueta V, Robinson LR, Aanensen KE, Lee B (2010) A quantitative and kinetic fusion protein-triggering assay can discern distinct steps in the Nipah virus membrane fusion Cascade. J Virol 84(16): 8033–8041

7. (a) Jiang SB, Lin K, Strick N, Neurath AR (1993) HIV-1 INHIBITION BY A PEPTIDE. Nature 365(6442):113–113; (b) Wild C, Greenwell T, Matthews T (1993) A synthetic peptide from HIV-1 GP41 is a potent inhibitor of virus-mediated cell-cell fusion. AIDS Res Hum Retrovir 9(11):1051–1053

8. (a) Johnson JB, Aguilar HC, Lee B, Parks GD (2011) Interactions of human complement with virus particles containing the Nipah virus glycoproteins. J Virol 85(12):5940–5948; (b) Erbar S, Maisner A (2010) Nipah virus infection and glycoprotein targeting in

endothelial cells. Virol J 7:10; (c) Whitt MA (2010) Generation of VSV pseudotypes using recombinant Delta G-VSV for studies on virus entry identification of entry inhibitors and immune responses to vaccines. J Virol Methods 169(2):365–374

9. Nakane S, Matsuda Z (2015) Dual Split protein (DSP) assay to monitor cell-cell membrane fusion. In: Pfannkuche K (ed) Cell fusion: overviews and methods, 2nd edn. Humana Press Inc, Totowa, pp 229–236

10. Schindelin J, Arganda-Carreras I, Frise E, Kaynig V, Longair M, Pietzsch T, Preibisch S, Rueden C, Saalfeld S, Schmid B, Tinevez JY, White DJ, Hartenstein V, Eliceiri K, Tomancak P, Cardona A (2012) Fiji: an open-source platform for biological-image analysis. Nat Methods 9(7):676–682

Part II

Studying Infectious Henipaviruses In Vitro

Chapter 5

Recombinant Cedar Virus: A Henipavirus Reverse Genetics Platform

Moushimi Amaya, Christopher C. Broder, and Eric D. Laing

Abstract

The isolation of Cedar virus, a nonpathogenic henipavirus that is closely related to the highly pathogenic Nipah virus and Hendra virus, provides a new platform for henipavirus experimentation and a tool to investigate biological differences among these viruses under less stringent biological containment. Here, we detail a reverse genetics system used to rescue two replication-competent, recombinant Cedar virus variants: a recombinant wild-type Cedar virus and a recombinant Cedar virus that express a green fluorescent protein from an open reading frame inserted between the phosphoprotein and matrix genes. This recombinant Cedar virus platform may be utilized to characterize the determinants of pathogenesis across the henipaviruses, investigate their receptor tropisms, and identify novel pan-henipavirus antivirals safely under biosafety level-2 conditions.

Key words Reverse genetics, Henipavirus, Cedar virus, Virus rescue, Virus titration, Virus plaque assay

1 Introduction

The known pathogenic members of the genus *Henipavirus*, *Nipah henipavirus* Nipah virus (NiV) and *Hendra henipavirus* Hendra virus (HeV), are zoonotic agents distinguished from the many paramyxoviruses that cause human and animal diseases by virtue of their uniquely broad host tropism and impressive lethality [1–3]. NiV and HeV can cause a systemic and often fatal respiratory and/or neurological disease in 11 mammalian species including humans [4–6]. NiV in Bangladesh and India is of particular concern where outbreaks occur annually with nearly 100% case fatality rates, no subclinical infections, and well-documented person-to-person transmission [1, 7]. Currently, there are no vaccines or therapeutics against NiV or HeV approved for human use, and they remain infectious disease transboundary threats to public health and economically important livestock throughout South and Southeast Asia, Oceania, and Australia [8, 9]. HeV and NiV are enveloped,

Alexander N. Freiberg and Barry Rockx (eds.), *Nipah Virus: Methods and Protocols*, Methods in Molecular Biology, vol. 2682, https://doi.org/10.1007/978-1-0716-3283-3_5,

single-stranded negative-sense RNA (-ssRNA) viruses, and a third bat-borne henipavirus, Cedar virus (CedV), was isolated and classified as a new species, *Cedar henipavirus*, in the genus *Henipavirus*. Whereas HeV and NiV are disease-causing zoonoses, CedV is nonpathogenic in four susceptible animal HeV and NiV disease models [10, 11].

The de novo production of replication-competent negative-sense RNA (-ssRNA) viruses from a cDNA template encoding the viral genome are commonly referred to as reverse genetics. This powerful technology has transformed the field of -ssRNA viruses and opened new avenues of research [12–14]. Modification of the viral genome through reverse genetics enables researchers to analyze the effects of specific mutations and gain a better understanding of all aspects of the viral life cycle, such as replication, tissue tropism, pathogenesis, and virus–host interactions [14, 15]. Moreover, the generation of recombinant viruses expressing fluorescent reporters allows researchers to monitor real-time viral replication and spread of the virus and identify infected cells or tissues in vitro or in vivo. The advent of reverse genetics systems has been instrumental in driving forward the development of vaccines, novel therapies, and antiviral screening assays.

Reverse genetics systems have been used to generate recombinant infectious and replication-competent viruses, particularly the henipaviruses: NiV, HeV, and CedV [14, 16–21]. The generation of recombinant henipaviruses by the use of reverse genetics has elucidated the role and functionality of individual genes and/or proteins to evade or antagonize the immune response, infectivity cycle, and pathogenesis [16, 18, 20, 22], investigate differences in receptor tropism [23], or characterize chimeric viruses by exchanging HeV and NiV genes [21]. The recovery of replication-competent -ssRNA viruses involves the co-transfection of cells with a plasmid expressing the positive sense, antigenome from a high-fidelity RNA polymerase promoter together with individual helper plasmids encoding the open reading frame of the nucleocapsid (N), phosphoprotein (P), and the RNA-dependent RNA polymerase (L). Genomic RNA requires encapsidation by the N protein before it can serve as a functional template to initiate transcription and replication [14]. Thus, in *trans* helper plasmid expression of N, P, and L proteins, which together form the virus polymerase complex, is required to initiate henipavirus replication and de novo protein synthesis.

Many factors are taken into consideration for a successful henipavirus rescue: (i) the antigenome must adhere to the "rule of 6"; (ii) the helper plasmid ratio must conform to the transcriptional gradient found in natural henipavirus infections; (iii) the ends of the viral genome must be cleaved precisely; and (iv) the inclusion of a T7 promoter to prevent the addition of the nonviral guanosine (G) residues [14]. Like other paramyxoviruses, to encapsulate the henipavirus genome, N proteins precisely bind to six nucleotides, so to promote replication initiation the genome length must remain a multiple of 6, thus obeying the "rule of 6" [24]. The transfected concentrations of each helper plasmid should follow the natural henipavirus N, P, and L expression ratio where N is present in the highest number, followed by P and then L. Expression of the antigenome by T7 polymerase must occur in the cytoplasm and can be achieved by either infecting cells with recombinant vaccinia expressing bacteriophage T7 polymerase, using cells stably expressing T7 polymerase, or transfection of a T7 polymerase expression plasmid. Buchholz et al. generated a BHK-derived cell line stably expressing T7 polymerase and BSR-T7/5 cells that remediated the cytotoxic effects of the vaccinia virus [25].

Here, we detail the methodology for the rescue of two recombinant CedV (rCedV) variants, one recombinant wild-type CedV (rCedV-wt) and one recombinant reporter CedV virus that express a green fluorescent protein (rCedV-GFP) from an additional open reading frame between the P and matrix (M) genes. While NiV and HeV are biosafety level 4 (BSL-4) pathogens, recombinant replication-competent CedV experimentation with rescued viruses can be conducted under BSL-2 containment settings [17]. The recombinant CedV antigenome was cloned into an expression plasmid (pOLTV5) [26] between a T7 polymerase promoter fused to the 5′ end of the CedV cDNA and an autocatalytic hepatitis delta virus (HDV)-derived ribozyme at the 3′ end of the cDNA followed by the T7 terminator. CedV N, P, and L open reading frames were sub-cloned into CMV promoter-driven expression plasmids (pCMV) [27]. BSR-T7/5 cells were co-transfected with the pOLTV5-rCedV antigenome plasmid and pCMV-N, pCMV-P, and pCMV-L helper plasmids in an optimal ratio for virus replication that was identical to the concentrations of N, P, and L helper plasmids used to rescue recombinant HeV [19]. A generalized schematic of a rCedV rescue system is illustrated in Fig. 1. The collected rCedV was purified over a sucrose cushion, tittered, and stored at −80 °C until used for infection assays.

2 Materials

All solutions are prepared using deionized water (diH_2O) and are stored at 4 °C unless otherwise stated. Prepare solutions in advance to maintain a streamlined workflow. Carefully dispose of waste as per the rules and regulations assigned by your institution.

2.1 Cells, Medium, Transfection Reagents, and Culture Vessels

1. BSR-T7/5 cells.
2. Vero E6 cells.

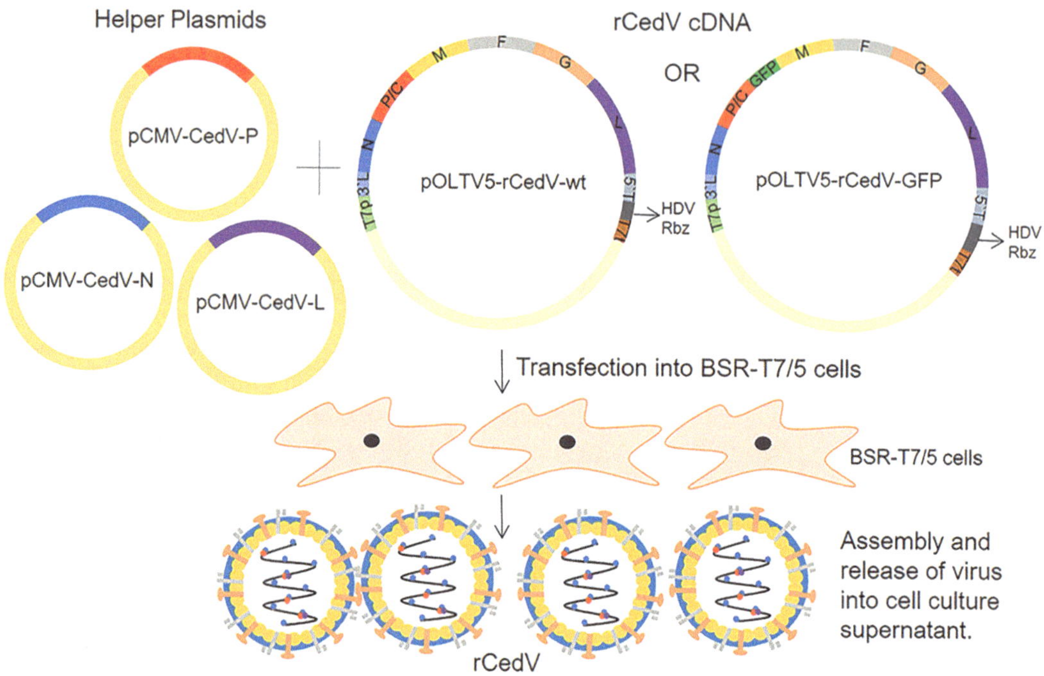

Fig. 1 Graphical representation of a CedV reverse genetics system. CedV N, P, and L gene open reading frames were cloned into CMV promoter-driven expression plasmids: helper plasmids. The full-length antigenome of CedV was ligated into the expression plasmid pOLTV5 between a T7 promoter at the 5′ end and a hepatitis delta virus ribozyme followed by a T7 terminator at the 3′ end of the cDNA. The helper plasmids, pCMV-CedV-N, pCMV-CedV-P, and pCMV-CedV-L, and the pOLTV5-rCedV antigenome plasmid were co-transfected into BSR-T7/5 cells, which constitutively express T7 polymerase. Successful rescue of replication-competent recombinant progeny CedV is dependent on transfection, T7 polymerase transcription of the full-length antigenome, and de novo replication and transcription of the CedV genome by the CedV polymerase complex

3. D-10: Dulbecco's modified Eagle's medium, 1% L-glutamine, 10% cosmic calf serum.
4. D-5: Dulbecco's modified Eagle's medium, 1% L-glutamine, 5% cosmic calf serum.
5. Opti-MEM Reduced Serum Medium.
6. Poly-D-Lysine (0.1 mg/mL).
7. Phosphate-buffered saline (PBS (1X)).
8. Trypsin-EDTA.
9. Lipofectamine LTX.
10. Sterile, 6-well culture plates.
11. Sterile, 12-well culture plates.
12. Sterile, 96-well culture plates.
13. Sterile, 50 mL polystyrene tubes.
14. Sterile, 15 mL polystyrene tubes.

15. Sterile, 2 mL screw cap freezer tubes.
16. Sterile, 1.5 mL Eppendorf tubes.
17. Ethanol (EtOH) 100% and 70%.
18. 37 °C water bath.
19. SW28 Ti Swinging-Bucket Beckman Rotor.
20. SW28 Ultra-Clear centrifuge tubes.
21. 20% (w/v) sucrose in TNE buffer: 20 mM Tris–HCl, 150 mM NaCl, 1 mM EDTA, pH 7.4.
22. 10% (w/v) sucrose in TNE buffer: 20 mM Tris–HCl, 150 mM NaCl, 1 mM EDTA, pH 7.4.
23. Fixing solution for plaque assay: 10% formaldehyde, diH_20. Store at room temperature.
24. Fixing solution for immunofluorescence: 4% paraformaldehyde, diH_20. Store at room temperature.
25. Permeabilizing solution: 0.5% Triton X-100, 1xPBS. Store at room temperature.
26. Blocking solution: 3% cosmic calf serum in 1xPBS.
27. 2% (w/v) carboxymethylcellulose (CMC) sodium salt (medium viscosity) in autoclaved diH_20 (*see* **Note 1**). Store at room temperature.
28. Crystal violet solution (CV): 0.5% (w/v) crystal violet, 25% methanol, autoclaved diH_20. Store at room temperature.

2.2 Plasmids

A schematic representation of the plasmids is shown in Fig. 2.

1. pOLTV5-rCedV-wt.
2. pOLTV5-rCedV-GFP.
3. pCMV-CedV-N.
4. pCMV-CedV-P.
5. pCMV-CedV-L.

3 Methods

The methods described below include those for the recovery, amplification, purification, and quantification of replication-competent infectious rCedV. Controls used to evaluate the efficiency of virus recovery are described. All work must be performed in a biosafety cabinet under BSL-2 conditions.

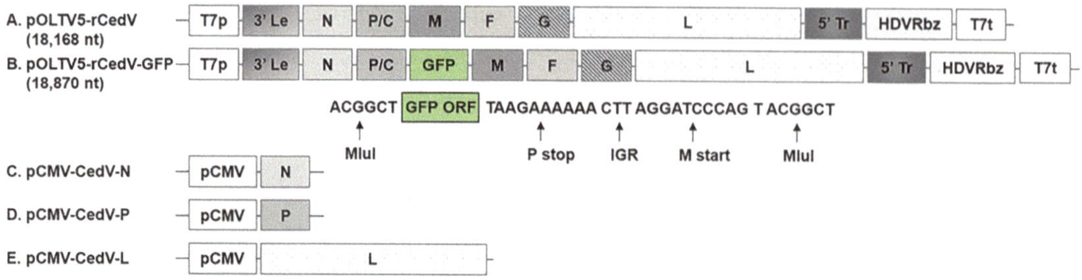

Fig. 2 Schematic representation of recombinant CedV genomes. (**a**) Cloned CedV DNA fragments were inserted between a T7 promoter at the 5′ end and a hepatitis delta virus ribozyme followed by a T7 terminator at the 3′ end of the cDNA in the pOLTV5 vector to yield pOLTV5-rCedV-wt. (**b**) A MluI restriction site was created between the P and M genes to facilitate the insertion of a modified turbo green fluorescent protein (GFP) gene to generate pOLTV5-rCedV-GFP. The 3′ terminus of the GFP gene is flanked by the P gene transcriptional stop, intergenic region (IGR), and M gene transcriptional stop sequences. A noncoding thymine (T) between the M gene transcriptional stop and MluI sequence was added to preserve the "rule of 6" necessary for replication. (**c**–**e**) pCMV-CedV-N, pCMV-CedV-P, and pCMV-CedV-L helper plasmids, respectively. T7p, T7 promoter; 3′ Le, 3′ leader; 5′ Tr, 5′ trailer; HDVRbz, hepatitis delta virus ribozyme; T7t, T7 terminator

3.1 Recovery of Replication-Competent rCedV from Plasmids

For successful recovery, it is important that the cells used for transfection be maintained at a low passage number (i.e., less than 30 passages) and that they are never allowed to reach 100% confluence. This ensures that the cells retain optimal transfectability.

1. Add 1 mL of poly-D-Lysine to each well of a 6-well plate and incubate at 37 °C for 10–15 min (*see* **Note 2**). Discard poly-D-Lysine and wash wells once with 1xPBS.
2. Seed BSR-T7/5 cells at a density of 2.5×10^5 cells/well in 2 mL D-10 (*see* **Note 3**).
3. Incubate the cells at 37 °C for 16–24 h in a humidified incubator containing 5% CO_2.
4. Check the confluence and viability of cells prior to beginning the assay.
5. At the time of transfection, the cells should be ~80% confluent.
6. Prepare the transfection mix. These concentrations are per well (*see* **Note 4**).
   6.1. pCMV-CedV-N (1.25 μg).
   6.2. pCMV-CedV-P (0.8 μg).
   6.3. pCMV-CedV-L (0.4 μg).
   6.4. pOLTV5 full-length CedV antigenome plasmid (3.5 μg).
   6.5. 12 μL of Lipofectamine LTX.
   6.6. 500 μL Opti-MEM.
7. Incubate at room temperature for 30 min.

8. As controls, include a helper plasmid-only well, a pOLTV5-rCedV plasmid-only well, and an untransfected well (*see* **Note 5**).
9. Remove the medium from the plate and add 1.5 mL of pre-warmed D-10.
10. Add the transfection complexes (500 μL) dropwise to the corresponding wells.
11. Following transfection, incubate the plate(s) at 37 °C in a humidified incubator containing 5% CO_2 for 4–5 days.
12. The day before harvesting the primary recovery wells, plate Vero E6 cells in a 6-well plate at a density of 5×10^5 cells/well in 2 mL of D-10.
13. Incubate the Vero E6 cells at 37 °C for 16–24 h in a humidified incubator containing 5% CO_2.
14. Place a beaker half filled with 100% EtOH at −80 °C.
15. The next day, check the confluence and viability of the Vero E6 cells prior to beginning the assay to ensure ~90–100% confluence.
16. Collect and reserve the supernatant in pre-labeled sterile screw cap tubes.
17. Gently wash the transfected cells once with 1 mL of 1xPBS.
18. Add 500 μL of trypsin-EDTA to each well and incubate at 37 °C for 5–10 min or until the cells detach. Tapping the side of the plate gently might help dislodge the cells if they are too adherent.
19. Use the collected supernatant to gather the trypsinized cells. Gently pipet the supernatant, up and down, into the corresponding wells to dislodge any still adherent cells and place the mixture in their appropriate screw cap tubes.
20. Complete three freeze–thaw cycles to release any cytosolic viruses from the transfected cells. Place the collected mixture tubes in a floating 1.5-mL microcentrifuge tube rack and place in the beaker of 100% EtOH at −80 °C for 15 min. Remove and place the rack in a 37 °C water bath for 5–10 min or until the mixture is thawed. Repeat the freeze–thaw cycle for a total of three times.
21. Replace the D-10 in the Vero E6 cell plate with 1.5 mL of D-5 and add 500 μL of the freeze/thawed cell culture supernatant to the Vero E6 cells and incubate at 37 °C in a humidified incubator containing 5% CO_2.
22. The Vero E6 cells should be monitored daily for the development of GFP reporter expression, or cytopathic effects (CPE),

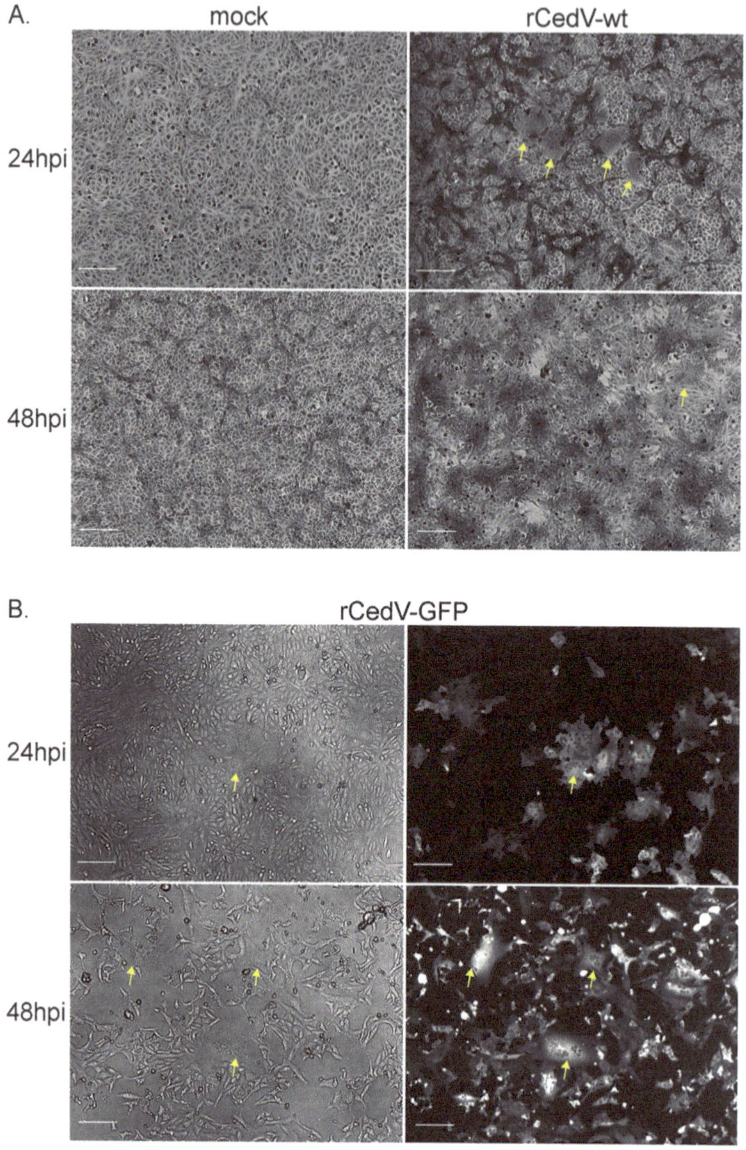

Fig. 3 Recombinant CedV forms syncytia in Vero E6 cells. Vero E6 cells were infected or not (mock) with rCedV-wt (**a**) and rCedV-GFP (**b**) from successful virus rescue wells. At 24 and 48 hpi, rCedV-infected cells were fixed with methanol and stained with 0.5% crystal violet-25% methanol. Images were captured with a Zeiss Axio Observer A1 inverted microscope using a 5X objective. Yellow arrows indicate giant cells, and the scale bar is 50 μm. (Reproduced from E.D. Laing et al., 2018 [17])

which are seen as areas of giant multinucleated cells or syncytia, a hallmark of henipavirus infections as shown in Fig. 3.

23. When 60–100% of the cells show signs of virus-induced CPE, harvest the supernatants.

24. Transfer the collected medium to a sterile 15 mL polystyrene tube(s) and centrifuge at 948 × g (2400 rpm) for 10 min to pellet cell debris.
25. Aliquot the cleared supernatants into appropriately labeled 2 mL sterile screw cap freezer tubes and store them at −80 °C. This is referred to as the first passage (P1) and can be stored indefinitely at −80 °C.
26. To amplify the virus for a large stock, confluent Vero E6 cells in fresh D-10 in cell culture flasks can be infected with rCedV-wt or rCedV-GFP at a multiplicity of infection (MOI) of 0.01.
27. Incubate ~3–4 days at 37 °C in a humidified incubator containing 5% CO_2.
28. When most cells are infected, this is when maximum GFP expression, CPE, or syncytia is observed, collect supernatant, and place in 50 mL conical tubes. These can be stored at −80 °C until ready to purify.

3.2 Virus Purification (See Notes 6 and 7)

1. Spin the collected supernatants at 948 × g (2600 rpm) for 10 min to pellet cell debris.
2. With a clean pipet, carefully transfer clarified supernatant to clean 50 mL polystyrene tubes on ice. Be careful not to disturb the pelleted cell debris.
3. Prepare sucrose cushion by transferring 8 mL of 20% (w/v) sucrose TNE buffer into SW28 ultracentrifuge tubes.
4. Slowly add clarified virus supernatant (27 mL/tube) to the sucrose cushion.
5. Centrifuge at 100,000 × g (27,000 rpm) with a SW28 rotor at 4 °C for 2 h.
6. Carefully aspirate supernatant without disturbing the virus pellet (*see* **Note 8**).
7. Resuspend pelleted virus in 400 μL of 10% (w/v) sucrose in TNE buffer at 4 °C overnight. Cover tubes with parafilm and wipe them down with 70% EtOH before removing them from the biosafety cabinet.
8. Next day, collect and combine all 400 μL resuspensions into a single tube. Then, sequentially wash the tubes by adding 500 μL of fresh 10% sucrose buffer to tube 1, withdrawing content, and transferring to tube 2, etc., to ensure the collection of all the resuspended virus pellets.
9. Store at −80 °C until ready to titer (*see* **Note 9**).

3.3 Titration of rCedV by Fluorescence

1. Seed Vero E6 cells at 1×10^4 cells/well in a 96-well plate in 100 μL of D-10.
2. Incubate the cells at 37 °C in a humidified incubator containing 5% CO_2.
3. Check the confluence and viability of cells prior to beginning the assay.
4. In sterile 1.5-mL Eppendorf tubes, prepare a ten-fold serial dilution of the virus sample using D-10 as the diluent, 10^{-1} to 10^{-8}, in triplicate, such that there will be 100 μL/well. Change tips between dilutions to prevent carryover.
5. Add to Vero E6 cells and incubate for 72 h at 37 °C in a humidified incubator containing 5% CO_2.
6. Enumerate rCedV-GFP foci using a ZEISS Axio Observer A1 inverted microscope with a 5X objective to calculate the infectious units/mL (IU/mL). In a 96-well plate well, ~5–10 GFP foci are adequate to count.

   6.1. IU/mL = (Ave # foci) × (well dilution) × (dilution factor).
7. For rCedV-wt, remove the medium from the 96-well plate and fix the cells with 4% paraformaldehyde for 1 h at room temperature.
8. Permeabilize cells with the permeabilizing solution for 20 min at room temperature (enough to cover the well).
9. Wash wells once with 1xPBS.
10. Block at room temperature for 10 min with blocking solution (enough to cover the well).
11. Incubate with a primary antibody against CedV-N-protein (1: 1000 dilution) in blocking solution for 1 h at room temperature.
12. Wash wells 3x with 1xPBS.
13. Add secondary antibody goat anti-rabbit 488 Alexa Fluor conjugate (Thermo Fisher Scientific) (1:1000 dilution) in blocking solution for 1 h in the dark at room temperature.
14. Wash wells 3x with 1xPBS.
15. Count fluorescent cells using a Zeiss Axio Observer A1 inverted microscope with a 5X objective and calculate the IU/mL as in step 5.

3.4 Titration of rCedV by Plaque Assay

1. Seed Vero E6 cells at 2.5×10^5 cells/well in a 12-well plate in 1 mL of D-10 such that they reach 90–100% confluency the next day.
2. Incubate the cells at 37 °C in a humidified incubator containing 5% CO_2.

3. Check the confluence and viability of cells prior to beginning the assay.
4. In sterile 1.5 mL Eppendorf tubes, prepare a ten-fold serial dilution of the virus sample using D-10 as the diluent, 10^{-1} to 10^{-8}, for duplicate wells, such that there will be 200 μL/well. Change tips between dilutions to prevent carryover.
5. Remove D-10 from the wells and add 200 μL/well of the diluted inoculums to their respective wells.
6. Incubate for 1 h at 37 °C while rocking plates every 20 min.
7. After infection, add 2 mL of the 2% CMC overlay to the inoculum using a 1:1 mix of D-5 + 2% CMC.
8. Incubate plates for 5–6 days at 37 °C in a humidified incubator containing 5% CO_2 (*see* **Note 10**).
9. Fix cells using 10% formaldehyde in diH_2O for 1 h at room temperature.
10. Discard formaldehyde and remove the CMC overlay.
11. Stain cells with the CV Stain for 15–30 min at room temperature.
12. Gently wash off the CV Stain with diH_2O and allow it to air dry (Fig. 4).

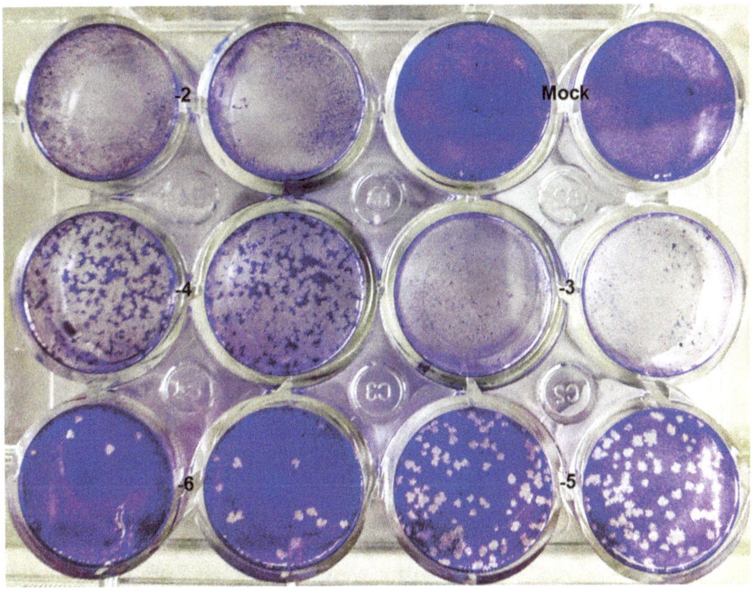

Fig. 4 Recombinant CedV forms plaques in Vero E6 cells. Vero E6 cells were inoculated with 200 μL of ten-fold serial dilutions of rCedV-wt in duplicate for 1 h. Two mL of a 1:1 mix of D-5 + 2% CMC was then added to each well and incubated for 5 days at 37 °C, 5% CO_2. The plates were fixed with 4% formaldehyde and then stained with 0.5% crystal violet-80% methanol in phosphate-buffered saline (1xPBS). Plaques were counted and calculated as PFU/mL

13. Calculate the plaque-forming units/mL (PFU/mL). A log drop should be noted between serial dilutions and the lower limit of detection should range between 25 and 50 plaques.

    13.1 PFU/mL = (Avg # Plaques) × (well dilution) × (dilution factor) (*see* **Note 11**).

4 Notes

1. Prepare in advance the 2% (w/v) carboxymethylcellulose (CMC) sodium salt (medium viscosity) in autoclaved diH_20. Slowly add CMC powder to water and stir/mix until dissolved. The solution can be left at room temperature overnight to dissolve completely. Do not autoclave. Store at room temperature. The product is ready to use and does not need to be warmed, open only in the hood, and keep sterile.
2. Coating the wells of 6-well plates with 1 mL of poly-D-Lysine helps the cells adhere to the plate and reduces cell loss during transfection.
3. Use cells that are of low passage number and not overgrown. When plating ensures that the cells are evenly dispersed in the well by rocking the plate back and forth and from side to side multiple times. Avoid swirling the plate as this will result in the cells accumulating in the middle of the well and will adversely affect transfection efficiencies.
4. A transfection master mix can be prepared. Ensure to add an extra well to accommodate for pipetting error.
5. The addition of helper plasmids only, rCedV antigenome plasmid-only, and untransfected wells in the rescue experiment will aid in identifying syncytia as a consequence of infection from "syncytia" due to the transfection. We recommend transfecting at least three wells per virus rescue attempt with rCedV antigenome plasmid and helper plasmids as rescue efficiency is not very high.
6. The day before virus purification, clean ultracentrifuge buckets (SW28 rotor) and ice buckets with 70% EtOH and UV overnight.
7. On the morning of virus purification, clean as many SW28 tubes as needed with 70% EtOH and dry them in the biosafety cabinet. Pre-cool the rotor to 4 °C before centrifugation.
8. Decanting the supernatant may offer less chance to disturb the pellet. If decanting is chosen, carefully pour the supernatant into a 10% bleach solution aspirating any residual liquid. A visible white pellet of the purified virus may be observable at this point.

9. We advise storing the virus in small volumes (~50 μL) to avoid freeze–thaw cycles of the viral stock as this may adversely affect the titers.
10. Avoid disturbing the plates as this will result in smeared plaques.
11. The dilution factor will be 5 = (1000 μL)/200 μL, if a different volume is used for the initial infection and adjusted in titer calculations.

Acknowledgments

The views expressed in the manuscript are solely those of the authors and do not represent official views or opinions of the Department of Defense or the Uniformed Services University of the Health Sciences.

Funding

Research support was provided by National Institutes of Health grants AI054715, AI077995, and AI142764 to C.C.B.

References

1. Luby SP (2013) The pandemic potential of Nipah virus. Antivir Res 100(1):38–43. https://doi.org/10.1016/j.antiviral.2013.07.011
2. Luby SP, Broder CC (2014) Paramyxoviruses: henipaviruses. In: Kaslow RA, Stanberry LR, Le Duc JW (eds) Viral infections of humans, epidemiology and control. Springer, New York, pp 519–536
3. Wang L-F, Mackenzie JS, Broder CC (2013) Henipaviruses. In: Knipe DM, Howley PM (eds) Fields virology, vol 1. Lippincott Williams & Wilkins, Philadelphia, pp 1070–1085
4. Broder CC, Weir DL, Reid PA (2016) Hendra virus and Nipah virus animal vaccines. Vaccine 34(30):3525–3534. https://doi.org/10.1016/j.vaccine.2016.03.075
5. Broder CC, Wong KT (2016) Henipaviruses. In: Reiss CS (ed) Neurotropic viral infections, 2nd edn, vol 1. Springer, Cham, pp 45–83
6. Geisbert TW, Feldmann H, Broder CC (2012) Animal challenge models of Henipavirus infection and pathogenesis. Curr Top Microbiol Immunol 359:153–177. https://doi.org/10.1007/82_2012_208
7. Arunkumar G, Chandni R, Mourya DT, Singh SK, Sadanandan R, Sudan P, Bhargava B, Nipah Investigators P, Health Study G (2019) Outbreak investigation of Nipah virus disease in Kerala, India, 2018. J Infect Dis 219(12): 1867–1878. https://doi.org/10.1093/infdis/jiy612
8. Broder CC, Xu K, Nikolov DB, Zhu Z, Dimitrov DS, Middleton D, Pallister J, Geisbert TW, Bossart KN, Wang LF (2013) A treatment for and vaccine against the deadly Hendra and Nipah viruses. Antivir Res 100(1):8–13. https://doi.org/10.1016/j.antiviral.2013.06.012
9. Amaya M, Broder CC (2020) Vaccines to emerging viruses: Nipah and Hendra. Annu Rev Virol 7(1):447–473. https://doi.org/10.1146/annurev-virology-021920-113833
10. Marsh GA, de Jong C, Barr JA, Tachedjian M, Smith C, Middleton D, Yu M, Todd S, Foord AJ, Haring V, Payne J, Robinson R, Broz I, Crameri G, Field HE, Wang LF (2012) Cedar virus: a novel Henipavirus isolated from Australian bats. PLoS Pathog 8(8):e1002836. https://doi.org/10.1371/journal.ppat.1002836

11. Schountz T, Campbell C, Wagner K, Rovnak J, Martellaro C, DeBuysscher BL, Feldmann H, Prescott J (2019) Differential innate immune responses elicited by Nipah virus and cedar virus correlate with disparate in vivo pathogenesis in hamsters. Viruses 11(3). https://doi.org/10.3390/v11030291
12. Beaty SM, Park A, Won ST, Hong P, Lyons M, Vigant F, Freiberg AN, tenOever BR, Duprex WP, Lee B (2017) Efficient and robust paramyxoviridae reverse genetics systems. mSphere 2(2). https://doi.org/10.1128/mSphere.00376-16
13. Conzelmann KK (2004) Reverse genetics of mononegavirales. Curr Top Microbiol Immunol 283:1–41. https://doi.org/10.1007/978-3-662-06099-5_1
14. Pfaller CK, Cattaneo R, Schnell MJ (2015) Reverse genetics of Mononegavirales: how they work, new vaccines, and new cancer therapeutics. Virology 479-480:331–344. https://doi.org/10.1016/j.virol.2015.01.029
15. Schmidt KM, Muhlberger E (2016) Marburg virus reverse genetics systems. Viruses 8(6). https://doi.org/10.3390/v8060178
16. Ciancanelli MJ, Volchkova VA, Shaw ML, Volchkov VE, Basler CF (2009) Nipah virus sequesters inactive STAT1 in the nucleus via a P gene-encoded mechanism. J Virol 83(16): 7828–7841. https://doi.org/10.1128/JVI.02610-08
17. Laing ED, Amaya M, Navaratnarajah CK, Feng YR, Cattaneo R, Wang LF, Broder CC (2018) Rescue and characterization of recombinant cedar virus, a non-pathogenic Henipavirus species. Virol J 15(1):56. https://doi.org/10.1186/s12985-018-0964-0
18. Lo MK, Peeples ME, Bellini WJ, Nichol ST, Rota PA, Spiropoulou CF (2012) Distinct and overlapping roles of Nipah virus P gene products in modulating the human endothelial cell antiviral response. PLoS One 7(10):e47790. https://doi.org/10.1371/journal.pone.0047790
19. Marsh GA, Virtue ER, Smith I, Todd S, Arkinstall R, Frazer L, Monaghan P, Smith GA, Broder CC, Middleton D, Wang LF (2013) Recombinant Hendra viruses expressing a reporter gene retain pathogenicity in ferrets. Virol J 10:95. https://doi.org/10.1186/1743-422X-10-95
20. Yoneda M, Guillaume V, Ikeda F, Sakuma Y, Sato H, Wild TF, Kai C (2006) Establishment of a Nipah virus rescue system. Proc Natl Acad Sci U S A 103(44):16508–16513. https://doi.org/10.1073/pnas.0606972103
21. Yun T, Park A, Hill TE, Pernet O, Beaty SM, Juelich TL, Smith JK, Zhang L, Wang YE, Vigant F, Gao J, Wu P, Lee B, Freiberg AN (2015) Efficient reverse genetics reveals genetic determinants of budding and fusogenic differences between Nipah and Hendra viruses and enables real-time monitoring of viral spread in small animal models of henipavirus infection. J Virol 89(2):1242–1253. https://doi.org/10.1128/JVI.02583-14
22. Satterfield BA, Cross RW, Fenton KA, Agans KN, Basler CF, Geisbert TW, Mire CE (2015) The immunomodulating V and W proteins of Nipah virus determine disease course. Nat Commun 6:7483. https://doi.org/10.1038/ncomms8483
23. Laing ED, Navaratnarajah CK, Cheliout Da Silva S, Petzing SR, Xu Y, Sterling SL, Marsh GA, Wang LF, Amaya M, Nikolov DB, Cattaneo R, Broder CC, Xu K (2019) Structural and functional analyses reveal promiscuous and species specific use of ephrin receptors by cedar virus. Proc Natl Acad Sci U S A 116(41):20707–20715. https://doi.org/10.1073/pnas.1911773116
24. Halpin K, Bankamp B, Harcourt BH, Bellini WJ, Rota PA (2004) Nipah virus conforms to the rule of six in a minigenome replication assay. J Gen Virol 85(Pt 3):701–707. https://doi.org/10.1099/vir.0.19685-0
25. Buchholz UJ, Finke S, Conzelmann KK (1999) Generation of bovine respiratory syncytial virus (BRSV) from cDNA: BRSV NS2 is not essential for virus replication in tissue culture, and the human RSV leader region acts as a functional BRSV genome promoter. J Virol 73(1):251–259
26. Peeters BP, de Leeuw OS, Koch G, Gielkens AL (1999) Rescue of Newcastle disease virus from cloned cDNA: evidence that cleavability of the fusion protein is a major determinant for virulence. J Virol 73(6):5001–5009
27. Chan YP, Yan L, Feng YR, Broder CC (2009) Preparation of recombinant viral glycoproteins for novel and therapeutic antibody discovery. Methods Mol biol 525:31-58, xiii. https://doi.org/10.1007/978-1-59745-554-1_2

Chapter 6

Utilizing Recombinant Reporter Henipaviruses to Conduct Antiviral Screening

Michael K. Lo

Abstract

Spillovers of Nipah virus (NiV) from its pteropid bat reservoir into the human population continue to cause near-annual outbreaks of fatal encephalitis and respiratory disease in Bangladesh and India since its emergence in Malaysia over 20 years ago. The current lack of effective antiviral therapeutics against NiV merits further testing of compound libraries against NiV using rapid quantitative antiviral assays. The development of recombinant henipaviruses expressing reporter fluorescence and/or luminescence proteins has facilitated the screening of such libraries. In this chapter, we provide a basic protocol for both types of reporter viruses. Utilizing these live NiV-based reporter assays requires modest instrumentation and side-steps the labor-intensive steps associated with traditional cytopathic effect or viral antigen-based assays.

Key words Recombinant Nipah virus, Reporter genes, Fluorescence, Luminescence, Antiviral screen

1 Introduction

Nipah virus (NiV) is a highly pathogenic paramyxovirus in the genus *Henipavirus* within the family *Paramyxoviridae* [1]. Humans are infected upon spillover of NiV from its bat reservoir host or by person-to-person transmission [2]. Due to its high pathogenicity, its potential use for bio-/agro-terrorism, and the current lack of approved therapeutics, NiV is designated as an overlap select agent requiring biosafety level-4 (BSL-4) containment. Although preventative measures have been studied [3], NiV continues to cause near-annual outbreaks of fatal encephalitis in Bangladesh for nearly two decades. While therapeutic monoclonal antibodies and soluble subunit vaccines against henipaviruses have shown great promise [4], screening available compound libraries for potentially efficacious therapeutics against NiV remains a high priority. Most high-throughput antiviral assays against NiV were developed to screen for inhibitors of virus entry and/or cell-to-cell fusion [5–8], while the NiV minigenome assay was used to screen for inhibitors of NiV replication [9]. A chemiluminescent immunodetection assay for

Alexander N. Freiberg and Barry Rockx (eds.), *Nipah Virus: Methods and Protocols*, Methods in Molecular Biology, vol. 2682, https://doi.org/10.1007/978-1-0716-3283-3_6,

live henipavirus infection significantly streamlined antiviral screening when compared with cytopathic effect or immune plaque-based assays, but had relatively limited signal-to-noise ratios (<100) and also required cell fixation and multiple incubation steps which are time and labor-intensive [10]. Alongside several independent groups, we have generated recombinant reporter henipaviruses which express green fluorescent (ZsGreen1) or bioluminescent (Renilla luciferase) proteins; such viruses facilitate high throughput assays to screen larger compound libraries, as well as in vivo/ex vivo studies in animal models [11–15]. Here, we have provided succinct in vitro antiviral assay protocols for these two types of reporter viruses.

2 Materials and Equipment

2.1 Cell Lines

The following list of commonly available immortalized cell lines has been used to evaluate antivirals against henipaviruses:

- Vero (CCL-81, ATCC®), HEK293T/17 (CRL-11268, ATCC®), HeLa (CCL-2, ATCC®), HT-1080 (CCL-121, ATCC®), NCI-H358 (CRL-5807, ATCC®), TIME (CRL-4025, ATCC®), HSAEC1-KT (CRL-4050, ATCC®) [11, 16–20].

2.2 Cell Culture Media

- Vascular Cell Basal Medium (ATCC® PCS-199-030™) supplemented with Microvascular Endothelial Cell Growth Kit-VEGF (ATCC® PCS-110-041). (Used for TIME cells).
- Airway Epithelial Cell Basal Medium (ATCC® PCS-300-030™) supplemented with Bronchial Epithelial Cell Growth Kit (ATCC® PCS-300-040™). (Used for HSAEC1-KT cells).
- RPMI 1640 with L-glutamine, without phenol red (Thermo Fisher 11835055), supplemented with 10% heat-inactivated fetal bovine serum (Hyclone/Cytiva Life Sciences SH30088.02HI) and penicillin/streptomycin (Thermo Fisher 15140122). (Used for NCI-H358 cells).
- Fluorobrite™ DMEM (Thermo Fisher A1896701) supplemented with 10% heat-inactivated fetal bovine serum and penicillin/streptomycin. (Used for all other abovementioned cell lines).

2.3 Cell Culture Plasticware

- 96-well flat-bottom black opaque (Costar 3916), clear-bottom black opaque (Costar 3603), white opaque (Costar 3917), clear (Costar 3598).

2.4 Assay Reagent

- Renilla-Glo™ Luciferase Assay System (Promega E2720).

2.5 Reporter Measurement Device

- BioTek H1 Synergy (or equivalent) fluorescence and luminescence microplate reader (*see* **Note 1**).

3 Methods

3.1 Fluorescence-Based Reporter Assay (ZsGreen1 Fluorescence Protein)

1. Seed 1–2 × 10^4 cells/well overnight in either a black opaque 96-well plate or black opaque clear-bottom 96-well plate to verify the approximate confluence of the plated cells.
2. Pretreat plated cells with desired compounds of interest at desired concentration(s) for at least 1 h (*see* **Note 2**).
3. Bring cells into BSL-4 laboratory containment. Conduct all cell manipulation in a class II biosafety cabinet.
4. Infect cells with rNiV-ZsG/NiV-GFP2AM virus at multiplicity of infection (MOI) = 0.25 (*see* **Note 3**).
5. Incubate plate(s) at 37 °C and 5% CO_2 for 48–72 h.
6. At the time of green fluorescence (excitation wavelength—488 nm, emission wavelength—518 nm) measurement, remove plates from incubator. Remove the plate cover, and proceed to place plate into microplate reader to obtain fluorescence intensity measurements.

3.2 Luminescence-Based Reporter Assay (Non-Secreted Renilla luciferase)

1. Seed 1–2 × 10^4 cells/well overnight in white opaque 96-well plates. Seed one clear plate to visually verify the approximate confluence of plated cells.
2. Pretreat plated cells with desired compounds of interest at desired concentration(s) for at least 1 h (*see* **Note 2**).
3. Bring cells into BSL-4 laboratory containment. Conduct all cell manipulation in a class II biosafety cabinet.
4. Infect cells with NiV-LUC2AM virus at MOI = 0.25 (*see* **Note 3**).
5. Incubate plate(s) at 37 °C and 5% CO_2 for ~24 h.
6. Within an hour of the expected time of assaying the infected plates, prepare Renilla-Glo™ assay reagent by diluting Renilla-Glo™ luciferase assay substrate into Renilla-Glo™ assay buffer at a ratio of 1:100.
7. Prior to adding assay reagent, remove plates from the incubator and allow them to equilibrate at room temperature (~5–10 min).
8. Using a multichannel pipette, add an equivalent volume of reagent into the wells of each plate (e.g., 100 μL of reagent

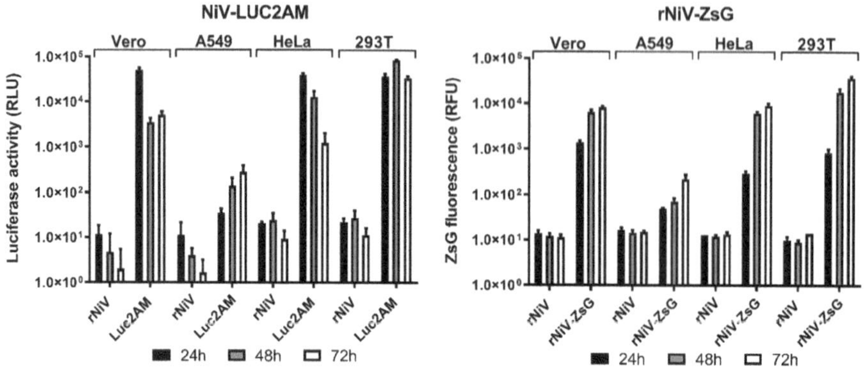

Fig. 1 Respective raw numbers reflecting the reporter activities of wild-type recombinant NiV (rNiV) or recombinant NiVs expressing either Renilla luciferase (NiV-LUC2AM) (left panel) or ZsGreen1 (rNiV-ZsG) (right panel) in different cell lines as indicated by annotated brackets. At 1, 2, and 3 days post-infection, relative light units (RLU) or relative fluorescence units (RFU) in the cells infected with reporter viruses were measured. (Figure is adapted from [11])

to 100 μL of cell culture media already present in well). Incubate plate at room temperature for at least 10 min.

9. Ensure that plate covers are removed; then proceed to place plate into microplate reader to obtain glow luminescence measurements (Fig. 1).

4 Notes

1. Prior to conducting antiviral assays on compound libraries, ensure that fluorescence and luminescence gain settings for microplate reader have been optimized so as not to exceed signal measurement bandwidth during sample measurement. Evaluate and optimize signal-to-noise (S:N) ratios for each type of reporter assay/virus by varying the amount of virus used for infection, as well as the amount of time allowed for infection prior to measurement of reporter activity. To ensure assay robustness for high-throughput utilization, evaluate reporter assays by calculating the Z′ factor. $Z' = 1 - [(3SD_C + 3SD_B)/(mean_C - mean_B)]$, where SD is the standard deviation, C is the control, and B is the background; when Z′ factor is >0.5, the assay is considered suitable for high throughput assays [21].
2. Leave at least 4 wells in each plate to serve as uninfected negative controls, in order to account for background fluorescence or luminescence from cells. In addition, allow for another 4 wells to serve as NiV-infected negative controls, by using a known inhibitor of NiV at a concentration known to completely ablate virus replication (e.g., 6-azauridine acetate at 20 μM) [11]. This control accounts for any background

fluorescence or luminescence introduced by the virus inoculum.

3. Utilizing reporter viruses expressing non-secreted luciferases and/or fluorescence proteins typically precludes the need to perform sterile phosphate-buffered saline washes to remove inoculum from infected cells, despite the presence of reporter protein in clarified virus supernatants due to infected cell lysis. However, when the reporter virus expresses a secreted luciferase (e.g., Gaussia luciferase), there will be significant reporter signal retained in supernatants from infected cells. In such contexts, washing infected cells 1 h post-infection may help retain optimal reporter signal-to-noise ratios.

References

1. Rota PA, Lo MK (2012) Molecular virology of the henipaviruses. Curr Top Microbiol Immunol 359:41–58
2. Luby SP (2013) The pandemic potential of Nipah virus. Antivir Res 100:38–43
3. Nahar N, Mondal UK, Sultana R, Hossain MJ, Khan MS, Gurley ES, Oliveras E, Luby SP (2013) Piloting the use of indigenous methods to prevent Nipah virus infection by interrupting bats' access to date palm sap in Bangladesh. Health Promot Int 28:378–386
4. Broder CC, Xu K, Nikolov DB, Zhu Z, Dimitrov DS, Middleton D, Pallister J, Geisbert TW, Bossart KN, Wang LF (2013) A treatment for and vaccine against the deadly Hendra and Nipah viruses. Antivir Res 100:8–13
5. Tamin A, Harcourt BH, Lo MK, Roth JA, Wolf MC, Lee B, Weingartl H, Audonnet JC, Bellini WJ, Rota PA (2009) Development of a neutralization assay for Nipah virus using pseudotype particles. J Virol Methods 160:1–6
6. Talekar A, Pessi A, Glickman F, Sengupta U, Briese T, Whitt MA, Mathieu C, Horvat B, Moscona A, Porotto M (2012) Rapid screening for entry inhibitors of highly pathogenic viruses under low-level biocontainment. PLoS One 7:e30538
7. Bossart KN, Mungall BA, Crameri G, Wang LF, Eaton BT, Broder CC (2005) Inhibition of Henipavirus fusion and infection by heptad-derived peptides of the Nipah virus fusion glycoprotein. Virol J 2:57
8. Porotto M, Orefice G, Yokoyama CC, Mungall BA, Realubit R, Sganga ML, Aljofan M, Whitt M, Glickman F, Moscona A (2009) Simulating henipavirus multicycle replication in a screening assay leads to identification of a promising candidate for therapy. J Virol 83: 5148–5155
9. Freiberg A, Dolores LK, Enterlein S, Flick R (2008) Establishment and characterization of plasmid-driven minigenome rescue systems for Nipah virus: RNA polymerase I- and T7-catalyzed generation of functional paramyxoviral RNA. Virology 370:33–44
10. Aljofan M, Porotto M, Moscona A, Mungall BA (2008) Development and validation of a chemiluminescent immunodetection assay amenable to high throughput screening of antiviral drugs for Nipah and Hendra virus. J Virol Methods 149:12–19
11. Lo MK, Nichol ST, Spiropoulou CF (2014) Evaluation of luciferase and GFP-expressing Nipah viruses for rapid quantitative antiviral screening. Antivir Res 106:53–60
12. Yun T, Park A, Hill TE, Pernet O, Beaty SM, Juelich TL, Smith JK, Zhang L, Wang YE, Vigant F, Gao J, Wu P, Lee B, Freiberg AN (2015) Efficient reverse genetics reveals genetic determinants of budding and fusogenic differences between Nipah and Hendra viruses and enables real-time monitoring of viral spread in small animal models of henipavirus infection. J Virol 89:1242–1253
13. Park A, Yun T, Hill TE, Ikegami T, Juelich TL, Smith JK, Zhang L, Freiberg AN, Lee B (2016) Optimized P2A for reporter gene insertion into Nipah virus results in efficient ribosomal skipping and wild-type lethality. J Gen Virol 97:839–843
14. Welch SR, Scholte FEM, Harmon JR, Coleman-McCray JD, Lo MK, Montgomery JM, Nichol ST, Spiropoulou CF, Spengler JR (2020) In situ imaging of fluorescent Nipah virus respiratory and neurological tissue tropism in the Syrian hamster model. J Infect Dis 221:S448–S453

15. Yoneda M, Guillaume V, Ikeda F, Sakuma Y, Sato H, Wild TF, Kai C (2006) Establishment of a Nipah virus rescue system. Proc Natl Acad Sci U S A 103:16508–16513
16. Lo MK, Amblard F, Flint M, Chatterjee P, Kasthuri M, Li C, Russell O, Verma K, Bassit L, Schinazi RF, Nichol ST, Spiropoulou CF (2020) Potent in vitro activity of beta-D-4′-chloromethyl-2′-deoxy-2′-fluorocytidine against Nipah virus. Antivir Res 175:104712
17. Lo MK, Spengler JR, Krumpe LRH, Welch SR, Chattopadhyay A, Harmon JR, Coleman-McCray JD, Scholte FEM, Hotard AL, Fuqua JL, Rose JK, Nichol ST, Palmer KE, O'Keefe BR, Spiropoulou CF (2020) Griffithsin inhibits Nipah virus entry and fusion and can protect Syrian Golden hamsters from lethal Nipah virus challenge. J Infect Dis 221:S480–S492
18. Hotard AL, He B, Nichol ST, Spiropoulou CF, Lo MK (2017) 4′-Azidocytidine (R1479) inhibits henipaviruses and other paramyxoviruses with high potency. Antivir Res 144:147–152
19. Lo MK, Jordan R, Arvey A, Sudhamsu J, Shrivastava-Ranjan P, Hotard AL, Flint M, McMullan LK, Siegel D, Clarke MO, Mackman RL, Hui HC, Perron M, Ray AS, Cihlar T, Nichol ST, Spiropoulou CF (2017) GS-5734 and its parent nucleoside analog inhibit Filo-, Pneumo-, and Paramyxoviruses. Sci Rep 7:43395
20. Siegel D, Hui HC, Doerffler E, Clarke MO, Chun K, Zhang L, Neville S, Carra E, Lew W, Ross B, Wang Q, Wolfe L, Jordan R, Soloveva V, Knox J, Perry J, Perron M, Stray KM, Barauskas O, Feng JY, Xu Y, Lee G, Rheingold AL, Ray AS, Bannister R, Strickley R, Swaminathan S, Lee WA, Bavari S, Cihlar T, Lo MK, Warren TK, Mackman RL (2017) Discovery and synthesis of a phosphoramidate prodrug of a pyrrolo[2,1-f][triazin-4-amino] adenine C-nucleoside (GS-5734) for the treatment of ebola and emerging viruses. *J Med Chem* 60:1648–1661
21. Zhang JH, Chung TD, Oldenburg KR (1999) A simple statistical parameter for use in evaluation and validation of high throughput screening assays. J Biomol Screen 4:67–73

Chapter 7

In Vitro Antiviral Screening for Henipaviruses at BSL4

Bruce A. Mungall

Abstract

In vitro screening for antivirals is an essential step in the development of effective treatments against new and emerging pathogens. Here, we describe a simple, cell-based screening assay for evaluating antiviral effectiveness against Hendra and Nipah live virus infection under BSL4 conditions.

Key words Antiviral screen, In vitro, Nipah virus, Hendra virus, Immunolabeling

1 Introduction

Hendra (HeV) and Nipah (NiV) viruses are two related paramyxoviruses classified into a new genus of the *Paramyxovirinae* called Henipavirus [1]. More than 20 and 25 years since NiV and HeV were first discovered, respectively [2, 3], there are still no approved therapeutics for treating henipavirus infection in humans. In recent years, there has been considerable progress in the development of immunotherapies and vaccines [4]. A number of subunit vaccine candidates utilizing either HeV or NiV F and G glycoproteins, expressed through recombinant viral vectors or as expressed soluble proteins, have been evaluated in vivo (reviewed in [4, 5]) with one formulation based on a recombinant soluble and oligomeric form of HeV G protein (sG) approved for use in horses (Equivac®) in Australia [6]. The Coalition of Epidemic Preparedness Innovation (CEPI) has recently selected four Nipah virus vaccine candidates to progress through phase I and II clinical trials (https://cepi.net/research_dev/priority-diseases/).

While prophylactic measures such as vaccines will always provide the most effective protection against disease, the development of vaccines for relatively small disease outbreaks comes with commercial challenges. Importantly, the small, sporadic nature of henipavirus outbreaks often means post-exposure antiviral therapy is the option available. In the absence of known henipavirus antivirals, broad-spectrum antivirals were initially evaluated and used.

Alexander N. Freiberg and Barry Rockx (eds.), *Nipah Virus: Methods and Protocols*, Methods in Molecular Biology, vol. 2682, https://doi.org/10.1007/978-1-0716-3283-3_7,

Ribavirin has been used for suspected viral infections, and the studies have demonstrated ribavirin effectiveness against both HeV and NiV in vitro [7, 8] but with limited effectiveness in vivo [9]. A limited non-randomized trial of ribavirin during the initial NiV outbreak in Malaysia showed ribavirin therapy was able to reduce mortality of acute NiV encephalitis [10], while during a recent outbreak in Kerala, India, the two surviving patients of the 23 infected cases were both given Ribavirin [11], while none of the healthcare worker contacts of a fatal case given Ribavirin post-exposure in that outbreak contracted NiV, despite documented transmission from that patient to another [12]. The antimalarial drug chloroquine has also been shown to inhibit NiV and HeV infection in vitro [13], but in vivo studies in hamsters showed no therapeutic impact on hamsters challenged with NiV or HeV [9] or against NiV in ferrets [14]. The effectiveness of a monoclonal antibody vaccine (m102.4) directed against the NiV recombinant viral envelope protein has also been demonstrated in vitro and in vivo with administration on compassionate grounds to critical NiV patients [5], while a recent Phase I study evaluated the safety, tolerability, pharmacokinetics, and immunogenicity of m102.4 in healthy adults [15]. Very recently, Griffithsin, a high-mannose oligosaccharide binding lectin that has shown in vivo broad-spectrum activity against a number of viruses, demonstrated potent in vitro activity and partial in vivo protection against NiV challenge [16].

Recent interest in a number of small molecule inhibitors has revealed potent in vitro and in vivo activity against henipaviruses. Balapiravir (R1479) and 4′-chloromethyl-2′-deoxy-2′-fluorocytidine (ALS-8112) are nucleoside analogs with demonstrated in vitro antiviral efficacy against NiV and HeV [17, 18]. Favipiravir (T-705), a purine analog inhibiting RNA-dependent RNA polymerase currently under evaluation for Ebola virus, has also demonstrated effectiveness against NiV in vitro and recently in vivo [19]. Additionally, another nucleotide analog prodrug remdesivir (GS-5734), also being evaluated for Ebola treatment, has shown broad-spectrum antiviral activity including potent in vitro and in vivo activity against NiV [20].

With repeated outbreaks of NiV in recent years [21], the ongoing development of potential post-exposure therapeutics is essential, requiring substantial screening and evaluation efforts. Due to the challenges inherent in conducting antiviral assays under BSL4 conditions, the vast majority of in vitro evaluations conducted use reporter assays or pseudo-virus replication assays, designed to mimic live virus. While these have traditionally demonstrated excellent utility, they do not always faithfully replicate natural virus infection and thus may not reflect the actual inhibition by specific compounds under natural conditions, necessitating the use of live virus assays under BSL4 containment. We describe here a simple, cell-based in vitro immunodetection-based screening protocol for evaluating the effectiveness and cytotoxicity of antivirals for the potential treatment of henipavirus infection at BSL4.

2 Materials

2.1 Viruses

1. HeV: Originally isolated in Vero cells from the lung of a horse infected in the Brisbane outbreak in October 1994 and was passaged five times in Vero cells followed by triple plaque purification and a further five passages in Vero cells as described previously [22].
2. NiV: Originally isolated in Vero cells from the brain of a human fatally infected in the 1998–1999 Malaysian outbreak and was passaged three times in Vero cells then double plaque purified and passaged a further three times in Vero cells as described previously [23]. HeV and NiV stock titers were adjusted to 1×10^6 $TCID_{50}$/mL.
3. The viruses were grown under Biohazard level 4 (BSL4) conditions in which laboratory workers wear positive pressure encapsulating suits supplied with breathing air.

2.2 Cells

1. African Green Monkey (Vero) Cells: Obtained from the American Type Culture Collection (ATCC CCL 81) and stored at −80 °C.

2.3 Media

1. Eagle's Minimal Essential Medium containing Earle's salts (EMEM): EMEM containing antibiotics (100 U/mL penicillin, 100 μg/mL streptomycin, and 500 μg/mL Fungizone) and 10% fetal calf serum.
2. Trypsin-EDTA solution: 1× trypsin-EDTA in phosphate-buffered saline (PBS) without calcium or magnesium, filter-sterilized.

2.4 Antibodies and Conjugates

1. Primary antibody: Rabbit polyclonal anti-nucleoprotein (N) antisera (complements of Brian Shiell, CSIRO, AAHL) [24].
2. Secondary antibodies: Anti-rabbit conjugated horse radish peroxidase (HRP, Sigma).

2.5 Other Reagents and Materials

1. Assay Plates: Flat-bottomed 96-well plates used for all dilutions/assays. Note that for chemiluminescent detection assays best results are achieved using opaque plates (black is preferable) to prevent cross-talk when measuring the signal.
2. Methanol: Laboratory-grade methanol for decontamination of assay plates from BSL4.

3. Plastic bags: Bags to contain assay plates immersed in methanol with an appropriate method for heat sealing.
4. Phosphate-buffered saline containing 0.05% Tween-20 (PBS-T).
5. 1% skim milk in PBS-T.
6. 1% H_2O_2.
7. Chemiluminescent assay buffer: 20 mM Tris–HCl, 1 mM $MgCl_2$, pH = 9.6.
8. Chemiluminescent peroxidase substrate: Chemiluminescent substrate for HRP (CPS-3, Sigma) diluted 1:10 in chemiluminescent assay buffer.
9. CellTiter-Glo® cytotoxicity kit (Promega, Madison, USA).

3 Methods

Preparation of cells and compounds to be tested is all prepared at BSL2 in a sterile, laminar flow hood, making sure that all equipment and solutions that come into contact with the cells are sterile. Once all assay components are ready, materials are transferred into the BSL4 laboratory (Subheading 3.2 below). All virus infection steps and subsequent incubations are conducted inside the BSL4 laboratory. Once complete, materials are appropriately decontaminated and removed from the BSL4 to a BSL2 laboratory where the remaining assay procedures take place (Subheading 3.4 below).

3.1 Cell and Compound Preparation (BSL2)

1. Protocols describing how to start growing Vero cells from frozen stock, maintain cultures, and split through trypsin subculture have been described elsewhere [25].
2. Vero cells are maintained in EMEM in 75 cm^2 flasks with vented caps to prepare the required quantity of cells.
3. The day before the assay is to be conducted, confluent monolayers of Vero cells are harvested and seeded at a density of 2×10^4 into individual wells of 96-well flat-bottomed microtiter plates and incubated at 37 °C and 5% CO_2 overnight in 100 μL EMEM.
4. Cells in 96-well plates should be >90% confluent when commencing the assay.
5. Compounds to be tested are prepared at BSL2 in preparation for the assay to reduce preparation time within BSL4. Stock dilutions of compounds are prepared in empty 96-well plates and diluted appropriately ready for transfer to cells when ready, preferably in the same media (EMEM) used to culture the cells used for the assay.

6. Depending on the number of compounds to be tested, initial prescreening experiments using a predefined concentration of compound may be necessary. For an initial screen of over 8000 compounds, we initially used all at 10 μM final concentration [26].
7. For final evaluation of compounds, it is necessary to screen across a range of concentrations to determine the 50% inhibitory concentration (IC_{50}). The simplest way to achieve this is to prepare ½ log dilutions over a suitable concentration range (e.g., 10 μM to 1 nM). Replicate wells for each compound concentration to ensure assay repeatability can be determined. Note also that it is necessary to include both positive and negative controls within each and every assay plate to ensure assay comparability and specificity (*see* **Note 1**).
8. Cytotoxicity testing should be conducted in parallel using the same stock dilutions of test compounds to determine the 50% cytotoxic concentration (CC_{50}), but instead of transferring to the BSL4 laboratory, compounds can be added to Vero cells in 96-well plates at BSL2 and assayed as below (Subheading 3.6 below).

3.2 Antiviral Screening (BSL4)

1. For antiviral titration experiments, medium is removed from the confluent Vero cells in 96-well plates and 100 μL of each dilution of each compound is added to cells prior to the addition of virus. Depending on the scale of compound testing to be conducted, a compromise between orienting dilutions using 8 cells (columns) or 12 cells (rows) of a 96-well plate may be required to achieve an appropriate dose dilution range.
2. Depending on the scope of the experiment being conducted, test compounds may require addition of cells prior to adding virus, combined with virus prior to addition of cells, or applied following adsorption of virus onto the cells. If compounds can be added prior to virus inoculation, it may be feasible to add the compounds to the Vero cell plates at BSL2 to reduce the time required in BSL4.

3.3 Hendra and Nipah Virus Infection of Cells (BSL4)

1. Under BSL4 conditions, HeV and NiV stock titers are adjusted to the appropriate multiplicity of infection (moi) (our assays used 1×10^6 $TCID_{50}$/mL) (*see* **Note 2**).
2. Medium is removed from the Vero cells in 96-well plates, and 100 μL of pre-prepared half-log dilutions of test compounds in EMEM is added to replicate wells of Vero cells.
3. 10,000 $TCID_{50}$ virus (moi = 0.25) of virus inoculum diluted in EMEM is added to replicate wells of cells in a total final volume of 200 μL.
4. Plates are incubated at 37 °C and 5% CO_2 for 18–24 h (*see* **Note 3**).

3.4 Assay Termination and Decontamination (BSL4)

1. The culture medium is then discarded into a container with disinfectant, and plates are inverted and tapped gently on tissue paper to remove excess media.
2. Media-free 96-well plates are immersed in a container of ice-cold absolute methanol and then enclosed in heat-sealed plastic bags filled with methanol.
3. Sealed bags are then sterilized with Microchem Plus during removal from the BSL4 laboratory (*see* **Note 4**).
4. Following removal from BSL4 to the BSL2 laboratory, methanol-fixed plates are air-dried at room temperature for a minimum of 30 min prior to immunolabeling.

3.5 Immunolabeling Assay for Viral Antigen (BLS2)

1. Viral N protein expressed by infected cells is quantified using a sandwich immunoassay utilizing a primary anti-NiV antibody (rabbit polyclonal anti-N [24] complements of Brian Shiell) combined with an anti-rabbit-HRP conjugate antibody and chemiluminescent detection.
2. Plates are washed three times with 0.01 M PBS-T.
3. Plates are then protein blocked with 100 μL of 1% skim milk in PBS-T and incubated at 37 °C for 30 min.
4. After protein blocking, plates are washed three times with PBS-T, followed by incubation with 100 μL anti-NiV antibody diluted 1:1000 in PBS-T containing 1% skim milk for 30 min at 37 °C and then washed three times with PBS-T.
5. Plates are incubated with 1% H_2O_2 for 15 min at room temperature then washed with PBS-T a further three times.
6. 100 μL of anti-rabbit conjugated-HRP diluted 1:2000 in PBS-T containing 1% skim milk is added to each well, and plates are incubated at 37 °C for 30 min and then washed a final three times with PBS-T.
7. For detection, 100 μL of CPS-3 diluted 1:10 in chemiluminescent assay buffer is added to each well.
8. Plates are incubated at room temperature for 15 min and then read using a Luminoskan Ascent luminometer (Thermo Fisher Scientific, Waltham, USA) using 100 mSec integration per well.
9. Raw data values for each infected well (signal) are then divided by an average of the raw data values for uninfected wells (noise) to produce signal:moise ratios for all wells (*see* **Note 1**).
10. Signal:noise values for drug-treated wells are converted to % inhibition (compared to untreated, infected wells), measurements are collated, and nonlinear regression analysis is performed using GraphPad Prism software (GraphPad Software, San Diego, CA USA) to determine the IC_{50}.

3.6 Cytotoxicity Assay (BSL2)

1. The CellTiter-Glo® Luminescent Cell Viability Assay is a homogeneous method of determining the number of viable cells in culture based on quantitation of the ATP present, which signals the presence of metabolically active cells.
2. Vero cell cytotoxicity was determined in monolayers (40,000 cells) in 96-well plates incubated with half-log dilutions of 200 μL final volume of each compound in EMEM overnight at 37 °C.
3. Media was removed, and 100 μL of CellTiter-Glo® Reagent, diluted 1:5 with chemiluminescent assay buffer, was added to each well, mixed well to lyse cells, equilibrated to room temperature for 10 min, and then read using a luminometer as described above.
4. Nonlinear regression analysis was performed using GraphPad Prism software to determine the concentration resulting in 50% cytotoxicity (CC_{50}).
5. To evaluate the margin of safety that exists between the dose needed for antiviral effects and the dose that produces unwanted and possibly dangerous side effects (cytotoxicity), the therapeutic index for each lead compound was then calculated from the efficacy and cytotoxicity data (CC_{50}/IC_{50}).

4 Notes

1. Example plate layout:

	NC	T1a	T2a	T3a	T1b	T2b	T3b	T1c	T2c	T3c	PCa	PCb
Dilutions > > > > > >												

NC, negative control (no compound, virus infected); T1, test compound 1; T2, test compound 2; T3, test compound 3; PC, positive control (known in vitro inhibitor, e.g., ribavirin); a, b, c, replicate wells.

- Signal:noise (S/N) calculations: Raw value of each well (signal)/average of all NC wells.
- IC_{50} or CC_{50} calculated by nonlinear regression of S/N replicate values for each compound dilution.

2. To determine the appropriate infective dose of virus, medium is removed from the pre-seeded 96-well plates and half-log dilutions (10^5–10^1 $TCID_{50}$/mL) of virus in EMEM are added to replicate wells of Vero cells in a total final volume of 100 μL and incubated or 24 h at 37 °C and 5% CO_2. Plates were incubated at 37 °C for 5–7 days, and wells displaying cytopathic effect were scored as infected. Virus titer was calculated using the Reed–Muench method [27], and the limit of detection was 126 $TCID_{50}$/mL virus. In parallel, cells infected with dilutions of virus are processed as per the immunodetection assay to determine the optimal N protein expression kinetics for detection.
3. 18–24 h represents an optimal balance between adequate viral replication and minimal drug toxicity. Given the majority of experimental library compounds to be tested are likely to be dissolved in DMSO (or similar diluent), it is likely that the increased cell toxicity of potential antiviral drugs over this period may complicate analyses. This is why it is important to conduct cytotoxicity assays in parallel.
4. Given the nature of these pathogens, rigorous microsecurity requirements are necessary to ensure all materials from BSL4 laboratories are thoroughly inactivated prior to removal. Previous experiments in our laboratory have shown that submersion in ice-cold methanol for 10 min reduces the infectious titer of NiV and HeV by more than six logs (data not shown). All BSL4 procedures, including inactivation steps, must follow approved institution protocols.

Acknowledgments

The author wishes to thank Dr. Mohammad Aljofan for assistance in developing and validating these assays.

References

1. Wang L, Harcourt BH, Yu M et al (2001) Molecular biology of Hendra and Nipah viruses. Microbes Infect 3:279–287. https://doi.org/10.1016/s1286-4579(01)01381-8
2. Murray K, Selleck P, Hooper P et al (1995) A morbillivirus that caused fatal disease in horses and humans. Science 268:94–97. https://doi.org/10.1126/science.7701348
3. Chua KB, Goh KJ, Wong KT et al (1999) Fatal encephalitis due to Nipah virus among pig-farmers in Malaysia. Lancet 354:1257–1259. https://doi.org/10.1016/S0140-6736(99)04299-3
4. Thakur N, Bailey D (2019) Advances in diagnostics, vaccines and therapeutics for Nipah virus. Microbes Infect 21:278–286. https://doi.org/10.1016/j.micinf.2019.02.002
5. Broder CC, Weir DL, Reid PA (2016) Hendra virus and Nipah virus animal vaccines. Vaccine 34:3525–3534. https://doi.org/10.1016/j.vaccine.2016.03.075
6. Khusro A, Aarti C, Pliego AB et al (2020) Hendra virus infection in horses: a review on emerging mystery paramyxovirus. J Equine Vet Sci 91:103149. https://doi.org/10.1016/j.jevs.2020.103149
7. Aljofan M, Porotto M, Moscona A et al (2008) Development and validation of a chemiluminescent immunodetection assay amenable to high throughput screening of antiviral drugs for Nipah and Hendra virus. J Virol Methods 149:12–19. https://doi.org/10.1016/j.jviromet.2008.01.016
8. Wright PJ, Crameri G, Eaton BT (2005) RNA synthesis during infection by Hendra virus: an examination by quantitative real-time PCR of RNA accumulation, the effect of ribavirin and the attenuation of transcription. Arch Virol 150:521–532. https://doi.org/10.1007/s00705-004-0417-5
9. Freiberg AN, Worthy MN, Lee B et al (2010) Combined chloroquine and ribavirin treatment does not prevent death in a hamster model of Nipah and Hendra virus infection. J Gen Virol 91:765–772. https://doi.org/10.1099/vir.0.017269-0
10. Chong HT, Kamarulzaman A, Tan CT et al (2001) Treatment of acute Nipah encephalitis with ribavirin. Ann Neurol 49:810–813. https://doi.org/10.1002/ana.1062
11. Arunkumar G, Devadiga S, McElroy AK et al (2019) Adaptive immune responses in humans during Nipah virus acute and convalescent phases of infection. Clin Infect Dis 69:1752–1756. https://doi.org/10.1093/cid/ciz010
12. Banerjee S, Niyas VKM, Soneja M et al (2019) First experience of ribavirin postexposure prophylaxis for Nipah virus, tried during the 2018 outbreak in Kerala, India. J Infect 78:491–503. https://doi.org/10.1016/j.jinf.2019.03.005
13. Porotto M, Orefice G, Yokoyama CC et al (2009) Simulating henipavirus multicycle replication in a screening assay leads to identification of a promising candidate for therapy. J Virol 83:5148–5155. https://doi.org/10.1128/JVI.00164-09
14. Pallister J, Middleton D, Crameri G et al (2009) Chloroquine administration does not prevent Nipah virus infection and disease in ferrets. J Virol 83:11979–11982. https://doi.org/10.1128/JVI.01847-09
15. Playford EG, Munro T, Mahler SM et al (2020) Safety, tolerability, pharmacokinetics, and immunogenicity of a human monoclonal antibody targeting the G glycoprotein of henipaviruses in healthy adults: a first-in-human, randomised, controlled, phase 1 study. Lancet Infect Dis 20:445–454. https://doi.org/10.1016/S1473-3099(19)30634-6
16. Lo MK, Spengler JR, Krumpe LRH et al (2020) Griffithsin inhibits Nipah virus entry and fusion and can protect Syrian Golden hamsters from lethal Nipah virus challenge. J Infect Dis 221:S480–S492. https://doi.org/10.1093/infdis/jiz630
17. Hotard AL, He B, Nichol ST et al (2017) 4′--Azidocytidine (R1479) inhibits henipaviruses and other paramyxoviruses with high potency. Antivir Res 144:147–152. https://doi.org/10.1016/j.antiviral.2017.06.011
18. Lo MK, Amblard F, Flint M et al (2020) Potent in vitro activity of beta-D-4′--chloromethyl-2′-deoxy-2′-fluorocytidine against Nipah virus. Antivir Res 175:104712. https://doi.org/10.1016/j.antiviral.2020.104712
19. Dawes BE, Kalveram B, Ikegami T et al (2018) Favipiravir (T-705) protects against Nipah virus infection in the hamster model. Sci Rep 8:7604. https://doi.org/10.1038/s41598-018-25780-3
20. Lo MK, Feldmann F, Gary JM et al (2019) Remdesivir (GS-5734) protects African green monkeys from Nipah virus challenge. Sci Transl Med 11. https://doi.org/10.1126/scitranslmed.aau9242
21. Donaldson H, Lucey D (2018) Enhancing preparation for large Nipah outbreaks beyond Bangladesh: preventing a tragedy like Ebola in West Africa. Int J Infect Dis 72:69–72. https://doi.org/10.1016/j.ijid.2018.05.015

22. Hyatt AD, Selleck PW (1996) Ultrastructure of equine morbillivirus. Virus Res 43:1–15. https://doi.org/10.1016/0168-1702(96)01307-x
23. Shiell BJ, Gardner DR, Crameri G et al (2003) Sites of phosphorylation of P and V proteins from Hendra and Nipah viruses: newly emerged members of Paramyxoviridae. Virus Res 92:55–65. https://doi.org/10.1016/s0168-1702(02)00313-1
24. Juozapaitis M, Serva A, Zvirbliene A et al (2007) Generation of henipavirus nucleocapsid proteins in yeast Saccharomyces cerevisiae. Virus Res 124:95–102. https://doi.org/10.1016/j.virusres.2006.10.008
25. Ammerman NC, Beier-Sexton M, Azad AF (2008) Growth and maintenance of Vero cell lines. Curr Protoc Microbiol Appendix 4: Appendix 4E. https://doi.org/10.1002/9780471729259.mca04es11
26. Aljofan M, Sganga ML, Lo MK et al (2009) Antiviral activity of gliotoxin, gentian violet and brilliant green against Nipah and Hendra virus in vitro. Virol J 6:187. https://doi.org/10.1186/1743-422X-6-187
27. Reed LJ, Muench H (1938) Simple method for estimating fifty percent end points. Am J Hygiene 27:493–497

Chapter 8

Isolation of Primary Porcine Bronchial Epithelial Cells for Nipah Virus Infections

Mareike Elvert, Lucie Sauerhering, Anja Heiner, and Andrea Maisner

Abstract

The Malaysian strain of Nipah virus (NiV) first emerged in 1998/99 and caused a major disease outbreak in pigs and humans. While humans developed fatal encephalitis due to a prominent infection of brain microvessels, NiV-infected pigs mostly suffered from an acute respiratory disease and efficiently spread the infection via airway secretions. To elucidate the molecular basis of the highly productive NiV replication in porcine airways in vitro, physiologically relevant cell models that have maintained functional characteristics of airway epithelia in vivo are needed. Here, we describe in detail the method of isolating bronchial epithelial cells (PBEpC) from pig lungs that can be used for NiV infection studies. After the dissection of primary bronchia and removal of the mucus and protease digestion, bronchi segments are cut open and epithelial cells are scraped off and seeded on collagen-coated cell culture flasks. With this method, it is possible to isolate about 2×10^6 primary cells from the primary bronchi of one pig lung which can be cryopreserved or further subcultured. PBEpC form polarized monolayers on Transwell membrane inserts as controlled by immunostainings of epithelial marker proteins. NiV infection causes rapid formation of syncytia, allowing productive NiV infections in living PBEpC cultures to be monitored by phase-contrast microscopy.

Key words Primary porcine bronchial epithelial cells, Nipah virus, Dissection of pig bronchi, Collagen coating, Epithelial marker, Syncytia

1 Introduction

Nipah virus (NiV) is a fruit bat-borne highly pathogenic henipavirus that is sporadically transmitted to humans and other mammalian species. Due to its ability to cause severe clinical diseases in humans and livestock, the high mortality rate in humans, and the lack of any prophylactic or therapeutic treatment, NiV is classified as biosafety level 4 (BSL-4) pathogen. So far, there are two genetically distinct NiV strains ($NiV_{Bangladesh}$ and $NiV_{Malaysia}$) which differ in their geographic distribution, in their transmission patterns, and

Both authors "Mareike Elvert" and "Lucie Sauerhering" equally contributed to this work.

Alexander N. Freiberg and Barry Rockx (eds.), *Nipah Virus: Methods and Protocols*, Methods in Molecular Biology, vol. 2682, https://doi.org/10.1007/978-1-0716-3283-3_8,

also in some aspects regarding the clinical disease in humans [1]. Since 2001, $NiV_{Bangladesh}$ strains cause repeated small outbreaks in humans in India and Bangladesh, where NiV transmission from fruit bats to humans is often linked to the consumption of virus-contaminated date palm sap followed by human-to-human transmissions [2–6]. In contrast, $NiV_{Malaysia}$ had so far caused only one large disease outbreak in pigs and humans in Malaysia and Singapore in 1998/99 [7, 8]. During this NiV outbreak, pigs that had probably been infected by eating fruits contaminated with NiV-containing bat secretions passed the infection to humans in close contact [1]. Though both, pigs and humans, were symptomatically infected with NiV, humans developed fatal encephalitis with high mortality rates, while pigs mostly suffered from a severe respiratory disease [7, 9–11]. The highly productive virus replication in pig lungs led to effective virus shedding in airway secretions which importantly contributed to the rapid and efficient spread of the infection within the pig population, thereby also amplifying the risk of zoonotic transmissions to humans in close contact [11].

To understand the molecular mechanisms underlying NiV replication in airway cells, cell culture models are needed that allow studying host factors either needed for virus replication or involved in antiviral defense. The cell model that is chosen for these studies is critically important. Since most commonly used tumor-derived and artificially immortalized cell lines only poorly reflect the situation in vivo, primary cells reflect the phenotype of healthy cells in vivo much better than cell lines. The use of freshly isolated primary cells from a healthy donor has the advantage that the isolated cells express most of the important cell properties and functions. However, their limited lifespan makes experiments challenging, especially if they need to be performed under BSL-4 conditions. Despite these limitations, some studies in primary human cultures were already done in vitro, giving molecular insights into NiV growth kinetics, the cell tropism, and cytokine profiles in NiV-infected human airway epithelia [12–16]. The successful conduction of these studies was clearly facilitated by the fact that primary human airway epithelial cells can be purchased from different sources. In contrast to human cells, primary porcine respiratory epithelia are not commercially available. To elucidate the molecular mechanisms by which NiV replication in airway epithelia cells causes clinical disease in pigs and leads to productive virus shedding via airway secretions in vivo [11, 17, 18], studies in appropriate cell culture models are required. We therefore established a protocol adapting methods described earlier [19, 20] in order to isolate primary porcine bronchial epithelial cells (PBEpC) from fresh pig lungs that can be used as a model for NiV infection studies in vitro.

2 Materials

2.1 Lung Tissue Dissection, Cell Seeding, Subculturing, and Cryopreservation

1. Scalpels with blades of different sizes (#11, #20, #22).
2. Broad-tipped forceps.
3. Metal dissecting board (autoclavable).
4. Beakers (5 L and 600 mL).
5. 10-cm Petri dishes.
6. 12-mL Polystyrene CELLSTAR™ Cell Culture Tubes.
7. 50-mL conical centrifuge tubes.
8. 2-mL round bottom cryogenic vials.
9. Screen mesh polyester monol, mesh width 250 μm (NeoLab) (*see* **Note 1**).
10. Hemocytometer (Neubauer counting chamber, non-sterile).

    All following solutions are sterile and stored at 4 °C unless otherwise indicated.
11. PBS_{def}: Dulbecco's Ca^{2+} and Mg^{2+} deficient phosphate-buffered saline pH 7.2 (PBS, 8 g/L NaCl, 0.2 g/L KCl, 0.2 g/L KH_2PO_4, 2.16 g/L Na_2HPO_4-$7H_2O$).
12. PBS^{++}: PBS additionally containing 0.1 g/L $CaCl_2$ and 0.1 g/L $MgCl_2$-$6H_2O$.
13. Isolation medium: Low-glucose (1.0 g/L) Dulbecco's Modified Eagle Medium (DMEM) supplemented with penicillin (50 U/mL), streptomycin (50 μg/mL), amphotericin B (2.5 μg/mL), kanamycin sulfate dissolved in H_2O (100 μg/mL), enrofloxacin dissolved in H_2O (10 μg/mL), clotrimazol dissolved in DMSO (1 μg/mL), and DL-dithiothreitol (DTT, 0.5 mg/mL).
14. Protease XIV from Streptomyces griseus (1 mg/mL). Store at −20 °C.
15. Airway Epithelial Cell Growth Medium (AEGM, ready-to-use, Promocell): Thaw the supplement pack (stored at −20 °C), and transfer the entire content to 500 mL basal medium. Swirl gently until a homogenous mixture is formed. Add the following: L-glutamine (4 mM), penicillin (50 U/mL), streptomycin (50 μg/mL); amphotericin B (2.5 μg/mL), and kanamycin sulfate dissolved in H_2O (50 μg/mL) (*see* **Note 2**).
16. Passage Kit 4 from Provitro (PBS and Detachment Solution).
17. Glycerine (≥99.5%, p.a.), autoclaved before use.

2.2 Collagen Coating of Cell Culture Dishes

Cell culture material used for PBEpC cultures (*see* **Note 3**):

- T25 flasks with vent caps.
- 6-well plates.
- 12 mm Transwell inserts: Transwell permeable, transparent membrane supports with filter pore sites of 0.4 μM in 12-well plates (12 mm Transwell® with 0.4 μm Pore Polyester Membrane Insert).

1. 0.2 M pure glacial acetic acid (HAc) in H_2O, sterile-filtered.
2. Collagen I rat protein, tail (*see* **Note 4**).

2.3 Immunostaining of Epithelial Cell Markers

1. Scalpels (blade size #11).
2. Thin-tipped forceps.
3. Cannula or needle.
4. Parafilm.
5. Whatman paper.
6. 24-well plate.
7. 15 cm Petri dish.
8. PBS^{++}.
9. 4% PFA (paraformaldehyde, extra pure) dissolved in DMEM, sterile-filtered, and stored at −20 °C. Only thaw on the day of use.
10. 0.2% TX-100 in PBS^{++} (Triton X-100), stored at room temperature.
11. 2% BSA blocking solution; 0.35% BSA in PBS^{++} (BSA; albumin bovine fraction V, protease-free, lyophil, SERVA). Store at 4 °C.
12. Mowiol mounting solution (Mowiol 4–88). 2.4 g Mowiol 4–88 and 6 g glycerol are mixed with 6 mL dH_2O. After soaking for 24 h, 12 mL of 0.2 M Tris–HCl, pH 8.5, is added. Incubate at 50–60 °C with constant mixing until Mowiol is completely dissolved. Clear by centrifugation for 15 min at 1000 × *g*. Transfer the supernatant to a new tube, and add DABCO (1,4-Diazabicyclo-[2,2,2]octan) at a final concentration of 10% (w/v). Store at −20 °C. Only thaw before use.
13. Primary antibodies directed against epithelial marker proteins are stored as recommended by the suppliers. The following antibodies are used and were diluted in 0.35% BSA directly before use (*see* **Note 5**):
    - Anti-cytokeratin: Mix equal volumes of antibodies against acidic cytokeratin (Mouse IgG1; Acris #AM10029PU-S) and antibodies against basic cytokeratin (Mouse IgG1; Acris #AM10030PU-S). Prepare a 1:10 dilution.

- Anti-ZO-3: Prepare a 1:10 dilution of antibodies against ZO-3/TJP3 (Rabbit IgG; Millipore #AB3220).
- Anti-E-cadherin: Prepare a 1:50 dilution of purified antibodies against the E-cadherin cytoplasmic tail (clone 36/E-cadherin, mouse IgG2a; BD Biosciences, #610181).

14. For detection of the primary antibodies, Alexa Fluor (AF)-conjugated secondary antibodies from goat are used: AF488-labeled anti-mouse IgG and AF568-labeled anti-rabbit IgG are diluted in 0.35% BSA at a ratio of 1:250 directly before use (*see* **Note 6**).

2.4 NiV Infection (Kept or Transferred to the BSL-4 Containment)

1. NiV Malaysia strain [21, 22] (*see* **Note 7**).
2. AEGM and PBS^{++}.
3. RLT buffer of RNeasy Mini-Kit.
4. ß-ME (2-mercaptoethanol).
5. EtOH (ethanol absolute).
6. 1.6 mL CryoPure tubes.
7. 1.5 mL PP tubes with screw caps.
8. 5 mL PP tube.
9. Cell scraper (16 cm, blade length: 1.35 cm).

3 Methods

After removal of the lung from the donor (pig), sterility needs to be maintained throughout the preparation. Therefore, the lung dissection and cell seeding are conducted under a laminar flow hood. All surgical equipment, other materials and surfaces need to be sterilized prior use. While pig bronchi dissection and culturing of primary porcine cells can be conducted in a biosafety level 1 or 2 laboratory, infection studies with NiV need to be performed under the highest biosafety level 4 (BSL-4) conditions strictly following all safety regulations regarding standard practices, safety equipment, and facility requirements. Accordingly, all infection experiments with NiV described here were performed in the BSL-4 containment laboratory at the Institute of Virology, Philipps University Marburg, Germany.

3.1 Isolation of Primary Bronchial Epithelial Cells (PBEpC)

To aid adherence and growth of primary bronchial epithelia in vitro, cell culture flask surfaces and other materials used for PBEpC culturing are precoated with collagen.

3.1.1 Collagen Coating of Cell Culture Materials

1. Prepare a 1:100 solution of collagen I in 0.02 M HAc.
2. Add 2–3 mL of the collagen solution to a T25 flask. For collagen coating of a 6-well or a 12 mm Transwell filter, use

1–2 mL or 500 μL of the collagen solution, respectively (*see* **Note 8**).

3. Sterilize the opened flasks, wells, or filters by a 60 min UV treatment (UV-C irradiators of the lamina flow hood).
4. Close the lids of the flasks, 6-well plates, or 12-well plates with the Transwell membrane supports.
5. Incubate at 37 °C for 1–2 h or at 4 °C for at least 18 h. Dishes with collagen solution can be kept at 4 °C for maximally 2 weeks (*see* **Note 9**).
6. Directly before use, remove the collagen solution and wash the flasks, wells, or Transwell inserts twice with PBS^{++} (*see* **Note 10**).

3.1.2 Preparation of Bronchi Segments and Removal of Mucus (Day 1)

Transport and dissect a fresh intact pig lung obtained from a local slaughterhouse as rapidly as possible. Fresh lungs are a necessity for a successful outcome of the cell isolation regarding total cell numbers and cell viability (*see* **Note 11**). Lung dissection and cell isolation are performed in biological safety cabinet in a Level 1 or 2 facility (*see* **Note 12**).

1. Carefully dissect the primary bronchi free from peripheral lung tissue using scalpels (Fig. 1a–c).
2. Cut the two primary bronchi into 4–6 segments of 2–4 cm.
3. Use forceps to hold the bronchi segments over a 5 L beaker and rinse each one with approx. 50–100 mL PBS_{def} (*see* **Note 13**).
4. Put the segments in a 600 mL beaker and add isolation medium with DTT (improves the removal of mucus from the bronchi lumens) until all bronchi pieces are completely covered. Cover the beaker with aluminum foil (Fig. 1d). Incubate for 24 h at 4 °C.

3.1.3 Protease Digestion of Bronchi Segments (Day 2), Cell Isolation and Seeding (Day 3), and PBEpC Cultivation (Days 4–9)

1. Add 500 mg Protease XIV to 500 mL isolation medium.
2. Transfer the segments to a new 600 mL beaker, and add Protease XIV-containing isolation medium until all pieces are completely covered. Cover the beaker with aluminum foil. Incubate for 36 h at 4 °C.
3. Wash the segments: To remove the protease-containing medium, hold the bronchi segment with forceps over a 5 L beaker and rinse with 50–100 mL PBS_{def}.
4. Transfer the segment to a 10 cm Petri dish, and open the bronchi longitudinally using a scalpel #11 (*see* **Note 14**).
5. Transfer the cut segment (Fig. 1e) to a fresh 10-cm Petri dish. Carefully scrape off the lumen of the bronchus 4–5 times with a scalpel #20 to isolate the epithelial cells (Fig. 1f) (*see* **Note 15**).

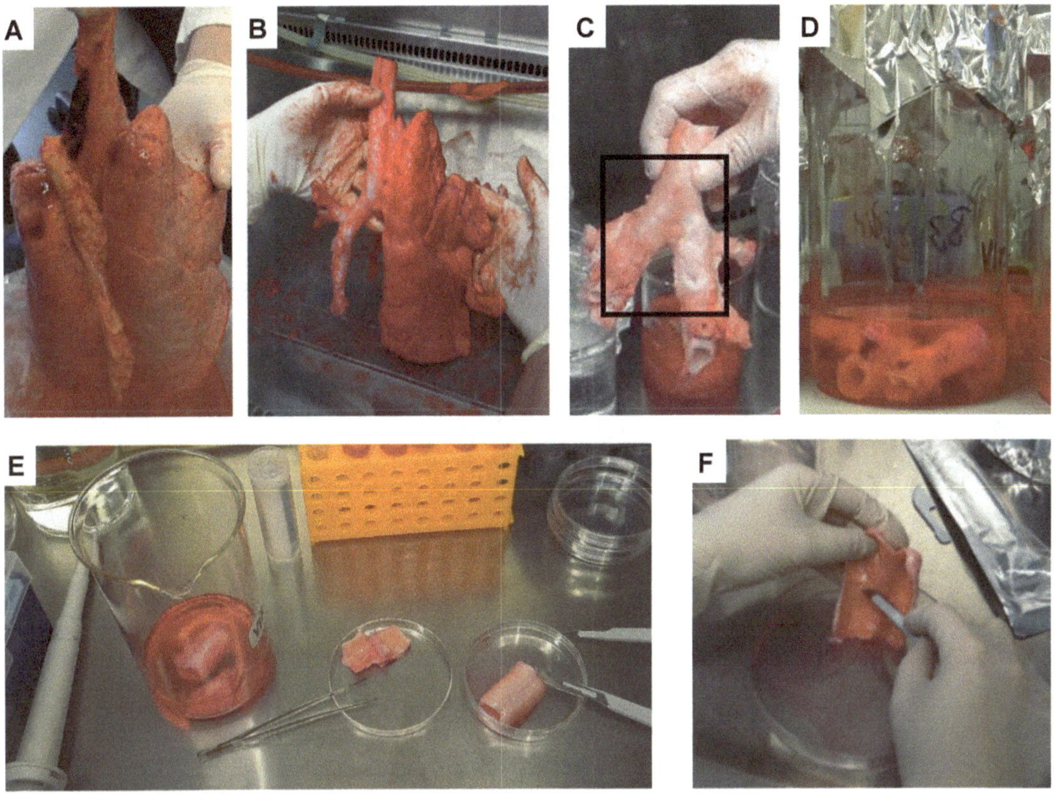

Fig. 1 Dissection of pig lungs to isolate primary porcine bronchial epithelial cells (PBEpC). The black box in (C) shows the parts of the bronchi from which the PBEpC are isolated (stem bronchus and left and right main bronchus down to the second segmentation)

6. Rinse the scalpel and the scraped-off epithelial cells in the cell culture dish with 1 mL PBS_{def}, and transfer the complete cell suspension to a 12 mL cell culture tube.
7. Continue with cell isolation from the next bronchi segment. Transfer the cell suspension to the cell culture tube (*see* **Note 16**).
8. After scrapping-off the cells from all segments, pellet the cells by low-speed centrifugation at 250 × *g* for 10 min at room temperature.
9. Carefully remove the supernatant from the cell pellet with a 1 mL pipette (*see* **Note 17**). Suspend the cell pellet carefully in a total volume of 4 mL AEGM.
10. Place a 10 × 10 cm pieces of screen mesh polyester monol in a 50-mL conical centrifuge tube. Filter the 4 mL cell suspension using a 1 mL pipette through the mesh to eliminate clumps and debris. Discard the mesh.
11. Add prewarmed AEGM to four collagen-coated T25 flasks (5 mL per flask). Transfer 1 mL of the filtrate to each of the

four T25 flasks, and gently swirl the suspension. Incubate the flasks at 37 °C and 5% CO_2 (*see* **Note 18**). Remove the cell culture medium 1 day after seeding on the T25 flasks, wash the cells carefully with 5 mL PBS_{def} to remove the mucus, and add 5 mL of fresh prewarmed AEGM (*see* **Note 19**).

12. Incubate the cultures at 37 °C at 5% CO_2, and examine cultures daily using an inverted microscope to ensure that the cells are growing. Cells should be passaged as soon as they have reached 80% confluence. This normally takes 4–5 days. Exchange the medium every 2 days.

3.2 PBEpC Cryopreservation and Subculturing

As soon as the isolated PBEpC cultures reach a confluence around 80% (Fig. 2), the cells must be detached from the collagen-coated T25 flask using a mild protease (*see* **Note 20**). PBEpC suspension can then be frozen for cryopreservation (Subheading 3.2.3) or can be split and subcultured on collagen-coated 6 wells (Subheading 3.2.4) or Transwell membrane inserts (Subheading 3.2.5).

3.2.1 Cell Detachment Using Passage Kit 4

1. Remove the cell culture supernatant from the T25 flask, and wash the cell monolayer with prewarmed 5 mL PBS (component of Passage Kit 4).
2. Remove the PBS, add 2.5 mL of the prewarmed detachment solution (Passage Kit 4), and incubate at 37 °C for approx. 10 min. Control cell detachment microscopically.
3. If the cells are completely detached, transfer the cell suspension into a 12 mL cell culture tube. Rinse the culture flask with 2 mL of AEGM, add the rinse to the tube, and centrifuge the suspension for 10 min at 250 × *g* at room temperature.

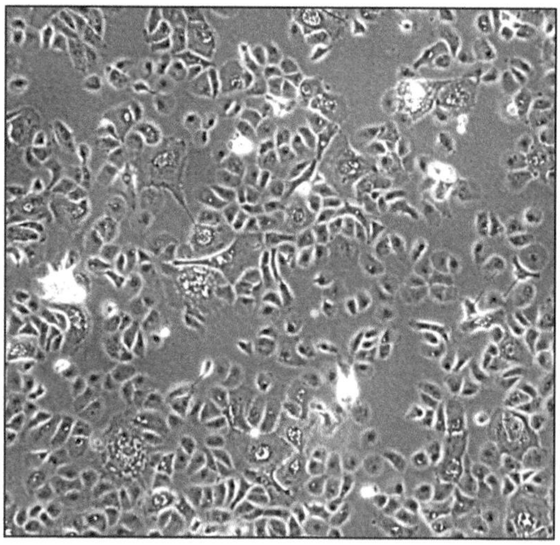

Fig. 2 PBEpC grown to 80% confluence on collagen-coated T25 flasks. Phase-contrast images of the live cell culture were recorded with a EVOS XL core microscope. Magnification, x100

4. Carefully remove the supernatant with a 1 mL pipette and resuspend the cell pellet in 1 mL AEGM (*see* **Note 21**).
5. After taking an aliquot for cell number determination (*see* Subheading 3.2.2), 1 mL cell suspension is mixed with 150 μL glycerine at a final concentration of 15% (v/v) and slowly frozen for cryopreservation (*see* Subheading 3.2.3). Alternatively, the cell suspension can be directly subcultured on collagen-coated 6 wells for infection studies (*see* Subheadings 3.2.4 and 3.4) or Transwell membrane inserts for epithelial cell characterization (*see* Subheadings 3.2.5 and 3.3).

3.2.2 Cell Counting

1. Clean the Neubauer counting chamber using 70% ethanol and a nonabrasive tissue.
2. Position the coverslip over the chamber so that Newton's rings appear.
3. Add 8 μL of the cell suspension to the edge of the coverslip.
4. Count the number of bright clear (viable) cells in all four edge quadrants and calculate the mean value.
5. Multiply the average cell number with 10^4 (chamber factor) and the volume of the cell suspension to calculate the cell number/mL (*see* **Note 22**).

3.2.3 Cryopreservation: Freezing and Thawing of PBEpC

1. Add 150 μL of sterile glycerine to a 2 mL cryogenic vial. Mix with 1 mL of the cell suspension detached from one 80% confluent T25 flask (approx. 1×10^6 cells/mL) by carefully pipetting.
2. Place the cells into a cryofreeze container with isopropanol. Transfer container to a −80 °C freezer for gradually freezing (*see* **Note 23**).
3. After 24–48 h, transfer the frozen vials into the vapor phase of liquid nitrogen.
4. Cell thawing: Put the frozen vials with PBEpC rapidly into a 37 °C warm water bath. Swivel the vial until the suspension is almost thawed (approx. 1 min). Dry and disinfect the vial outside, put the vial under a lamina flow, open the lid, and add 500 μL of prewarmed AEGM. Suspend the cells, and transfer the suspension to a 12 mL cell culture tube. Rinse the cryogenic vial twice with 1 mL AEGM to collect all cells, and add both suspensions to the cell culture tube.
5. Centrifuge at 250 × *g* for 10 min at room temperature (*see* **Note 21**). During centrifugation, add 5 mL prewarmed AEGM to two collagen-coated T25 flasks.
6. Remove the supernatant from the cell pellet with a pipette. Suspend the cells in 2 mL prewarmed AEGM (approx. 5×10^5 cells/mL).

7. Add 1 mL of the cell suspension to each collagen-coated T25 flask (*see* **Note 24**).
8. Incubate at 37 °C and 5% CO_2, and change the medium the next day.
9. Examine cultures daily using an inverted microscope to ensure that the cells are growing. Exchange the medium every second day. Cells are split and subcultured if they have reached a cell confluence of about 80% (*see* **Note 25**).

3.2.4 Subculturing PBEpC on 6-Well Plates

1. Detach the cells from the T25 flask as described above (Subheading 3.2.1), and suspend the cell pellet in 600 μL AEGM.
2. Add 2 mL of prewarmed AEGM to six collagen-coated 6 wells in a 6-well plate and add 100 μL of the cell suspension (approx. 1.5×10^5 cells per 6 wells). Gently swivel the plate to distribute the cells in the 6 wells. Incubate at 37 °C and 5% CO_2 overnight. Change AEGM medium the next day and then every 48 h, and examine cultures daily using an inverted microscope to ensure that the cells are growing.

3.2.5 Subculturing PBEpC on Transwell Membrane Inserts

For immunostainings (Subheading 3.3), PBEpC are cultivated on Transwell membrane inserts. These permeable supports permit cells to uptake molecules also from their basal surfaces. Thereby, metabolic activities can be carried out that are needed for cell polarization and the formation of apical and basolateral membrane domains separated by tight junctions (*see* **Note 26**).

1. Prepare the 12 mm Transwell membrane inserts for cell seeding: Wash with PBS^{++} twice. Remove the buffer. Add 250 μL AEGM to the apical filter chamber and 800 μL AEGM to the basal chamber. Incubate at 37 °C and 5% CO_2 for 30 min to equilibrate the filter membrane.
2. Remove the medium, and add 250 μL AEGM to the apical and 800 μL AEGM to the basal chamber (*see* **Note 27**).
3. PBEpC from an 80% confluent T25 flask were detached as described in Subheading 3.2.1 and suspended in 600 μL AEGM.
4. Add 50 μL of the cell suspension (approx. 7×10^4 cells per insert) on the apical filter chamber, and incubate the cells at 37 °C and 5% CO_2.
5. Change the medium from both sides the next day and then every 48 h. Check the cell growth microscopically daily (*see* **Note 28**).
6. Cultivate the cells until they are fully confluent. Then, incubate the cultures for another 4 days to allow polarization (*see* **Note 29**).

3.3 Epithelial Cell Marker Staining in PBEpC Grown on Transwell Membrane Inserts

To ensure that the PBEpC cultures are not "contaminated" with non-epithelial cell types such as fibroblasts, the cells are cultured on Transwell membrane inserts and characterized by immunostaining of cytokeratin (intermediate filament) which is generally expressed in epithelial cells, and detection of ZO-3 and E-cadherin, a tight junction and an adherens junction protein, which are expressed by airway epithelial cells after they have formed a polarized cell monolayer.

1. Remove the medium from the basal chamber of the 12 mm Transwell membrane insert.
2. Put the insert on a parafilm using a forceps, and remove the filter membrane from the Transwell insert by carefully cutting around the membrane edges with a scalpel #11.
3. Place the cutout membrane in a 24-well plate (cell monolayer on top).
4. Wash three times with 500 μL PBS^{++}. After the last washing step, remove the PBS^{++} completely (*see* **Note 30**).
5. Add 300 μL of 4% PFA and fix the cells for 15 min at room temperature.
6. Wash three times with 500 μL PBS^{++}, and remove the buffer.
7. Add 300 μL of 0.2% TX-100 and permeabilize the cells for 30 min at 37 °C.
8. Wash three times with 500 μL PBS^{++}, and remove the buffer.
9. Add 300 μL of 2% BSA blocking buffer for at least 1 h at room temperature.
10. Wash three times with 500 μL PBS^{++}, and remove the buffer.
11. Prepare primary antibody dilutions in 0.35% BSA (anti-cytokeratin, anti-ZO-3, anti-E-cadherin).
12. Prepare a "wet chamber." Put a Whatman paper (14 × 14 cm) into a 15 cm Petri dish. Moisten the paper with sterile H_2O, and cover it with parafilm (10 × 10 cm).
13. Drop 40 μL of the primary antibody solution on the parafilm. Place the cutout membrane on the drop (with the basal side contacting the liquid) using a forceps and a cannula.
14. Add 60 μL of the primary antibody dilution on the apical side, directly on top of the cell monolayer (*see* **Note 31**).
15. Close the lid of the "wet chamber," and incubate for 2 h at 4 °C.
16. Transfer the membranes back into the 24 well using forceps (*see* **Note 32**).
17. Wash three times with 500 μL PBS^{++}, and remove the buffer.

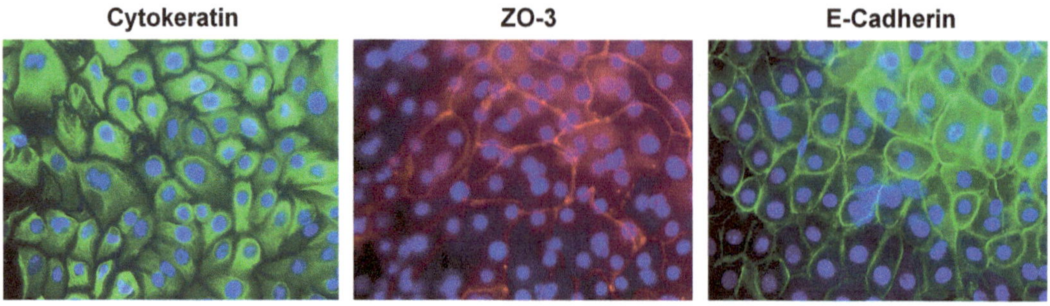

Fig. 3 Immunofluorescence analysis of epithelial marker protein expression in PBEpC. Polarized PBEpC cultured on Transwell membrane inserts were fixed, permeabilized, and incubated with primary antibodies directed against acidic and basic cytokeratins (Cytokeratin), or antibodies directed against the tight and adherens junction proteins ZO-3 and E-cadherin, respectively. Primary antibodies were detected with AF488- or AF468-labeled secondary antibodies. Images were recorded with a Axiovert 200 M (Zeiss). Magnification ×400

18. Prepare secondary antibody dilutions in 0.35% BSA (AF488-labeled anti-mouse IgG; AF568-labeled anti-rabbit IgG).
19. Add 300 μL of the appropriate secondary antibody on top of the membrane in the 24 well. Incubate at 4 °C for 2 h.
20. Remove the antibody solution. Wash three times with 500 μL PBS^{++}. Remove the buffer, and add 500 μL dH_2O (*see* **Note 33**).
21. Mounting the membrane: Add 20 μL Mowiol mounting solution on a slide, and place the membrane on top (basal side contacting the drop). Add 20 μL Mowiol solution to the cell monolayer. Put a cover slip on top (*see* **Note 34**).
22. Let the sample fully harden at 4 °C before imaging (Fig. 3).

3.4 NiV Infection of PBEpC

The growth of PBEpC cultivated on 6 wells (*see* Subheading 3.2.4) is daily controlled microscopically. If the cells have reached 80–90% confluence, one of the 6 wells is detached using the Passage Kit 4 (*see* Subheading 3.2.1) to determine the cell number (*see* Subheading 3.2.2). Then, the 6-well plate is transferred to the BSL-4 containment.

Infections studies with NiV are only performed in an approved BSL-4 containment with strict adherence to all biosafety requirements. Work is done by persons that are thoroughly trained in all practices and techniques required for handling selected agents and are proficient in the safety regulations and decontamination techniques according to the laboratory-specific biosafety manual.

3.4.1 NiV Infection

1. Thaw NiV stock virus solution at 37 °C (*see* **Note 35**).
2. Prepare a virus dilution in prewarmed AEGM in a 5 mL PP tube (*see* **Note 36**).

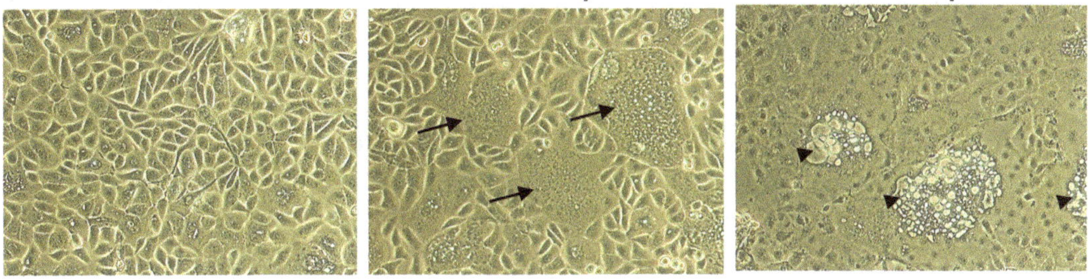

Fig. 4 Syncytia formation in NiV-infected PBEpC. PBEpC grown on collagen-coated 6 wells were kept uninfected (Mock) or were infected with a total virus dose of 3 × 10^4 $TCID_{50}$ for one (NiV 24 h p.i.) or 2 days (NiV 48 h p.i.). Live cell cultures were monitored by phase-contrast microscopy using a Nikon TS100 microscope. Magnification, x100. Large syncytia are already detectable at 24 h p.i. (arrows). At 48 h p.i., the cytopathic effect is very pronounced in the complete cell monolayer. Syncytia begin to disintegrate and detach (arrowheads)

3. Wash the 6 wells with 1 mL prewarmed AEGM. Remove the medium, and add 500 μL virus dilution. For mock controls, add 500 μL AEGM.
4. Incubate 1 h at 37 °C and 5% CO_2 (*see* **Note 37**).
5. Remove the virus inoculum, and wash the cells 4 times with prewarmed PBS^{++} (1 mL per well and washing step).
6. Remove the washing buffer and add 2–3 mL prewarmed AEGM. Incubate at 37 °C and 5% CO_2.
7. Examine NiV-infected cells microscopically at least once a day to monitor the formation of syncytia (*see* **Note 38**). Due to the ability to rapidly cause cell–cell fusion, syncytia are a major characteristic of an NiV infection in confluent primary airway cell cultures [14]. Syncytia can be monitored by light microscopy in live cell cultures (Fig. 4) to check whether the infection was successful and further downstream analyses are justified.

3.4.2 Sampling Virus Supernatants

If syncytia formation indicates that a PBEpC culture is successfully infected by NiV, cell supernatants and cell lysates are sampled at different time points after infection and stored for qualitative and quantitative analyses later on.

1. Transfer 1.4 mL of the infected cell supernatant to a 1.5 mL PP tube (*see* **Note 39**).
2. Centrifuge the supernatant at 1800*g* for 5 min at 4 °C to clear from cell debris.
3. Transfer 1 mL of the cleared supernatant to a 1.6 mL CryoPure tube, and store at −80 °C for virus titration by the $TCID_{50}$ method (*see* **Note 40**).
4. Mix 350 μL RLT buffer with 3.5 μL ß-ME in a 1.5 mL PP tube with a screw cap.

5. Transfer 100 μL of the cleared supernatant to the tube and mix by gently swiveling.
6. Incubate for 10 min at room temperature.
7. Add 250 μL EtOH, mix by gently swiveling, and store at 4 °C until RNA isolation (*see* **Note 41**).

3.4.3 Harvesting NiV-Infected Cell Lysates for RNA Isolation

1. Completely remove the supernatant from the NiV-infected 6 well.
2. Mix 600 μL RLT and 6 μL ß-ME. Add the mix to the 6 wells. Lyse the cells for 10 min at room temperature.
3. Scrape the lysed cells of the plate with a cell scraper.
4. Transfer 600 μL of the cell lysate to a 1.5 mL PP tube, and add 600 μL EtOH. Close the tube by tightening the screw cap, mix by gently swiveling, and store at 4 °C until RNA isolation (*see* **Note 41**).

4 Notes

1. The mesh is provided at a size of 100 × 115 cm, cut 10 × 10 cm pieces, and autoclave.
2. AEGM with additives stored at 4 °C can be used for maximally 4 weeks.
3. Corning culture dishes have proven best for culturing PBEpC. Transwell inserts with Polyester membranes can also be used without coating.
4. Collagen I is provided as 20 mL vial at 3 mg/mL and must be stored at 2–8 °C in the dark. Diluted collagen solution can be stored at 4 °C for approx. 2 weeks.
5. Prepare 100 μL primary antibody dilution for each membrane cut out from a 12 mm Transwell insert.
6. Prepare 300 μL primary antibody dilution for each Transwell membrane.
7. NiV stock virus is prepared from cleared supernatants of NiV-infected Vero 76 cells, stored in 1.5 mL Cryogenic vials at −80 °C in the BSL-4 containment of the Philipps University Marburg, Germany.
8. Culture dish surfaces must be completely covered by collagen solution. Transwell membrane inserts are only coated on the upper, apical side.
9. If incubated 4 °C in the fridge, enwrap the culture dishes in sterile plastic to prevent drying or contamination.
10. Collagen-coated material must be washed with sufficient volumes PBS^{++} to completely remove the acetic acid. Transwell

membrane inserts must be washed from the apical and basal sides.

11. The pig lung should be removed completely including the trachea. After packaging in a sterile plastic bag, the fresh lungs must be rapidly transported at room temperature (not on ice!).
12. All work surfaces within the cabinet should be decontaminated with an appropriate solution; 70% ethanol or isopropanol is routinely used for this purpose. Any materials required for the procedure should be similarly decontaminated and placed in or near the cabinet. As lungs and bronchi segments need to be handled by hands, gloves also need to be sterilized.
13. Washing is necessary to already remove some of the mucus from the bronchi lumens.
14. Hold the segment with one hand covered with a sterilized glove while cutting with the other hand.
15. Hold the segment with one hand covered with a sterilized glove in an upright position while you scrape with the other hand. Avoid scraping off any underlying connective tissue.
16. The cells from all 4–6 bronchi segments are collected in one cell culture tube.
17. The isolated cells do not form a clearly defined pellet.
18. Cells isolated from bronchi segments from one pig lung are always seeded onto four T25 flasks at an approx. cell density of $4–5 \times 10^5$ cells/flask.
19. Send the removed cell culture supernatant to a clinical microbiology laboratory for testing for any bacterial or fungal contamination.
20. At 80% confluence, PBEpC are still in the log phase of growth. If cell confluence is nearing 100%, cell passaging is often difficult because primary cells stop growing and undergo cell-cycle arrest when they have reached confluence (contact inhibition).
21. If there are visible "mucus filaments" in the supernatant, the centrifugation step is repeated.
22. The chamber factor is the number required to convert the volume of 0.1 mm^3 into mL.
23. Use polycarbonate freezing containers filled with isopropyl alcohol and with a high-density polyethylene closure to ensure freezing at a 1 °C/min cooling rate.
24. Splitting the cell suspension into two T25 flasks ensures cell seeding at max. 40% density.
25. PBEpC can be passaged up to 5 times and used for studies in subconfluent monolayers.

26. Polarization and expression of epithelial markers can also be detected if PBEpC of higher passage numbers are seeded on Transwell inserts. However, if it is planned to establish differentiated air–liquid interface cultures on Transwells, only PBEpC from passage 1 or passage 2 should be used.
27. If medium or buffers are added to a Transwell membrane insert always add 250–300 μL of the solution to apical side first, and then add 800–1000 μL to the basal filter chamber. For medium removal, aspirate in the opposite order. Remove the medium from the basal chamber first, and then remove the fluid from the apical side.
28. As PBEpC are cultivated on transparent Transwell membrane inserts, cell monolayers can be monitored by phase-contrast microscopy in the 12-well plate using an inverted microscope.
29. Within the four days, confluent PBEpC monolayers form a polarized monolayer with a moderate TEER (transepithelial resistance). Yet, they do not begin differentiate into ciliated, non-ciliated, and mucus-producing cells because this would require a specialized growth medium and cultivation under air–liquid conditions for several weeks.
30. Membranes need to be washed thoroughly to completely remove any mucus from the surface of the cell monolayer. Mucus components can prevent subsequent antibody binding.
31. By adding the antibody solution below and on top of the membrane, the primary antibodies can reach the target proteins from both cell sides.
32. To facilitate the lifting of the membrane from the parafilm with forceps, use a thin cannula to raise the membrane.
33. Final washing with H_2O prevents the salts in PBS to from crystals interfering with microscopic analysis after mounting.
34. Eventual air bubbles can be removed by gently pressing the coverslip down on the membrane with a pipette tip.
35. NiV stock virus is only thawed once and used the same day.
36. NiV dilution depends on the stock virus titer and the required infection dose. For example, to infect PBEpC in a 6 well with an infection dose of 3×10^4 $TCID_{50}$, mix 1 μL of an NiV stock with a titer of 3×10^7 $TCID_{50}$/mL with 500 μL AEGM.
37. Swivel the 6-well plates every 15 min to ensure an even distribution of the virus inoculum.
38. The lids of virus-infected 6-well plates must never be removed outside the lamina flow in BSL-4 containment. Therefore, microscopic examination can only be done with an inverted phase-contrast microscope at low magnifications.

39. Tubes with infectious material handled outside the lamina flow must have a closed screw cap.
40. If supernatants are frozen again after thawing, the infectious virus titers usually drop by at least one log step.
41. To quantitate viral RNA in cell supernatants or cell lysates, RNA is isolated according to the protocol of the manufacturer. The protocol and the primers used for cDNA synthesis and quantitative NiV-N real-time PCR have been described earlier [14, 23].

Acknowledgements

The authors thank Markus Eickmann, Gotthard Ludwig, and Michael Schmidt for their excellent support in the BSL-4 containment. This work was funded by the Deutsche Forschungsgemeinschaft (DFG, German Research Foundation)—Projektnummer 197785619—SFB 1021. M.E. and L.S. were supported by a fellowship of the Jürgen-Manchot-Stiftung.

References

1. Ang BSP, Lim TCC, Wang L (2018) Nipah virus infection. J Clin Microbiol 56(6): e01875-17. https://doi.org/10.1128/JCM.01875-17
2. Gurley ES, Montgomery JM, Hossain MJ, Bell M, Azad AK, Islam MR et al (2007) Person-to-person transmission of Nipah virus in a Bangladeshi community. Emerg Infect Dis 13(7):1031–1037
3. Luby SP, Hossain MJ, Gurley ES, Ahmed BN, Banu S, Khan SU et al (2009) Recurrent zoonotic transmission of Nipah virus into humans, Bangladesh, 2001–2007. Emerg Infect Dis 15(8):1229–1235
4. Lo MK, Lowe L, Hummel KB, Sazzad HM, Gurley ES, Hossain MJ et al (2012) Characterization of Nipah virus from outbreaks in Bangladesh, 2008–2010. Emerg Infect Dis 18(2):248–255. https://doi.org/10.3201/eid1802.111492
5. Gurley ES, Hegde ST, Hossain K, Sazzad HMS, Hossain MJ, Rahman M et al (2017) Convergence of humans, bats, trees, and culture in Nipah virus transmission, Bangladesh. Emerg Infect Dis 23(9):1446–1453. https://doi.org/10.3201/eid2309.161922
6. Islam MS, Sazzad HM, Satter SM, Sultana S, Hossain MJ, Hasan M et al (2016) Nipah virus transmission from bats to humans associated with drinking traditional liquor made from date palm sap, Bangladesh, 2011–2014. Emerg Infect Dis 22(4):664–670. https://doi.org/10.3201/eid2204.151747
7. Chua KB, Goh KJ, Wong KT, Kamarulzaman A, Tan PS, Ksiazek TG et al (1999) Fatal encephalitis due to Nipah virus among pig-farmers in Malaysia. Lancet 354(9186):1257–1259
8. Chua KB, Bellini WJ, Rota PA, Harcourt BH, Tamin A, Lam SK et al (2000) Nipah virus: a recently emergent deadly paramyxovirus. Science 288(5470):1432–1435
9. Goh KJ, Tan CT, Chew NK, Tan PS, Kamarulzaman A, Sarji SA et al (2000) Clinical features of Nipah virus encephalitis among pig farmers in Malaysia. N Engl J Med 342(17): 1229–1235
10. Wong KT, Shieh WJ, Kumar S, Norain K, Abdullah W, Guarner J et al (2002) Nipah virus infection: pathology and pathogenesis of an emerging paramyxoviral zoonosis. Am J Pathol 161(6):2153–2167
11. Mohd Nor MN, Gan CH, Ong BL (2000) Nipah virus infection of pigs in peninsular Malaysia. Rev Sci Tech 19(1):160–165
12. Escaffre O, Borisevich V, Carmical JR, Prusak D, Prescott J, Feldmann H et al (2013) Henipavirus pathogenesis in human respiratory epithelial cells. J Virol 87(6):

3284–3294. https://doi.org/10.1128/JVI.02576-12

13. Escaffre O, Borisevich V, Vergara LA, Wen JW, Long D, Rockx B (2016) Characterization of Nipah virus infection in a model of human airway epithelial cells cultured at an air-liquid interface. J Gen Virol 97(5):1077–1086. https://doi.org/10.1099/jgv.0.000441
14. Sauerhering L, Zickler M, Elvert M, Behner L, Matrosovich T, Erbar S et al (2016) Species-specific and individual differences in Nipah virus replication in porcine and human airway epithelial cells. J Gen Virol 97:1511–1519. https://doi.org/10.1099/jgv.0.000483
15. Sauerhering L, Müller H, Behner L, Elvert M, Fehling SK, Strecker T et al (2017) Variability of interferon-λ induction and antiviral activity in Nipah virus infected differentiated human bronchial epithelial cells of two human donors. J Gen Virol 98(10):2447–2453. https://doi.org/10.1099/jgv.0.000934
16. Borisevich V, Ozdener MH, Malik B, Rockx B (2017) Hendra and Nipah virus infection in cultured human olfactory epithelial cells. mSphere 2(3). https://doi.org/10.1128/mSphere.00252-17
17. Middleton DJ, Weingartl HM (2012) Henipaviruses in their natural animal hosts. Curr Top Microbiol Immunol 359:105–121. https://doi.org/10.1007/82_2012_210
18. Pickering BS, Hardham JM, Smith G, Weingartl ET, Dominowski PJ, Foss DL et al (2016) Protection against henipaviruses in swine requires both, cell-mediated and humoral immune response. Vaccine 34(40):4777–4786. https://doi.org/10.1016/j.vaccine.2016.08.028
19. Bals R, Beisswenger C, Blouquit S, Chinet T (2004) Isolation and air-liquid interface culture of human large airway and bronchiolar epithelial cells. J Cyst Fibros 3(Suppl 2):49–51. https://doi.org/10.1016/j.jcf.2004.05.010
20. Goris K, Uhlenbruck S, Schwegmann-Wessels-C, Köhl W, Niedorf F, Stern M et al (2009) Differential sensitivity of differentiated epithelial cells to respiratory viruses reveals different viral strategies of host infection. J Virol 83(4):1962–1968. https://doi.org/10.1128/JVI.01271-08
21. Moll M, Diederich S, Klenk HD, Czub M, Maisner A (2004) Ubiquitous activation of the Nipah virus fusion protein does not require a basic amino acid at the cleavage site. J Virol 78(18):9705–9712
22. Diederich S, Sauerhering L, Weis M, Altmeppen H, Schaschke N, Reinheckel T et al (2012) Activation of the Nipah virus fusion protein in MDCK cells is mediated by cathepsin B within the endosome-recycling compartment. J Virol 86(7):3736–3745. https://doi.org/10.1128/jvi.06628.11
23. Freitag TC, Maisner A (2015) Early activation of primary brain microvascular endothelial cells by Nipah virus glycoprotein-containing particles. J Virol 90(5):2706–2709. https://doi.org/10.1128/JVI.02825-15

Chapter 9

Primary Culture of the Human Olfactory Neuroepithelium and Utilization for Henipavirus Infection In Vitro

Mehmet Hakan Ozdener, Barry Rockx, and Nancy E. Rawson

Abstract

The olfactory receptor neurons (ORNs) are a unique cell type involved in the initial perception of odors. These specialized epithelial cells are located in the neuroepithelium of the nasal cavities and directly connect the nasal cavity with the central nervous system (CNS) via axons, which traverse the cribriform plate to synapse within the olfactory bulb. ORNs are derived from precursor cells that lie adjacent to the basal lamina of the olfactory epithelium. These precursor cells divide several times and their progeny differentiate into mature sensory neurons throughout life. In addition to its major and critical role in sensory transduction, the olfactory neuroepithelium may be an important tissue for viral replication and represents a potential site for viral entry into the CNS. In general, to gain access to the CNS, neurotropic viruses such as henipaviruses can use peripheral neural pathways or the circulatory system. However, the olfactory system has been reported to provide a portal of entry to the CNS for henipaviruses. The ability to obtain biopsies from living human subjects and culture these cells in the laboratory provides the opportunity to examine viral replication and effects on a neuronal cell population. As the most exposed and unprotected segment of the nervous system, the olfactory neuroepithelium may have an important role in neuropathology and systemic dissemination of viruses with established CNS effects. This chapter presents methods for primary culture of human ORNs, which have been used successfully by multiple investigators. The protocol provides a consistent, heterogeneous olfactory epithelial cell population, which demonstrates functional responses to odorant mixtures and exhibits several key features of the olfactory receptor neuron phenotype, encompassing olfactory receptors and signaling pathways.

Key words Olfactory, Smell, Odor, Virus, Viral disorders

1 Introduction

Olfactory receptor neuronal cells are highly specialized cells with unique histological, molecular, and physiological characteristics that permit detection of a wide range of both simple and structurally complex volatile molecules. Human olfactory mucosa is a specialized neuroepithelium in the superior reaches of the nasal cavity. The sensory epithelium, roughly the area of a postage stamp, occupies the olfactory cleft and projects onto the dorsal portion of the superior turbinate. In humans, the extent of the

Alexander N. Freiberg and Barry Rockx (eds.), *Nipah Virus: Methods and Protocols*, Methods in Molecular Biology, vol. 2682, https://doi.org/10.1007/978-1-0716-3283-3_9, © Springer Science+Business Media, LLC, part of Springer Nature 2023

neuroepithelial sheet varies within and among individuals and can become patchy and interspersed with respiratory or fibrotic tissue with age or disease [1–3]. The olfactory neuroepithelium is a pseudostratified epithelium comprised of multiple cell types. Mature olfactory sensory neurons (OSNs) are bipolar cells classically identified by the expression of olfactory marker protein [4]. These cells are derived from a population of proliferative basal cells that produce precursors which differentiate into immature neurons expressing Gap-43 and neuron-specific tubulin [3, 5]. In addition, supporting cells including microvillar and sustentacular cells provide trophic and protective support, expressing detoxification enzymes such as cytochrome P450 [6]. These differentiated cell types sit on a layer of horizontal and globose basal cells. Horizontal basal cells may represent a function comparable to a blood–brain barrier. While little is known about their physiological properties, they are molecularly defined by the expression of specific cytokeratins (e.g., CK-18), and in humans, (but not rodent) olfactory epithelium, express p75-nerve growth factor receptor [7, 8]. Unlike the very orderly layers of OMP immunoreactive OSNs observed in rodent olfactory epithelium, the frequency of OMP immunoreactive OSNs in the human middle turbinate tends to be sparse and scattered. This accounts for the approximately 60% success rate in obtaining sensory epithelium from biopsies obtained from this region [9–11].

The epithelium is a self-renewing tissue that can generate new neurons from stem and progenitor cells within the basal layers [12, 13]. Mesenchymal-like stem cells are present in the underlying lamina propria and are also likely to participate in regeneration [2, 14]. As a regenerative tissue, the olfactory epithelium contains a population of progenitor cells capable of replicating and differentiating to replace mature neurons as they are lost due to injury, infection, or normal senescence [15]. Our understanding of olfactory receptor neuronal cell function has arisen largely from studies of dissociated cells and tissues. In humans, the olfactory neuroepithelium is accessible via biopsy using relatively simple procedures, and olfactory epithelial biopsies have been established as a viable approach to obtain fresh sensory epithelial tissue for physiological and molecular studies [16, 17]. In view of this, several laboratories have developed protocols to establish primary cultures of the human olfactory epithelium (hOE) using biopsies from the sensory epithelium as a starting point. Olfactory-specific functional and molecular properties are retained by cells in these preparations, although the classic bipolar morphology is generally lost, particularly with extended passaging. A number of neuronal and non-neuronal markers identified in human olfactory epithelium have been used for culture characterization [15]. Key among these is as follows: olfactory marker protein, neuron-specific tubulin, neural cell adhesion molecule, and adenylate cyclase III

(ACIII), an element of the olfactory transduction pathway [18, 19]. Olfactory marker protein is a prototypical and specific marker for mature olfactory receptor neurons [20], while neuron-specific tubulin and neural cell adhesion molecule are found in the immature and mature olfactory neurons in vivo and *in vitro* [16, 18, 21]. Adenylate cyclase and other components of the signal transduction pathway are key markers of function both for odorant receptors and for neurotransmitter response. Unfortunately, no reliable antibodies for human odorant receptors (ORs) are presently available, so molecular methods are required to verify the presence and population of ORs that are expressed in vitro. In addition, cultured olfactory receptor neuronal cells express receptors and transduction elements for several neurotransmitters including dopamine (D2R), serotonin (5HT2C), and glutamate (NMDA subtypes 1 and 2A/2B) [22]. The development of odorant sensitivity and the expression of olfactory-specific marker molecules was related to structural maturation of cultured olfactory cells [18]. Several studies have demonstrated that the olfactory system can provide a direct route for entry of certain pathogens into the CNS, in spite of protection from most common infections via mucosal and immunological components [23, 24]. There is evidence that HSV-1, vesicular stomatitis virus (VSV), Borna disease virus (BDV), rabies virus (RABV), influenza A virus, parainfluenza viruses, and prions can enter the CNS through an olfactory route [25–28]. We have recently shown that human olfactory neurons are highly susceptible to infection with henipaviruses, supporting in vivo data showing that henipaviruses can infect the olfactory epithelium in the nasal turbinates and that infected neurons extend through the cribriform plate and into the olfactory bulb [29, 30]. Primary olfactory neuronal cultures provide a tool to improve our understanding of viral neuropathology and transit into the CNS.

The methods described here provide for the generation, maintenance, and characterization of primary hOE cultures as used in our laboratory. Factors contributing to variability and success are noted.

2 Materials

2.1 Human Olfactory Epithelial Biopsy

The main sensory region is located within the olfactory cleft, separated from the cranial cavity by a thin, porous bone called the cribriform plate, and the fragility of this has led current investigators to obtain tissue from the superior aspect of the middle turbinate and apposed septum rather than the olfactory cleft. Detection thresholds for one or more odorants may be obtained unilaterally to insure that the individual's sense of smell is normal on the side from which the biopsy is obtained [17]. However, it must be noted that there is only a minimal association between the likelihood of obtaining OSNs from a biopsy and that individual's olfactory performance, given that the biopsy represents only a tiny fraction of the total epithelial sheet. Hundreds of biopsies from healthy subjects and a variety of patient populations have been obtained using this technique without severe adverse events [12, 14, 17, 18, 31–33].

1. 0.5% phenylephrine hydrochloride and 0.5% tetracaine hydrochloride spray to facilitate visualization and anesthetization.
2. Small sponge plaget such as a Merocel® Otic Wick.
3. Xylocaine (e.g., lidocaine, 4%).
4. Sterile giraffe forceps or similar instrument.

2.2 Cell Culture

1. T25 (25 cm^2) and T75 (75 cm^2) tissue culture flasks.
2. Phosphate-buffered saline (PBS, with calcium and magnesium, 137 mM sodium chloride, 10 mM disodium phosphate, 2.7 mM potassium chloride, 1.8 mM monopotassium phosphate, 1 mM calcium chloride, and 0.5 mM magnesium chloride).
3. Trypsin/EDTA (0.05% Trypsin 0.53 mM EDTA, Gibco®/BRL).
4. Iscove's Modified Eagle's Medium (IMEM) (Gibco®/BRL) supplemented with 10% fetal bovine serum (FBS, HyClone) and a triple cocktail of antibiotics (100 U/mL/100 μg/mL, penicillin/streptomycin, and 0.5 μg/mL amphotericin B). Alternatively, DMEM, low glucose (1 gm/mL, Gibco/Thermo Fisher) supplemented with extra 2 mM L-glutamine, 10% fetal bovine serum (FBS, Sigma), and a triple cocktail of antibiotics (100 U/mL/100 μg/mL, penicillin/streptomycin, and 0.5 μg/mL amphotericin B).
5. Preparation of coverslips: Prior to use, treat coverslips with 2 M NaOH for 1 h and leave overnight in 70% nitric acid (HNO_3). Wash with 9 M HCl acid for 1 h and autoclave coverslips in water and rinse with 70% ethanol and 100% ethanol, and then air dry.
6. Isolation solution (Hank's buffer): (145 mM NaCl, 5 mM KCl, 2 mM EDTA, 1 mM Na-pyruvate, 20 mM HEPES, 100 μg/mL gentamicin).
7. 15 mL conical tubes.
8. Cryovials.
9. Freezer containers, e.g., Nalge Nunc Cryo 1 °C Mr. Frosty Freezing Container.
10. Freezing medium for cryopreservation: 5% DMSO, 95% FBS.

2.3 Immunocytochemistry

1. 4% paraformaldehyde in PBS.
2. Peroxidase blocking solution: 4 mL PBS, 0.5 mL 100% methanol (4 °C), 0.5 mL 30% H_2O_2 (4 °C).
3. Blocking and antibody diluting solution: 3% normal goat serum, 3% bovine serum albumin, 0.3% Triton X-100 in PBS.
4. Primary antibodies: polyclonal antibody against olfactory marker protein (OMP) made in goat (Wako), 1:100 dilution, and polyclonal anti-adenylate cyclase III (ACIII) made in rabbit (Santa Cruz Biotechnology®) at 1:200 dilution and monoclonal antibody against cyclic nucleotide gated channel alpha 2 (CNGA2) protein generated in mouse (LSBio), at 1:100 dilutions.
5. Secondary antibodies were as follows: Alexa Fluor® 488-conjugated anti-goat IgG made in donkey (Molecular Probes®) or Alexa Fluor® 633-conjugated anti-rabbit IgG made in goat (Molecular Probes®).
6. Mounting medium and nuclear stain: VectaShield® with DAPI (4,6-diamidino-2-phenylindole) (Vector Labs).

2.4 Calcium Imaging

1. Mammalian Ringer's solution: 145 mM NaCl, 5 mM KCl, 1 mM $CaCl_2$, 1 mM $MgCl_2$, 1 mM sodium pyruvate, and 20 mM Na HEPES; adjust pH to 7.1–7.2 and osmolarity to 300–310 mOsmol/L using 5 M NaCl, and then filter sterilize.
2. For high K^+ stimulation, 40 mM of NaCl is replaced with KCl. For Ca^{2+}-free Ringer's, $CaCl_2$ is removed and replaced with 1 mM ethylene glycol tetraacetic acid (EGTA).
3. For the isolation solution, $CaCl_2$ and $MgCl_2$ are omitted from the mammalian Ringer's and replaced with 2 mM ethylenediaminetetraacetic acid (EDTA).
4. Cell loading solution: 1 mM Fura-2 AM (Molecular Probes®) in 10 mg/mL Pluronic F127 (Molecular Probes®) in Ringer's solution.
5. Odors: A variety of odor stimuli have been used in functional assays. Odors should be the purest available and stored in amber, air-tight vials, frozen, and/or under liquid nitrogen to minimize deterioration. Some odors exhibit autofluorescence, and negative controls should always be used to avoid artifacts. For general culture characterization, a mixture of odors is typically used to increase the likelihood of finding responsive cells. In our studies, eugenol, lyral, and heptanal were prepared as 1 M stock in DMSO and freshly dissolved at 100 μM in Ringer's Solution with sonication. Oxidation products may exhibit an odor different from the fresh compound, so experiments aiming to relate molecular features to a particular odorant response require assurance of the odor identity and purity using an appropriate analytical technique.

2.5 Henipavirus Infection

1. Nipah virus (NiV) Malaysia strain, NiV Bangladesh strain, and Hendra virus (HeV) stocks.
2. PBS.
3. Iscove's Modified Eagle's Medium (IMEM) (Gibco®/BRL) supplemented with 10% fetal bovine serum (FBS, HyClone) and a triple cocktail of antibiotics (100 U/mL/100 μg/mL, penicillin/streptomycin, and 0.5 μg/mL amphotericin B).
4. Sterile tubes for preparing inoculum.

3 Methods

3.1 Harvest, Isolation, Culture, and Maintenance of Human Olfactory Cells

1. Spray the anterior portion of the superior turbinate and apposed nasal septum (*see* **Note 1**) with 0.5% phenylephrine hydrochloride and 0.5% tetracaine hydrochloride spray to facilitate visualization and anesthetization (*see* **Note 2**).
2. Wait 10–15 min. For anesthesia of the biopsy site. After anesthetization, biopsies of approximately 1 mm^3 are obtained using a giraffe forceps or similar instrument from the turbinate and apposed septum and are immediately transferred to IMEM on ice for transport to the laboratory (*see* **Note 3**).
3. Subjects are observed for 10–15 min after the procedure in the event of nosebleed and are asked to refrain from strenuous activity or blowing their nose for several hours after the procedure.
4. Biopsy specimens are transferred into isolation solution (Hank's Buffer) and minced finely with iridectomy scissors.
5. The minced tissue is incubated for ~30 min at room temperature inside cell culture hood.
6. Cells are dissociated by trituration with a fire-polished pipette and centrifugation at 600×*g* for 5 min at room temperature.
7. The pellet is resuspended in 3 mL IMEM and transferred to a 25 cm^2 culture flask.
8. Flasks are maintained in a humidified incubator (37 °C, 5% CO_2).
9. Allow to grow for 2–4 weeks until cell growth is sufficient (80–90% confluence) for transfer to continuous culture.

3.2 Propagation of Human Olfactory Cells

1. Replace 1/3 of the IMEM every 6–7 days until cultured cells have reached 80–90% confluence (*see* **Note 4**).
2. To passage cells, wash cells once with sterile PBS and then trypsinize cells using 0.25% w/v trypsin/EDTA for 2–3 min at 36 °C, and gently collect detached cells into a centrifuge tube.

3. After centrifugation at 600 × *g* for 5 min at room temperature, resuspend cells in Iscove's medium and transfer them to fresh T75 flasks (passage 1). Split cells at a 1:4 dilution in a T75 flask for maintaining adequate growth of the cells over time (*see* **Note 5**). At this stage, aliquots may be frozen for future use or used for experimental analysis.
4. Replace 1/3 of medium every 6–7 days.
5. Repeat **steps 2** and **3** when cells have reached 80–90% confluence.
6. Cells are now ready to be processed for immunohistochemistry, RNA isolation, calcium imaging, or other applications.
7. For growth on coverslips for functional assays or immunocytochemistry, transfer approximately 2000–4000 suspended cells to cleaned, sterilized uncoated coverslips and maintain them in culture media for up to 3–5 days (90% confluence).

3.3 Freezing and Thawing Cultured Human Olfactory Cells

1. To freeze stocks of primary olfactory cells, after trypsinization, add 5 mL of complete Iscove's medium and transfer cells to sterile 15 mL conical centrifuge tubes. Centrifuge at 160–200*g* for 5 min at room temperature.
2. Carefully discard the supernatant and gently resuspend cells with appropriate volume of freezing medium.
3. Transfer cells to labeled, sterile cryovials, cap tightly, and place in a freezing container containing isopropanol. Place into a −80 °C freezer for at least 1 day prior to transferring indefinitely to liquid nitrogen or −80 °C freezer. We did not observe significant differences in viability of cells stored at −80 °C or liquid nitrogen for up to 6 months.
4. For thawing, transfer cryovial directly to 37 °C water bath and swirl vial to thaw as quickly as possible.
5. Spray vial with ethanol. Transfer cells into a sterile T25 or T75 cell culture flask with cell IMEM (5 mL for T25 and 15 mL for T75 flask).
6. Continue to culture cells according to Subheading 3.2.

3.4 Confocal Immunofluorescence for Olfactory Cell Markers

1. Human olfactory cells grown on sterile, uncoated coverslips for 3–5 days are fixed with 4% paraformaldehyde in PBS (pH 7.2) for 10 min at room temperature.
2. After washing in PBS, the cells are treated with peroxidase solution to remove endogenous peroxidase activity.
3. Cells are blocked with blocking solution for 30–60 min and then incubated with primary antibodies diluted in blocking solution (OMP at 1:100; CNGA2 at 1:100; ACIII at 1:200) overnight at 4 °C.

4. After washing with PBS, cells are then incubated with the appropriate secondary antibody diluted 1:500 in blocking buffer for 30 h at room temperature.
5. After washing in PBS (3 × 15 min) and water (3 × 20 min), coverslips are mounted with Vectashield® with DAPI.
6. Fluorescent images are captured with a Leica TCS SP2 Spectral Confocal Microscope (*see* Fig. 1c–h, **Note 6**).

3.5 Calcium Imaging for Functional Assays

1. Aliquots of 2000–4000 suspended cells are transferred onto sterile, uncoated coverslips in petri dishes and grown for 2–4 days in a humidified incubator to achieve 80–90% confluence.
2. Cells are loaded calcium sensitive dye by applying ~0.5 mL loading solution and incubating for 1 h at 36 °C.
3. Cells are first superfused with Ringer's solution and then exposed to odorant stimuli via superfusion, with each stimulus applied for 30–60 s and washed with Ringer's solution for at least 2 min (*see* Fig. 2 and **Note** 7).
4. Tracking of changes in cytosolic fluorescence is performed using standard imaging equipment and data analysis procedures (*see* **Note 8**).
5. Intracellular calcium may either increase or decrease in response to odor stimulation, although the mechanism and role of odorant-induced calcium decreases in odorant signaling are unclear. Following a response, calcium levels should return to baseline. Odor stimulation should be organized to minimize repetitive exposures to the extent possible to minimize adaptation. Individual cells rarely respond to multiple odors, and the proportion of odor-responsive cells may vary across cultures and days in culture (*see* **Note 8**).

3.6 Henipavirus Infection of hOEC

The growth of hOEC grown on coverslips (*see* Subheading 3.2) is checked daily microscopically. If the cells have reached 80–90% confluence, the coverslips are transferred to the BSL-4 laboratory.

All infectious work with henipaviruses should be performed in a class II biological safety cabinet in a BSL4 laboratory.

1. Thaw henipavirus stock virus solution at 37 °C.
2. Prepare an appropriate virus dilution in culture media, depending on the required multiplicity of infection (*see* **Note 9**).
3. Remove the medium and add 200 μL virus dilution. For mock controls, add 200 μL IMEM.
4. Incubate 1 h at 37 °C and 5% CO_2, while gently rocking the plate every 10–15 min to ensure even distribution of the inoculum.

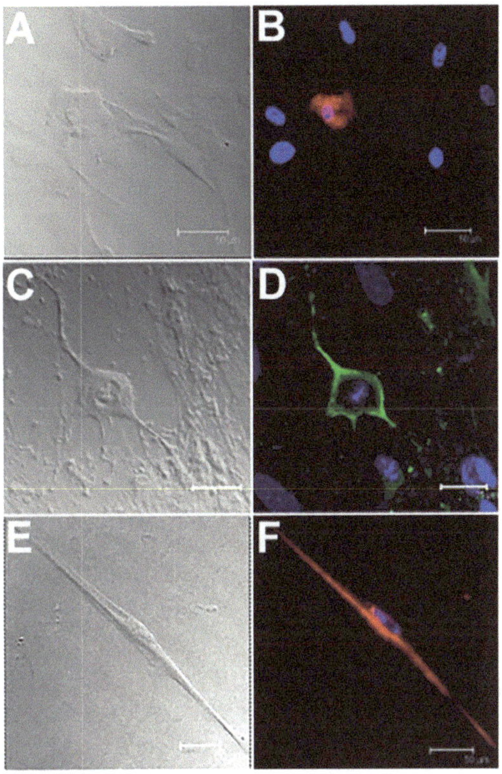

Fig. 1 Immunostaining of cultured human olfactory cells. Cultured human olfactory cells maintain their immunologic and physiological properties. Immunostaining of cultured human olfactory cells showed the presence of specific biomarkers. (**a**, **c**, and **e**) Transmission images of corresponding fields are shown on the left. (**b**) Immunoreactivity was observed for olfactory marker protein (OMP, red) in cultured human olfactory cells. (**d** and **f**) Immunoreactivity for adenylate cyclase III (green) and cyclic-nucleotide-gated alpha 2 (CNGA2, red) channels was also observed in cultured human olfactory cells. Nuclei of cells were stained blue with DAPI. Scale bars = 50 μm

5. Remove the virus inoculum, and wash the cells 3 times with PBS (1 mL per well for each washing step).
6. Remove PBS, and add 2 mL prewarmed IMEM. Incubate at 37 °C and 5% CO_2.
7. Examine henipavirus-infected cells microscopically to monitor the formation of syncytia.
8. Take the required samples for downstream analysis using pre-approved methods of inactivation.

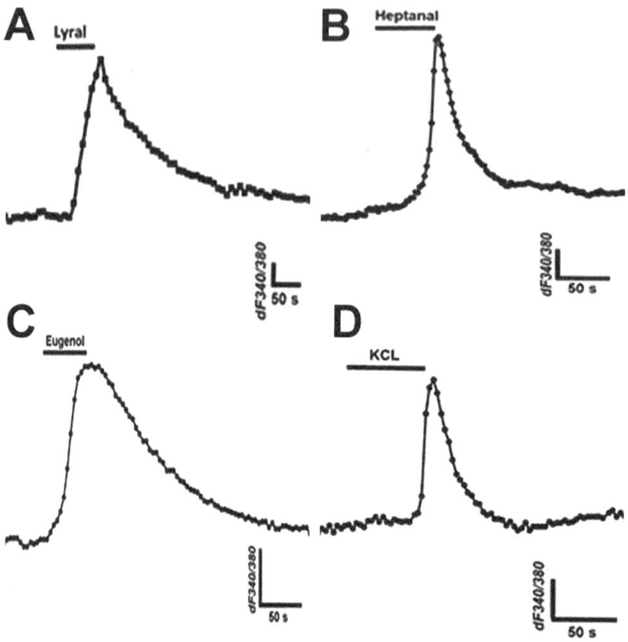

Fig. 2 Cultured human olfactory cells respond to odor stimuli. Changes in intracellular calcium levels ($[Ca^{2+}]_i$) in cultured human olfactory cell were measured using Fura-2. Graphs illustrate representative changes in $[Ca^{+2}]_i$ levels in individual cells during exposure to (**a**) lyral, (**b**) heptenal, (**c**) eugenol, and (**d**) potassium chloride (KCL 40 mM)

4 Notes

1. This region contains olfactory epithelium in approximately 60% of healthy subjects [31]. Subjects are asked to refrain from taking anti-coagulants such as aspirin prior to biopsy, and a medical history is obtained to insure that other health criteria are met. These medical criteria may vary depending on the purpose of the study, and viable olfactory neurons have been obtained from individuals ranging in age from 12 to 84, smokers and non-smokers, subjects with various psychological or neurological disorders [1, 9, 10, 15, 17, 19, 31, 34, 35].
2. Alternately, following the epinephrine/tetracaine spray, additional anesthetic may be applied by placing a small sponge plaget such as a Merocel® Otic Wick between the middle turbinate and nasal septum and injecting xylocaine into the wick to deliver anesthetic. This procedure reduces the degree of pressure sensed by the subject during the procedure, but also increases the risk of tissue damage from the sponge plaget and potential adverse effects of the xylocaine on the OE cells (care must be taken by the surgeon to inspect the nasal cavity for any signs of infection or inflammation and for adequate access to

the region to be biopsied). We have observed that samples containing blood tend to be less viable. Nosebleed constitutes the most likely difficulty and has been readily addressed with standard office procedures.

3. In our hands, this process typically takes about 20–30 min, but longer delays of up to 2 h were not found to significantly impact viability.
4. Cell growth rates vary, likely in relation to the proportion of proliferating precursors in the biopsy sample. In some cases, 2 weeks may be sufficient to attain 80% confluence, while other samples grow more slowly and 4–5 weeks were required (*see* Fig. 1a, b). Either culture type could generate odorant-responsive cells and could be propagated further, although comparative studies of the impact of this difference on the proportion of cells expressing olfactory marker protein or responding to odor stimuli have not been examined.
5. The culture protocol described here takes advantage of the mixed cell population and the use of serum to promote growth and differentiation. The full complement of growth factors required for this process remains unknown, but a variety of conditions and factors have been investigated to determine whether a more defined medium may be achieved. Among these are as follows: basic fibroblast growth factor, nerve growth factor, and dopamine [22, 36, 37]. While some features of growth or differentiation are influenced modestly by these factors, a sufficiently comprehensive analysis of the complex OE environment governing proliferation and differentiation has yet to be achieved to construct a defined media that may be considered a true reflection of that environment.
6. The proportion of cells expressing proteins for neuronal markers varies among biopsies and across passages. The proliferation rate generally declines across passages and days post-plating, but the specific rates of proliferation vary greatly across cultures.
7. As activation of odorant receptors triggers the influx of extracellular calcium [18], calcium imaging has been widely used to evaluate odorant responsiveness. Ratiometric imaging has the advantage of minimizing effects due to leaching of dye. Values obtained from such experiments are not absolute intracellular calcium concentrations unless a calibration is performed for each field of cells imaged.
8. The prevalence of odorant responsive cells typically peaks between day 2 and day 4 of culture when cells are plated on coverslips and declines thereafter. In contrast, the prevalence of cells exhibiting voltage-sensitive calcium channels is typically lower initially and increases to day 5–6 post-plating

(unpublished data). It is critical to characterize the cultures using both molecular and functional measures to insure that cells expressing the phenotype of interest are present. Rather than attempting to achieve homogeneity in these parameters, one may exploit the individuality of each culture to provide insight into the donor.

9. In order to determine the required amount of virus for a specific multiplicity of infection, the number of cells present in the culture should be quantified. In order to do this, 1 extra culture should be trypsinized using 0.25% w/v trypsin/EDTA for 2–3 min at 36 °C, and detached cells are gently collected into a centrifuge tube and are quantified.

References

1. Paik S, Lehman M, Seiden AM, Duncan HJ (1992) Olfactory biopsy. Arch Otolaryngol Head Neck Surg 118(7):731–738
2. Trojanowski JQ, Newman PD, Hill WD, Lee VM (1991) Human olfactory epithelium in normal aging, Alzheimer's disease, and other neurodegenerative disorders. J Comp Neurol. https://doi.org/10.1002/cne.903100307
3. Leopold DA, Hummel T, Schwob JE et al (2000) Anterior distribution of human olfactory epithelium. Laryngoscope. https://doi.org/10.1097/00005537-200003000-00016
4. Kream RM, Margolis FL (1984) Olfactory marker protein: turnover and transport in normal and regenerating neurons. J Neurosci 4(3):868–879
5. Monti Graziadei GA, Margolis FL, Harding JW, Gradiadei PPC (1977) Immunocytochemistry of the olfactory marker protein. J Histochem Cytochem. https://doi.org/10.1177/25.12.336785
6. Ling G, Gu J, Genter MB et al (2004) Regulation of cytochrome P450 gene expression in the olfactory mucosa. Chem Biol Interact 147(3):247–258
7. Schlage WK, Bülles H, Friedrichs D et al (1998) Cytokeratin expression patterns in the rat respiratory tract as markers of epithelial differentiation in inhalation toxicology. I. Determination of normal cytokeratin expression patterns in nose, larynx, trachea, and lung. Toxicol Pathol. https://doi.org/10.1177/019262339802600307
8. Feron F, Bianco J, Ferguson I, Mackay-Sim A (2008) Neurotrophin expression in the adult olfactory epithelium. Brain Res. https://doi.org/10.1016/j.brainres.2007.12.003
9. Lane AP, Gomez G, Dankulich T et al (2002) The superior turbinate as a source of functional human olfactory receptor neurons. Laryngoscope. https://doi.org/10.1097/00005537-200207000-00007
10. Lovell MA, Jafek BW, Moran DT, Rowley JC (1982) Biopsy of human olfactory mucosa: an instrument and a technique. Arch Otolaryngol. https://doi.org/10.1001/archotol.1982.00790520047013
11. Lanza DC, Deems DA, Doty RL et al (1994) The effect of human olfactory biopsy on olfaction: a preliminary report. Laryngoscope. https://doi.org/10.1288/00005537-199407000-00010
12. Hahn CG, Gomez G, Restrepo D et al (2005) Aberrant intracellular calcium signaling in olfactory neurons from patients with bipolar disorder. Am J Psychiatry. https://doi.org/10.1176/appi.ajp.162.3.616
13. Matigian N, Abrahamsen G, Sutharsan R et al (2010) Disease-specific, neurosphere-derived cells as models for brain disorders. Dis Model Mech. https://doi.org/10.1242/dmm.005447
14. McCurdy RD, Féron F, Perry C et al (2006) Cell cycle alterations in biopsied olfactory neuroepithelium in schizophrenia and bipolar I disorder using cell culture and gene expression analyses. Schizophr Res. https://doi.org/10.1016/j.schres.2005.10.012
15. Hahn CG, Han LY, Rawson NE et al (2005) In vivo and in vitro neurogenesis in human olfactory epithelium. J Comp Neurol. https://doi.org/10.1002/cne.20424
16. Borgmann-Winter KE, Rawson NE, Wang H-Y et al (2009) Human olfactory epithelial cells generated in vitro express diverse neuronal characteristics. Neuroscience 158. https://doi.org/10.1016/j.neuroscience.2008.09.059

17. Rawson NE, Gomez G, Cowart B et al (1997) Selectivity and response characteristics of human olfactory neurons. J Neurophysiol 77: 1606–1613
18. Gomez G, Rawson NE, Hahn CG et al (2000) Characteristics of odorant elicited calcium changes in cultured human olfactory neurons. J Neurosci Res 62:737–749. https://doi.org/10.1002/1097-4547(20001201)62:5<737::AID-JNR14>3.0.CO;2-A
19. Wolozin B, Sunderland T, Zheng B et al (1992) Continuous culture of neuronal cells from adult human olfactory epithelium. J Mol Neurosci 3:137–146. https://doi.org/10.1007/BF02919405
20. Danciger E, Mettling C, Vidal M et al (1989) Olfactory marker protein gene: its structure and olfactory neuron- specific expression in transgenic mice. Proc Natl Acad Sci U S A. https://doi.org/10.1073/pnas.86.21.8565
21. Yee KK, Pribitkin EA, Cowart BJ et al (2010) Neuropathology of the olfactory mucosa in chronic rhinosinusitis. Am J Rhinol Allergy. https://doi.org/10.2500/ajra.2010.24.3435
22. Ensoli F, Fiorelli V, Vannelli B et al (1998) Basic fibroblast growth factor supports human olfactory neurogenesis by autocrine/paracrine mechanisms. Neuroscience. https://doi.org/10.1016/S0306-4522(98)00104-3
23. van Riel D, Verdijk R, Kuiken T (2014) The olfactory nerve: a shortcut for influenza and other viral diseases into the central nervous system. J Pathol 235:277–287. https://doi.org/10.1002/path.4461
24. Durrant DM, Ghosh S, Klein RS (2016) The olfactory bulb: an immunosensory effector organ during neurotropic viral infections. ACS Chem Neurosci 7(4):464–469
25. Borisevich V, Ozdener MH, Malik B, Rockx B (2017) Hendra and Nipah virus infection in cultured human olfactory epithelial cells. mSphere. https://doi.org/10.1128/mSphere.00252-17
26. Durrant DM, Ghosh S, Klein RS (2016) The olfactory bulb: an immunosensory effector organ during neurotropic viral infections. ACS Chem Neurosci 7:464–469. https://doi.org/10.1021/acschemneuro.6b00043
27. Koyuncu OO, Hogue IB, Enquist LW (2013) Virus infections in the nervous system. Cell Host Microbe 13:379–393. https://doi.org/10.1016/j.chom.2013.03.010
28. Van Riel D, Verdijk R, Kuiken T (2015) The olfactory nerve: a shortcut for influenza and other viral diseases into the central nervous system. J Pathol. https://doi.org/10.1002/path.4461
29. Borisevich V, Ozdener MH, Malik B, Rockx B (2017) Hendra and Nipah virus infection in cultured human olfactory epithelial cells. mSphere 2. https://doi.org/10.1128/mSphere.00252-17
30. Munster VJ, Prescott JB, Bushmaker T et al (2012) Rapid Nipah virus entry into the central nervous system of hamsters via the olfactory route. Sci Rep 2:736. https://doi.org/10.1038/srep00736
31. Féron F, Perry C, McGrath JJ, Mackay-Sim A (1998) New techniques for biopsy and culture of human olfactory epithelial neurons. Arch Otolaryngol Head Neck Surg. https://doi.org/10.1001/archotol.124.8.861
32. Restrepo D, Okada Y, Teeter JH et al (1993) Human olfactory neurons respond to odor stimuli with an increase in cytoplasmic Ca2+. Biophys J. https://doi.org/10.1016/S0006-3495(93)81565-0
33. Rawson NE, Brand JG, Cowart BJ et al (1995) Functionally mature olfactory neurons from two anosmic patients with Kallmann syndrome. Brain Res. https://doi.org/10.1016/0006-8993(95)00283-V
34. Ronnett GV, Leopold D, Cai X et al (2003) Olfactory biopsies demonstrate a defect in neuronal development in Rett's syndrome. Ann Neurol. https://doi.org/10.1002/ana.10633
35. Johnson GS, Basaric-Keys J, Ghanbari HA et al (1994) Protein alterations in olfactory neuroblasts from Alzheimer donors. Neurobiol Aging. https://doi.org/10.1016/0197-4580(94)90048-5
36. Féron F, Vincent A, Mackay-Sim A (1999) Dopamine promotes differentiation of olfactory neuron in vitro. Brain Res. https://doi.org/10.1016/S0006-8993(99)01959-9
37. Vawter MP, Basaric-Keys J, Yunhua L et al (1996) Human olfactory neuroepithelial cells: tyrosine phosphorylation and process extension are increased by the combination of IL-1β, IL-6, NGF, and bFGF. Exp Neurol. https://doi.org/10.1006/exnr.1996.0189

Part III

Studying Infectious Henipaviruses In Vivo

Chapter 10

Mouse Models of Henipavirus Infection

Mathieu Iampietro, Stéphane Barron, Aurélie Duthey, and Branka Horvat

Abstract

The Nipah and Hendra viruses, belonging to *henipavirus* genus, are recently emerged zoonotic pathogens that cause severe and often fatal, neurologic, and/or respiratory diseases in both humans and various animals. As mice represent a small animal model convenient to study viral infections and provide a well-developed experimental toolbox for analysis in immunovirology, we describe in this chapter a few basic methods used in biosafety 4 level (BSL4) conditions to study *henipavirus* infection in mice.

Key words Henipavirus, Emerging infection, Transgenic mice, Murine model, Seroneutralization, BSL4, Clinical scoring, Type I interferon

1 Introduction

Hendra virus (HeV) and Nipah virus (NiV) are two paramyxoviruses recently identified from two emerged zoonotic episodes, belonging to *henipavirus* genus. Unlike other paramyxoviruses, they can cause severe diseases in a wide range of animals and humans [1]. The receptors associated with henipaviruses infections are Ephrin B2 and Ephrin B3 proteins that are highly conserved across vertebrate species including mice [2]; however, mice were described to be resistant to infection through different routes such as intranasal [3], intraperitoneal [3, 4], or subcutaneous [5].

Two novel murine models were identified as susceptible to HeV and NiV infection. Elderly mice (12 months old) from C57BL/6 and BALB/c strains have been shown to be susceptible to HeV-induced disease when inoculated intranasally, presenting neurological symptoms similar to those observed in humans, whereas subcutaneously injected mice and juveniles (8 weeks old) are resistant [6]. Histopathological studies demonstrated severe encephalitis associated with neuronal loss, gliosis, perivascular cuffing, and non-suppurative meningitis. However, no virus was isolated from infected brains, and seroneutralizing antibodies were sometimes detected, but at very low levels. In contrast to

Alexander N. Freiberg and Barry Rockx (eds.), *Nipah Virus: Methods and Protocols*, Methods in Molecular Biology, vol. 2682, https://doi.org/10.1007/978-1-0716-3283-3_10, © Springer Science+Business Media, LLC, part of Springer Nature 2023

HeV infection, NiV-infection of aged mice (with either Malaysia or Bangladesh strain, administrated intranasally) did not lead to the development of encephalitis, but rather to subclinical self-limiting infection of lower respiratory tract [7].

Genetic modifications in mice represent well-characterized and effective tools allowing the study of specific biological mechanisms by the addition of exogenous genes (transgenic or knock-in) or the inactivation/deletion of endogenous genes (knock-out, KO). Transgenic mice thus present important animal models as they can be generated to evaluate individual roles for different genes. Moreover, such animal models have already contributed to very important findings in the fields of virology and immunology. As one of the most important mechanisms of host defense triggered by viruses is the type I interferon (IFN-I) pathway, transgenic C57BL/6 mice knocked-out for IFN-I receptor (IFNAR KO) gene [8] were generated and analyzed for the susceptibility to henipavirus infection [9]. While intracranial, intraperitoneal, and intranasal infection of IFNAR KO mice resulted in high mortality, only intracranial inoculation resulted in fatal outcomes in wild-type (WT) mice demonstrating the crucial role of IFN-I system in the protection against henipaviruses. Indeed, IFNAR KO mice developed similar clinical manifestations to those described in other animal models and humans such as lack of grooming associated with agitation, followed by pain-related symptoms, prostration, and finally disability and paralysis. Following infection through the peritoneal route with 10^6 pfu, all mice died within a period from 6 to 9 days post-infection. Interestingly, IFNAR KO animals infected with a lower dose of NiV or HeV developed high titers of neutralizing antibodies in a period of 3 weeks, highlighting the existence of a strong and powerful antiviral humoral response. This murine model has been subsequently used for real-time monitoring of recombinant NIV and HeV spread in vivo [10]. Globally, IFNAR KO mice helped to demonstrate the involvement of IFN-I system in the control of henipaviruses and highlight the essential role of transgenic animals in the development of countermeasures against HeV or NiV infections.

In murine models described so far, infection using NiV and HeV viruses did not require previous adaptation of the virus to mice, as it has been necessary for some other highly pathogenic viruses, emerged from bats, such as Ebola virus [11]. This avoids the introduction of mutations in viral genome during the adaptation to the new host, but requires utilization of either genetically modified hosts or aged mice, where different defects of the immune system appear during aging. Finally, transgenic mice represent a robust animal model as numerous and various tools already exist, particularly with specific modifications allowing the study of the innate or adaptive immune system, and will help in the development of new antiviral treatments or preventive strategies.

2 Materials

1. *Mice:* Four- to 12-week-old wild-type C57BL/6 mice or type I IFN Receptor Knock-Out (IFNAR1-KO) mice [8] (B6.129S2-*Ifnar1*^{tm1Agt}/Mmjax, catalog no. 032045; The Jackson Laboratory) as well as the other types of either wild-type or transgenic mice could be used within the protocol described in this chapter. Before moving mice into BSL4, animals are individually marked (injection of paste to tattoo under the skin of the palms of animal's legs, according to a defined pattern, although other type of mouse labeling could be applied). Mice are then placed in cages, separating males from females. Food and water are provided ad libitum, and cages are cleaned at least once a week, depending on the number of mice.
2. *Nipah and Hendra Viruses:* NiV strain Malaysia (isolate UMMC1, GenBank AY029767) [12] and HeV [13] obtained from Porton Down laboratory, UK, were prepared and isolated from infection of Vero E6 cells, in the INSERM P4 Jean Mérieux laboratory. Virus stocks were prepared in the BSL4 laboratory by infecting Vero E6 cells with a multiplicity of infection (MOI) of 0.01 plaque-forming units (pfu) and cell and virus are recovered 24 h post-infection, as described previously [14].
3. *Biosafety Level 4 (BSL4) Animal Room:* All experiments are performed in BSL4 animal room equipped and maintained according to the national and international guidelines [15].
4. *Experimental Protocol:* Animal procedure is performed as described in Fig. 1. All animals need to be handled in strict accordance with good animal practice, and protocol needs to be approved by regional and national ethical committees.
5. *Clinical Scoring System:* Animals are monitored daily, and different parameters are followed: weight, activity in the cage, animal behavior, and presence of pain and neurological signs. The different number of points is attributed to each parameter, and clinical scores of infected animals are evaluated as presented in Table 1.

   Temperature could be measured in mice using temperature transponders (e.g., model IPTT 300, PLEXX). Transponder needs to be injected subcutaneously into mice, before moving them into BSL4. It allows direct reading of temperature and error-free animal identification via adequate interface, leading to direct data transfer to computer.

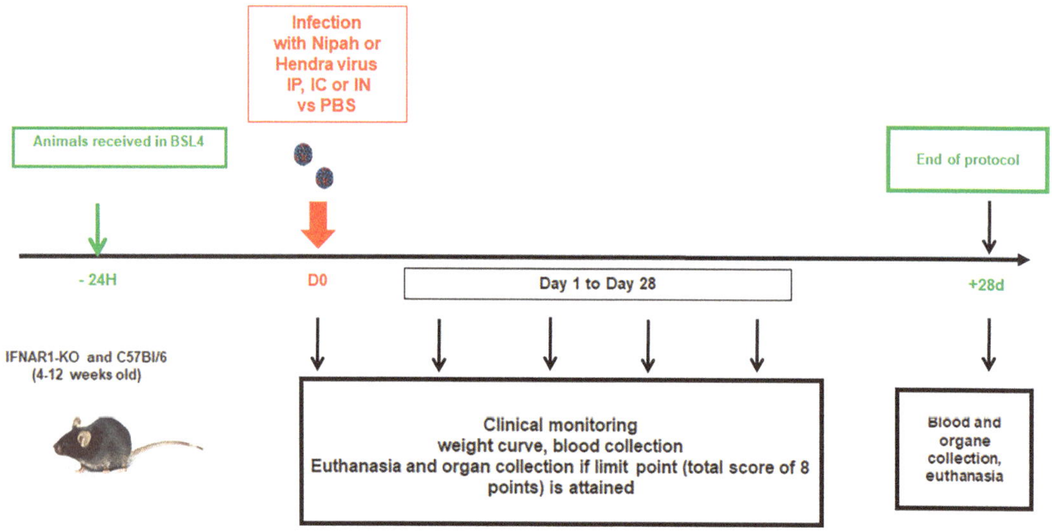

Fig. 1 Schematic presentation of animal experimental protocol to study henipavirus infection in mice. Mice are moved into BSL4 animal room 24 h before infection. After infection, different parameters are followed as described in the text

3 Methods

3.1 Manipulation of Mice in BSL4

Groups of maximum 6 mice per cage, 4–12 weeks old (age homogenous within an experimental group), are received into BSL4 animal room and hosted at least 24 h prior to infection. All manipulation is performed according to the strict rule of security within BSL4 containment, requiring the utilization of 3 pairs of protective gloves and manipulation of infected animals with forceps (Fig. 2). (**Note 1**)

3.2 Anesthesia

Prior to infection and any further manipulation, mice are anesthetized using inhaled anesthetic isoflurane (Fig. 3). (**Note 2**)

1. Place the animal in the induction chamber.
2. Adjust the oxygen flowmeter to approximately 0.5–1.0 L/min.
3. Adjust the isoflurane vaporizer to approximately 3–5% for induction and approximately 1–3% for maintenance.
4. During recovery from anesthesia, the following clinical parameters must be monitored at a minimum of 5 min intervals until the animal is ambulatory: respiratory rate, movement, and the ability to maintain sternal recumbency.
5. To protect the animal from hypothermia, they should be placed in a heating blanket, to conserve body temperature. Anesthetized animal should never be placed on metal surfaces.
6. It is estimated that animals will recover from isoflurane anesthesia within 5 min.

Table 1
Scoring system used for evaluating henipavirus infection in mice, showing a number of points attributed to different criteria linked to the observed clinical signs

Group/ ID of mouse	Weight loss (ΔW, %)	Aspect related to weight loss	State of animal hair	Behavior	Activity	Total score
	0 pt.[a]: $\Delta W \leq 10\%$ 1 pt.: $10\% < \Delta W \leq 15\%$ 2 pts.: $15\% < \Delta W \leq 20\%$ 5 pts.: $\Delta W > 20\%$	0 pt.: NTR[b] 1 pt.: emaciation 2 pts.: severe emaciation/ wasting	0 pt.: NTR 1 pt.: disheveled 2 pts.: very disheveled	0 pt.: NTR 1 pt.: hyperreactivity to external stimuli	0 pt.: NTR 1 pt.: slight loss of tone 2 pts.: significant loss of tone/ prostrate	(If the total score is equal to or higher than 8 pts., the animal has reached the limit point and has to be euthanized)
	Facies pain	**Demarche pain**	**Paralysis**	**Moribund**		
	0 pt.: NTR 1 pt.: pointed snout 2 pts.: pointed snout + eyes closed set	0 pt.: NTR 1 pt.: slightly spine arched/slightly demarche of pain 2 pts.: severely arched spine/severely demarche of pain	0 pt.: NTR 8 pts.: paralysis of one or more members	0 pt.: NTR 8 pts.: animal lying without reaction, about to die		

[a] *pt.* point
[b] *NTR* nothing to report

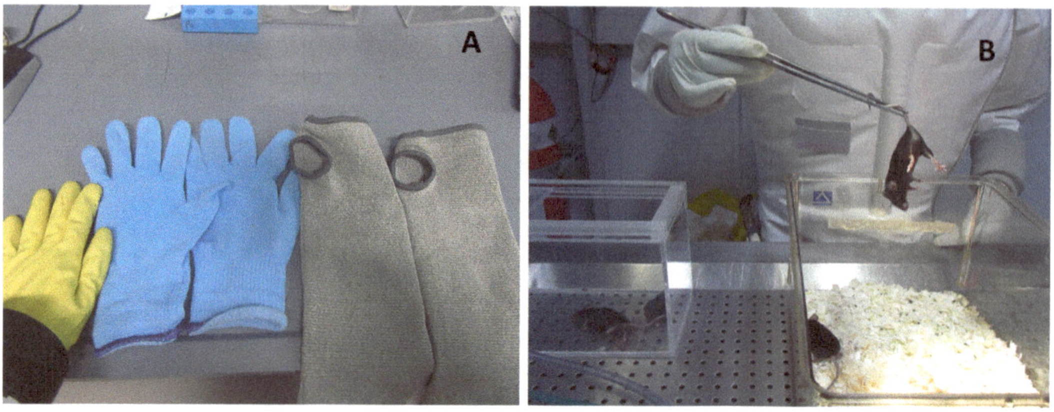

Fig. 2 Equipment used to manipulate mice in the BSL4 containment. (**a**) Three pairs of different types of gloves are regularly used for the protection of experimenter in all animal manipulations. (**b**) Mice are manipulated using a forceps and direct contact with experimenter's hands is never applied with awake animals

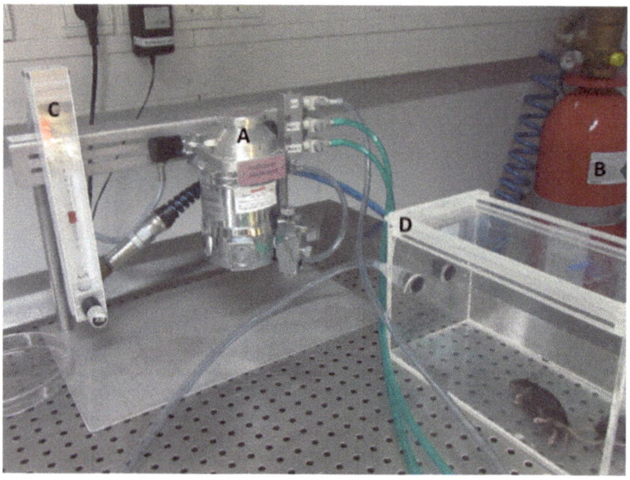

Fig. 3 Volatile anesthetic equipment used for the isoflurane anesthesia of mice in BSL4 animal room. (*A*) Anesthetic vaporizer; (*B*) oxygen tank and air room compressor; (*C*) oxygen flow meter; (*D*) induction chamber for mice. Oxygen arrives through the blue hookah that is seen behind; isoflurane tank is at the level of the violet label. Gas mixture is transmitted to the induction chamber by the transparent pipe. The green tubes conduct the anesthetic to mouse-adapted masks, that are used for the anesthesia during intracardiac blood sampling

3.3 Infection

1. Mice anesthetized with isoflurane as described above are infected using different routes and not exceeding the max volume as described previously [16], either intraperitoneally with 0.4 mL of virus, intranasally with 30 μL of virus, or intracerebrally with 50 μL of virus.
2. Equivalent volumes of phosphate-buffered saline (PBS) 1× are used as a control for each route of inoculation.

3. Animals are monitored daily and their clinical scores are established by evaluating temperature, weight curves, and clinical signs (described in Table 1). Animals are euthanized when clinical score equal or higher than 8 is attained.

3.4 Blood Collection and Serum Preparation

Blood collection is performed by retro-orbital bleeding of anesthetized mice during the experimental protocol or by cardiac puncture at the end of the protocol, before the necropsy. (**Note 3**)

Retro-Orbital Bleeding

1. Standard heparinized or non-heparinized micro-hematocrit capillary tubes can be used for blood collection.
2. A drop of tetracaine is applied to the eye 5 min before bleeding to prevent pain caused by this action.
3. The animal is positioned in profile on the table, and the loose skin of the head is tightened between the thumb and middle finger.
4. The tip of the capillary tube is placed at the medial canthus of the eye under the nictitating membrane.
5. A short thrust past the eyeball will enter the slightly resistant membrane of the sinus. The eyeball itself remains uninjured.
6. As soon as the sinus is punctured, blood enters the tubing by capillary action. It may be helpful to retract the tube to facilitate blood flow.
7. When the allowable amount of blood is collected, the tube is withdrawn and slight pressure with a piece of gauze on the eyeball is used to prevent further bleeding.

Blood Collection Parameters

1. The maximum amount of blood that may be withdrawn at one time from this location is 1% of the animal's body weight (e.g., 0.2 mL from a 20 g adult mouse).
2. Blood can only be collected once per week from one eye. Subsequent bleeds should use alternate eyes.
3. The maximum number of bleeds allowed for each animal is two bleeds per eye.

Cardiac Puncture

1. This approach is used to collect blood at the end of the protocol from surviving euthanized mouse or a mouse under deep terminal anesthesia.
2. Blood is collected by introducing a needle and pushing forward in the sagittal plan at the posterior extremity of the sternum. The length of the needle allows reaching and crossing the myocardium. 0.1–1 mL of blood can be obtained depending on the size of the mouse and whether the heart is beating.

Blood samples are taken from the heart, preferably the ventricle, which can be accessed either via the left side of the chest, through the diaphragm, from the top of the sternum or by performing a thoracotomy. Blood should be withdrawn slowly to prevent the heart collapsing.

3. Pull gently the syringe plunger to puncture blood (from 0.5 to 1 mL).
4. Remove the needle from the syringe before ejecting punctured blood into hemolysis tube. NB: For serum collection, the puncture is done by "dry needling." For whole blood collection, the puncture is carried out with anticoagulant (heparin, sodium citrate, etc.).

Serum Preparation

1. Harvest collected blood in a glass tube.
2. Agitate tubes and put them at 37 ° C for 30 min to allow coagulation.
3. Put the tubes at 4 °C.
4. Centrifuge the tubes at 3000 rpm for 5 min at 4 °C.
5. Harvest supernatant into 1.5-ml Eppendorf tube.
6. Centrifuge the tube at 10,000 g for 10 min at 4 °C in order to remove non-soluble material.
7. Keep serum at −80 °C until use.

3.5 Virus Titration from Murine Tissues

To determine the presence and titer of infectious virus in different organs and characterize virus adaptation to the murine tissue, virus isolation and titration could be performed.

1. A small fragment (30 mg) of different tissues is mechanically crashed twice for 30 s each in tubes containing sterile glass beads and 0.5 mL of DMEM.
2. Centrifuge the samples at 3000 rpm for 5 min at 4 °C.
3. Supernatants are harvested and are ready for titration.
4. Subconfluent Vero E6 cells, plated in 6-well plates, are used for the titration in subsequent steps.
5. Cells are incubated for 1 h at 37 °C in a 5% CO_2 incubator with 1 mL of serial dilutions of virus stocks using 1:10 as the starting dilution.
6. Cells are washed twice with DMEM without FCS.
7. Cells are covered with 2 mL of 1.6% carboxymethylcellulose in DMEM containing 5% FCS and incubated for 5 days at 37 °C.
8. Then, cells are stained with 0.2% crystal violet, as described below.
9. After rinsing the excess of dye with water, whitish plaques corresponding to the development of virus-induced cytopathic effect are counted and the titer is expressed as pfu/mL.

3.6 Seroneutralization

Determination of the presence of seroneutralizing antibodies in the serum of infected animals is a commonly used procedure, performed to determine the development of the adaptive humoral immune response in mice.

1. Serum samples prepared as described above are diluted in Dulbecco's modified Eagle's medium supplemented with 2% FCS (DMEM), by performing twofold dilutions.
2. Diluted serum samples are then incubated with HeV or NiV (10–30 pfu/well in 96-well microtiter plates) for 60 min at 37 °C in 96-well microtiter plates in the final volume of 100 μL.
3. A total of 2.5×10^4 Vero cells in 100 μL medium are added to each well as indicator cells and plates are incubated for 5 days at 37 °C.
4. After 5 days of culture, supernatants are aspirated and 100 μL of 0.2% crystal violet (containing 10% formaldehyde and 10% ethanol) is added to each well. Crystal violet dye stains attached cells in culture through the binding to cellular DNA and proteins. Cells that undergo cell death following virus infection lose their adherence and are subsequently lost from the cell population, reducing the amount of crystal violet staining in a culture (Fig. 4).

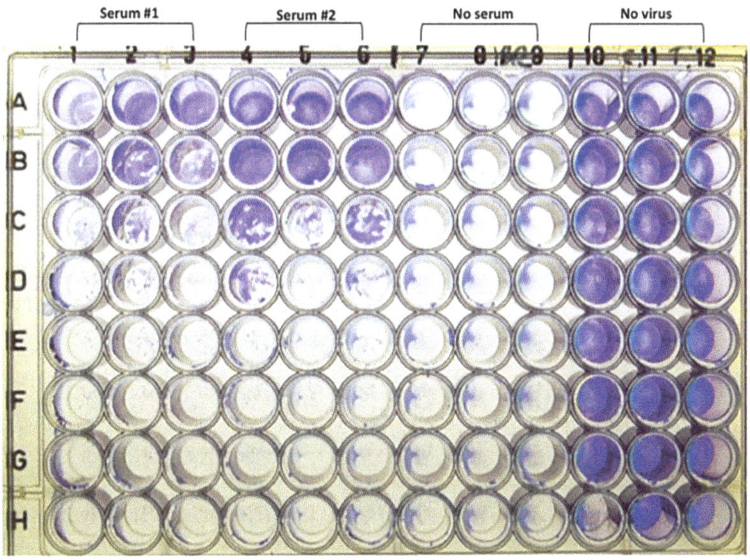

Fig. 4 Example of seroneutralization assay performed in 96-well microtiter plate format. Following Crystal violet staining, we note the absence of cytopathic effects in cells cultured in columns 10–12, corresponding to negative control (absence of virus), while the positive control in columns 7–9 (cells infected with NiV in the absence of seroneutralizing antibodies) displayed full cytopathic effects. Samples tested in columns 1–3 were diluted by one log compared to samples from columns 4–6 and both series exhibited moderate cytopathic effects

5. Neutralizing titers are expressed as the reciprocal dilution of the last serum dilution which completely inhibits virus-induced cytopathic effects.

3.7 Euthanasia and Collection of Organs for RNA Isolation and Immunocytochemistry

1. Mice which attained the score of 8 points or mice at the end of the protocol are euthanized by cervical dislocation, after anesthesia by isoflurane according to paragraph 3.2.
2. Different organs (lungs, brain, kidneys, spleen, liver, lymph nodes, heart, and bladder) are taken during necropsy, put into petri dishes, inspected macroscopically for the presence of bleeding, visible inflammation, or any anomalies, and photographed to preserve observations.
3. For the RNA isolation, 10–30 mg of organs are collected into cryotubes and frozen at −80 °C. RNA isolation can be processed in any later time point, using Trizol or Qiagen kit according to manufacturer's instructions.
4. For immunohistochemistry, organs are cut into small pieces (around 0.5 cm) to achieve the max efficiency of virus inactivation and fixed in 10% neutral buffer formalin (corresponding to the 4% buffered formaldehyde, diluted in PBS). Alternatively, 4% paraformaldehyde diluted in PBS could be used. In both cases, the fixation is performed during 2 weeks, with one change of the bath after the first week.

4 Notes

1. Manipulation in BSL4 containment is associated with many restrictions linked to very particular work conditions, necessity to wear particular suites, several pairs of gloves, etc. Utilization of the BSL4 animal room is usually planned many months in advance, requiring the organization of experiments in all details well in advance.
2. Utilization of anesthesia is the point which needs to be monitored with particular precautions. Isoflurane is a vasodilator, and its use can result in fatal hypotension. Administer isoflurane with caution in animals that may be dehydrated or otherwise at risk for hypotension. Maintaining animals with isoflurane concentrations in excess of the recommended levels may result in death of both healthy and compromised animals.
3. Retro-orbital blood sampling under BSL4 conditions is a delicate gesture, which requires special attention. The lack of sensation of the manipulator due to the utilization of 3 pairs of gloves increases the risk of asphyxiation of the animal. Finally, the risk of animal bite remains present during the induction of anesthesia and weighing or changing animals, so constant precautions need to be taken during handling of mice in BSL4.

Acknowledgement

The authors acknowledge the contribution of all the members of INSERM Laboratory P4 Jean Mérieux, particularly Audrey Vallve, and Immunobiology of viral infection team at CIRI for the realization of the manuscript. The work was supported by INSERM, LABEX ECOFECT (ANR-11-LABX-0048) of Lyon University, within the program "Investissements d'Avenir" (ANR-11-IDEX-0007) and Aviesan Nipah virus study project.

References

1. Eaton BT, Broder CC, Middleton D, Wang L-F (2006) Hendra and Nipah viruses: different and dangerous. Nat Rev Microbiol 4:23–35. https://doi.org/10.1038/nrmicro1323
2. Bossart K (2008) Functional studies of host-specific ephrin-B ligands as Henipavirus receptors. Virology 372:357–371. https://doi.org/10.1016/j.virol.2007.11.011
3. Wong KT, Grosjean I, Brisson C, Blanquier B, Fevre-Montange M, Bernard A et al (2003) A golden hamster model for human acute Nipah virus infection. Am J Pathol 163:2127–2137
4. Westbury HA, Hooper PT, Selleck PW, Murray PK (1995) Equine morbillivirus pneumonia: susceptibility of laboratory animals to the virus. Aust Vet J 72:278–279
5. Bossart KN, Bingham J, Middleton D (2007) Targeted strategies for Henipavirus therapeutics. Open Virol J 1:14–25. https://doi.org/10.2174/1874357900701010014
6. Dups J, Middleton D, Yamada M, Monaghan P, Long F, Robinson R et al (2012) A new model for Hendra virus encephalitis in the mouse. PLoS One 7:e40308. https://doi.org/10.1371/journal.pone.0040308
7. Dups J, Middleton D, Long F, Arkinstall R, Marsh GA, Wang L-F (2014) Subclinical infection without encephalitis in mice following intranasal exposure to Nipah virus-Malaysia and Nipah virus-Bangladesh. Virol J 11:11. https://doi.org/10.1186/1743-422X-11-102
8. Müller U, Steinhoff U, Reis LF, Hemmi S, Pavlovic J, Zinkernagel RM et al (1994) Functional role of type I and type II interferons in antiviral defense. Science 264:1918–1921
9. Dhondt KP, Mathieu C, Chalons M, Reynaud JM, Vallve A, Raoul H et al (2012) Type I interferon signaling protects mice from lethal Henipavirus infection. J Infect Dis. https://doi.org/10.1093/infdis/jis653
10. Yun T, Park A, Hill TE, Pernet O, Beaty SM, Juelich TL et al (2015) Efficient reverse genetics reveals genetic determinants of budding and fusogenic differences between Nipah and Hendra viruses and enables real-time monitoring of viral spread in small animal models of henipavirus infection. J Virol 89:1242–1253. https://doi.org/10.1128/JVI.02583-14
11. Bray M, Davis K, Geisbert T, Schmaljohn C, Huggins J (1998) A mouse model for evaluation of prophylaxis and therapy of Ebola hemorrhagic fever. J Infect Dis 178:651–661
12. Chan YP, Chua KB, Koh CL, Lim ME, Lam SK (2001) Complete nucleotide sequences of Nipah virus isolates from Malaysia. J Gen Virol 82:2151–2155
13. Guillaume V, Wong KT, Looi RY, Georges-Courbot M-C, Barrot L, Buckland R et al (2009) Acute Hendra virus infection: analysis of the pathogenesis and passive antibody protection in the hamster model. Virology 387: 459–465. https://doi.org/10.1016/j.virol.2009.03.001
14. Guillaume-Vasselin V, Lemaitre L, Dhondt KP, Tedeschi L, Poulard A, Charreyre C et al (2016) Protection from Hendra virus infection with canarypox recombinant vaccine. Npj Vaccines 1:16003
15. Frasier D, Talka J (2005) Facility design considerations for select agent animal research. ILAR J 46:23–33
16. Turner PV, Brabb T, Pekow C, Vasbinder MA (2011) Administration of substances to laboratory animals: routes of administration and factors to consider. J Am Assoc Lab Anim Sci 50: 600–613

Chapter 11

In Vivo Imaging of Nipah Virus Infection in Small Animal Rodent Models

Kendra Johnson, Terry Juelich, Jennifer Smith, Benhur Lee, and Alexander N. Freiberg

Abstract

In vivo imaging system (IVIS) is a powerful tool for the study of infectious diseases, providing the ability to non-invasively follow viral infection in an individual animal over time. Recombinant henipaviruses expressing bioluminescent or fluorescent reporter proteins can be used both to monitor the spatial and temporal progression of Nipah virus (NiV) infection in vivo as well as in ex vivo tissues. Virally produced luciferases react with systemically administered substrate to produce bioluminescence that can then be detected via IVIS imaging, while fluorescent reporters inherently generate detectable fluorescence without a substrate. Here we describe protocols applying bioluminescent or fluorescent reporter expressing recombinant viruses to in vivo or ex vivo imaging of NiV infection.

Key words In vivo imaging, Recombinant Nipah virus, Reporter genes, Luminescence, Fluorescence, Rodent animal model

1 Introduction

In vivo imaging system (IVIS) technology is a powerful tool and qualitative non-invasive approach that allows for real-time monitoring of disease progression in the same living animal over time [1, 2]. Insertion of a luminescent or fluorescent reporter gene into a viral genome leads to expression of these reporters at sites of viral replication and allows to determine viral load, tissue tropism, and gene expression patterns in certain tissues after infection with a recombinant virus. Both types of reporter proteins are detectable using IVIS technology; bioluminescence is produced by luciferase enzymes reacting with their substrate (such as D-luciferin) and fluorescent reporters emit light after excitation with specific wavelengths.

Nipah virus (NiV) is a highly pathogenic zoonotic bat-borne paramyxovirus (genus henipavirus) that causes severe encephalitis and respiratory disease with high-fatality rates in humans

Alexander N. Freiberg and Barry Rockx (eds.), *Nipah Virus: Methods and Protocols*, Methods in Molecular Biology, vol. 2682, https://doi.org/10.1007/978-1-0716-3283-3_11,

[3, 4]. Most of our understanding on spread of NiV in tissues and virus-induced pathogenesis has mainly resulted from natural history of disease studies of experimentally infected animals or to a minor extend from end-stage histopathology findings from fatal human cases [5]. Small animal models, such as immune-compromised mouse and hamster models, have shown to develop aspects of the clinical disease observed in patients, with both models developing encephalitis and severe respiratory disease. Histologically they show systemic vasculitis, perivascular cuffing, meningeal inflammation, and bronchointerstitial pneumonia [6].

The availability of reverse genetics systems for henipaviruses allows for the generation of recombinant viruses encoding reporter genes suitable for IVIS imaging to monitor the spatial and temporal progression of NiV infection in vivo as well as in ex vivo tissues [7–13]. Using a T7 polymerase-driven reverse genetics system for NiV Malaysia strain (NiV-M), reporter viruses have been generated expressing luminescent or fluorescent proteins [8, 14]. The procedures used to image NiV infection in mouse and hamster models are outlined.

2 Materials

NiV is a biosafety level 4 (BSL-4) agent and should be handled in accordance with the guidelines stipulated in the "Biosafety in Microbiological and Biomedical Laboratories" (BMBL) (https://www.cdc.gov/labs/BMBL.html).

Work with NiV in hamsters requires animal biosafety level 4 (ABSL-4) space approved by the U.S. Centers for Disease Control and Prevention (CDC) or equivalent and approval from the Institution or University, or equivalent, to work with NiV in hamsters at ABSL-4. Furthermore, approval from the Institutional Animal Care and Use Committee (IACUC) to work with hamsters at ABSL-4 is required.

2.1 IVIS Equipment

1. IVIS Spectrum platform with charge-coupled device camera system (Perkin Elmer) (*see* **Note 1**).
2. Plexiglas anesthesia system.
3. Animal isolation chamber (Perkins Elmer XIC-3) and anesthesia manifold (Perkins Elmer RAS-4) for use during imaging (*see* **Notes 2** and **3**).
4. Living Image software.
5. Class II Biosafety Cabinet (BSC).

2.2 Materials and Supplies

1. Balance and container to weigh animals.
2. Appropriate anesthetic (for example, isoflurane).
3. Small-animal electric hair clipper.
4. Recombinant virus stock expressing fluorescent or luminescent reporter.
5. Substrate for bioluminescent imaging (for example, D-luciferin, Caliper Life Sciences).
6. Sterile Dulbecco's phosphate-buffered saline (DPBS).
7. 26 gauge 1 mL syringe for IP injection (BD syringe).
8. Appropriate disinfectant (5% quaternary ammonium, 70% ethanol, etc.).
9. Plasticware for ex vivo imaging (for example, 6 well plates, black bottom plates/dishes).

3 Methods

3.1 In Vivo Bioluminescence Imaging

1. Three to four days before inoculation, shave animal (for example, mouse or hamster) to maximize detection of bioluminescent signal. Animals should be placed on an alfalfa-free diet 14 days prior to study start to reduce background during fluorescence imaging. Bioluminescence is not affected by diet (*see* **Note 4**).
2. On day of infection, thaw NiV stock at room temperature and prepare the challenge concentration by diluting a pre-calculated NiV stock volume into Dulbecco's Modified Eagle Medium with 2% Fetal Bovine Serum inside BSC (*see* **Note 5**).
3. Anesthetize animal and verify sedation level (either inside BSC or on downdraft table—depending on laboratory set up) according to approved animal study protocol.
4. Inoculate animal with recombinant NiV encoding reporter genes.
   (a) According to the experimental design, different viral doses and routes of administration can be used (e.g., intraperitoneal (IP), intranasal, and aerosol exposure). Detailed information about inoculation protocols can be found elsewhere.
5. Substrate Administration.
   (a) Weigh animals (*see* **Note 6**).
   (b) Thaw aliquot of D-luciferin solution at room temperature (*see* **Note 7**).

(c) Calculate volume of D-luciferin (30 mg/mL) to be administered to each animal for a final concentration of 150 mg/kg body weight.

(d) Fully anesthetize animals with isoflurane and inject IP with individually calculated volume of D-luciferin substrate. Volume varies per animal to allow for administration of 150 mg/kg of substrate per animal (*see* **Note 8**).

(e) Allow animals to wake up and allow for the D-luciferin substrate to disperse throughout the body (optimally 10 min). Waiting too long will allow the D-luciferin to become completely dispersed and will no longer be visible during imaging.

(f) Fully anesthetize animals with isoflurane, and place and arrange animals in imaging box. If multiple animals are being imaged at the same time, plastic dividers must be used in the chamber to prevent signal interference between animals.

6. Imaging.

(a) Use LivingImage software to initialize IVIS platform for luminescence imaging (*see* **Note 9**).

(b) Ensure acquisition settings are as desired (e.g., auto acquisition time setting with fixed f/stop at F1 and medium binning).

(c) Place imaging box in IVIS imaging chamber and connect hoses to anesthesia hoses in chamber. Center box in chamber (*see* **Notes 2**, **3**, and **10**).

(d) Click acquire image-software will first obtain a greyscale photographic image and then use a longer exposure to obtain the luminescent image (*see* **Note 11**).

(e) The overlaid images will be displayed after capture—luciferase activity is displayed as radiance using a rainbow log scale where red represents the highest and blue the lowest photon flux.

(f) Enter experimental details, such as the day post-infection, animal Identification Number, etc., and save the data.

(g) Depending on the study design, images can be obtained from both dorsal and ventral sides of each animal, ensuring that the order of orientations imaged remains the same between sequential animals (*see* **Note 12**).

(h) After imaging, return animals to their cages and monitor until they have recovered from anesthesia.

(i) Disinfect all equipment with appropriate disinfectant after completion of imaging (*see* **Note 13**).

3.2 In Vivo Fluorescence Imaging

While it is possible to perform fluorescence in vivo imaging, no data have been published for NiV infection using a fluorescent reporter. High levels of tissue autofluorescene and background can complicate whole animal in vivo imaging. The procedure follows the same basic steps as bioluminescent imaging, excluding administration of a luciferin substrate, and would require adjustment of IVIS settings accordingly.

3.3 Ex Vivo Bioluminescent Imaging

Luminescence: Follow **steps 1–4** as described in Subheading 3.1. Depending on the study design, individual (non-fixed) tissues can be utilized for ex vivo IVIS imaging immediately after necropsy (*see* **Note 14**).

1. Once necropsy has been completed, rinse tissue of interest in cold PBS.
2. Place tissue(s) in 6 well tissue culture plates and cover in 0.5 mM D-luciferin substrate for 10 min at room temperature.
3. Rinse tissues with cold PBS and transfer to a new plate for imaging (*see* **Note 14**).
4. Place plate in the center of the IVIS imaging chamber and image. The process of image acquisition is the same as for in vivo bioluminescence, aside from using plates rather than the animal isolation imaging box.
5. After imaging of an entire tissue has been completed, tissues can be processed for further analysis according to study protocol.
6. Once imaging is complete, properly disinfect all equipment with appropriate disinfectant.

Fluorescence: Because fluorescence is an inherent property of the expressed reporter gene and independent of a substrate, the step of D-luciferin administration before imaging is not required and tissues can be imaged directly after necropsy (*see* **Note 15**).

1. Initialize the IVIS platform for fluorescence imaging and adjust settings according to the reporter used (e.g., emission filter is set to 570 nm and the excitation filter 620 nm for red fluorescent reporter proteins).
2. Rinse tissues in PBS and place in a 6-well plate for imaging (*see* **Note 14**).
3. Place plate in the center of the IVIS imaging chamber and image. Images will be displayed as a brightfield image overlaid with fluorescence as represented by radiant efficiency on a color scale of dark red (low) to yellow (high).

4. After desired imaging is complete, tissues can be processed for further analysis according to study protocol.
5. Properly disinfect all equipment with appropriate disinfectant.

3.4 Analysis of Data

The LivingImage software contains a variety of tools that can be used to analyze the raw data. Detailed description of all the functions can be found in the LivingImage software manual [15]. Standard steps to process data are as follows:

1. Image clean up and optimization: Especially with fluorescent IVIS, background from either tissue or culture plate autofluorescence can affect data analysis.
2. ROI quantification: LivingImage software can be used to quantify the light signal in user-defined specific regions of interest (ROI).
   (a) For bioluminescent imaging, make sure the units are set to photon flux (photons/s/cm^2/steradian). For fluorescent imaging, make sure units are set to radiant efficiency.
   (b) Designate ROI for quantification and adjust size within the organ of interest to the size of the area exhibiting bioluminescent signal.
   (c) Apply the ROI to other images in the series—location can be adjusted but keep the area inside the ROI the same.
   (d) Values from a sequence of images will be displayed in a table that can be saved in a .csv format that can be exported into Excel for further analysis.
   (e) Normalize the data by subtracting the value of the non-infected time point.

4 Notes

1. Verify that the IVIS platform is working properly at least 1 week before initiating an experiment. This will provide time to address potential problems.
2. Due to the BSL4 containment requirements, anesthetized animals must be enclosed in an isolation box during imaging. The box we use allows for imaging of up to three mice or young hamsters at a time. It comes as one large chamber but also includes a sheet of black plastic that can be cut to form dividers. We added two black plastic dividers (creating three equally sized sections) using black electrical tape to reduce the background signal between animals while imaging.
3. Depending on the laboratory set-up and location of the IVIS platform, slightly different requirements for anesthesia may be

required. If the IVIS platform is located in a separate room than the animal housing and/or procedure room and anesthetized animals must be transported between rooms for imaging, ensuring that the hoses on the box are attached to each other, resulting in a closed air circulation.

4. Animals should be shaved no more than 7 days before imaging, as hair will begin to grow back. Shaving 3–4 days before inoculation allows the procedure to be done at lower containment before animals are transferred to BSL4 for infection. This also allows the animals to recover from the shaving process. Diamond dry cellulose bedding should be used if possible, to maintain animal comfort.
5. All dilutions of viral stocks are performed under sterile conditions in a high-containment BSL4 environment within a Class II BSC.
6. Because the D-luciferin substrate dose is based on a weight ratio, it is necessary to obtain an animal weight before each imaging session.
7. D-luciferin is stored as a powder at −20 °C. Aliquots of D-lucifierin reconstituted in DPBS (30 mg/mL stock) can be stored at −80 °C, although efficacy should be verified before beginning an experiment if stored for a long time without being used. Aliquots should be thawed and warmed to room temperature immediately before use.
8. Anesthesia is required at this step due to working at BSL4.
9. IVIS platform should be left turned on in standby mode at all times. Initialization is done through the attached computer to prepare the platform for imaging and should be done prior to beginning manipulation if animals, as it can take time.
10. If more than one animal will be imaged at a time, it may be necessary to reduce background signals. For example, if one animal has very strong bioluminesence, it may be necessary to cover that animal with a piece of black paper to detect a weaker signal in other animals.
11. A typical exposure for a 2D image is 1 min. Some IVIS models also have the ability to take a series of images at different wavelengths to reconstruct a 3D model that can be used to identify individual organs using a mouse template. For generating a 3D reconstruction, a 5-min exposure is required. However, if the longer exposure is desired, only one side of the animal (ventral/dorsal) can be imaged. Due to potential side effects from extended anesthesia, especially during advanced stages of disease, total time in the IVIS should be limited to no more than 5–6 min.

12. Flipping of animals within the box must be done inside BSC or on downdraft table, which requires to factor in the time for transport to and from the BSC or downdraft table in between imaging sessions. Try to safely move as quickly as possible to minimize the time the animals are under anesthesia.
13. Cleaning the imaging box with approved disinfectants at BSL4 (such as 5% quaternary ammonium) can interfere with imaging capabilities and result in high-background signals. The glass top box should be cleaned only with a special glasses cleaner, using kimwipes or a soft cloth. The interior can be carefully wiped down (not the glass) with a cloth wetted with 70% ethanol.
14. After necropsy, the signal remains relatively stable. Unlike in vivo imaging, where time under anesthesia must be considered, ex vivo imaging does not have to be done as quickly.
15. Autofluorescence from plastic plates can be particularly problematic. Ideally, use black bottom plates to reduce background. It may also be necessary to tape the edges of the plate with black electrical tape if the background is too high.

Acknowledgments

This work was supported by National Institutes of Health (grant numbers R33 AI102267 to A.N.F. and B.L., RO1 AI123449 to B.L., and R21 AI138233 to A.N.F.) and by the University of Texas Medical Branch Department of Pathology start-up funds (to A.N.F.).

References

1. Andreu N, Zelmer A, Wiles S (2011) Noninvasive biophotonic imaging for studies of infectious disease. FEMS Microbiol Rev 35(2): 360–394
2. Hutchens M, Luker GD (2007) Applications of bioluminescence imaging to the study of infectious diseases. Cell Microbiol 9(10): 2315–2322
3. Hayman DTS, Johnson N (2014) Nipah virus: a virus with multiple pathways of emergence. In: The role of animals in emerging viral diseases. Elsevier, Amsterdam
4. Kenmoe S, Demanou M, Bigna JJ et al (2019) Case fatality rate and risk factors for Nipah virus encephalitis: a systematic review and meta-analysis. J Clin Virol 117:19–26
5. Escaffre O, Borisevich V, Rockx B (2013) Pathogenesis of Hendra and Nipah virus infection in humans. J Infect Dev Ctries 7(4): 308–311
6. de Wit E, Munster VJ (2015) Animal models of disease shed light on Nipah virus pathogenesis and transmission. J Pathol 235(2):196–205
7. Griffin BD, Leung A, Chan M et al (2019) Establishment of an RNA polymerase II-driven reverse genetics system for Nipah virus strains from Malaysia and Bangladesh. Sci Rep 9(1):11171
8. Yun T, Park A, Hill TE et al (2015) Efficient reverse genetics reveals genetic determinants of budding and fusogenic differences between Nipah and Hendra viruses and enables real-time monitoring of viral spread in small animal models of henipavirus infection. J Virol 89(2): 1242–1253
9. Yoneda M, Guillaume V, Ikeda F et al (2006) Establishment of a Nipah virus rescue system.

Proc Natl Acad Sci U S A 103(44): 16508–16513
10. Beaty SM, Park A, Won ST et al (2017) Efficient and robust paramyxoviridae reverse genetics systems. mSphere 2(2):e00376-16
11. Marsh GA, Virtue ER, Smith I et al (2013) Recombinant Hendra viruses expressing a reporter gene retain pathogenicity in ferrets. Virol J 10:95
12. Laing ED, Amaya M, Navaratnarajah CK et al (2018) Rescue and characterization of recombinant cedar virus, a non-pathogenic Henipavirus species. Virol J 15(1):56
13. Lo MK, Nichol ST, Spiropoulou CF (2014) Evaluation of luciferase and GFP-expressing Nipah viruses for rapid quantitative antiviral screening. Antivir Res 106:53–60
14. Escaffre O, Hill T, Ikegami T et al (2018) Experimental infection of Syrian hamsters with aerosolized Nipah virus. J Infect Dis 218(10):1602–1610
15. Living Image softtware user's manual (2012). Caliper Life Sciences, Inc.

Chapter 12

Nonhuman Primate Models for Nipah and Hendra Virus Countermeasure Evaluation

Chad E. Mire, Benjamin A. Satterfield, and Thomas W. Geisbert

Abstract

Hendra and Nipah viruses are henipaviruses that have caused lethal human disease in Australia and Malaysia, Bangladesh, India, and the Philippines, respectively. These viruses are considered Category C pathogens by the US Centers for Disease Control. Nipah virus was recently placed on the World Health Organization Research and Development Blueprint Roadmaps for vaccine and therapeutic development. Given the infrequent and unpredictable nature of henipavirus outbreaks licensure of vaccines and therapeutics will likely require an animal model to demonstrate protective efficacy against henipavirus disease. Studies have shown that nonhuman primates are the most accurate model of human henipavirus disease and would be an important component of any application for licensure of a vaccine or antiviral drug under the US FDA Animal Rule. Nonhuman primate model selection and dosing are discussed regarding vaccine and therapeutic studies against henipaviruses.

Key words Henipavirus, African green monkey, Vaccination, Treatment

1 Introduction

Hendra (HeV) and Nipah (NiV) viruses are zoonotic viruses within the genus henipavirus, in the family *Paramyxoviridae*, which have been re-emerging since they were initially discovered in 1994 [1] and 1998 [2], respectively. Henipaviruses can cause lethal disease in humans presenting with severe acute pulmonary disease and/or encephalitis with a case-fatality rate from 40% to 100% [3]. The reservoir for these viruses has been identified as mainly the pteropid bats as they have been associated with spillover leading to cases of human henipavirus disease [4, 5]. This spillover into humans can occur through direct contact with infected animals (pigs, horse) which serve as amplifying hosts, through consumption of NiV-contaminated unpasteurized date palm sap, and direct contact with infected humans [6]. Currently, there are no licensed vaccines or therapeutics for human use; however, there are several candidate

Alexander N. Freiberg and Barry Rockx (eds.), *Nipah Virus: Methods and Protocols*, Methods in Molecular Biology, vol. 2682, https://doi.org/10.1007/978-1-0716-3283-3_12,

interventions under development including recombinant protein-based vaccines, viral vectored vaccines, and human monoclonal antibodies.

To evaluate vaccines and therapeutics for emerging highly virulent viruses, there is often a need for relevant animal models that recapitulate the disease signs in humans since human efficacy trials are difficult to conduct with the sporadic nature of the outbreaks. The United States Food and Drug Administration (FDA) has established an "Animal Rule" (described in the FDA Code of Federal Regulations CFR 21314.600), which states that a new drug or biological product can be licensed through substantial evidence of efficacy shown in one or more well-characterized animal models that recapitulate the disease seen in humans [7].

To date there have been eight animal models used in henipavirus studies which include: the Interferon alpha receptor knockout (IFNAR-KO) mouse model [8]; the guinea pig model [9]; the pig model [10, 11]; the cat model [12]; the golden Syrian hamster model [13]; the ferret model [14]; and two nonhuman primate (NHP) models, one in squirrel monkeys [15] and the other in African green monkeys (AGM) [16]. Each of these models has at least one or more aspects of henipavirus disease observed in human cases; however, Syrian hamsters, ferrets, and AGM develop both severe respiratory and neurological disease. Hamsters recapitulate respiratory signs of disease at high-infectious doses and neurological signs of disease at low-infectious doses [17], while the ferret model can present with respiratory and neurologic disease from a similar infectious dose [18]. Both models are important for the initial evaluation of a vaccine or therapeutic efficacy; however, evaluating responses to vaccines and therapeutics is limited due to a lack of reagents. After an initial triage of vaccine and therapeutics in these models, the AGM model of disease is considered the "gold-standard" for final vaccine and therapeutic efficacy studies. Here, we describe the use of the AGM model from mode of infection to considerations for how to conduct therapeutic or vaccine studies in this model that recapitulates human henipavirus disease.

2 Materials

2.1 Requirements to Work with Henipaviruses in AGMs

1. Approved Animal Biosafety Level (ABSL)-4 facility for work with AGMs exposed to henipaviruses; approval from the U.S. Centers for Disease Control and Prevention (CDC) or equivalent.
2. Approval from the Institution/University biosafety committee, or equivalent, to work with henipaviruses in AGMs at ABSL-4.

3. Institutional Animal Care and Use Committee (IACUC), or equivalent, approval to work with AGMs exposed to henipaviruses at ABSL-4.
4. Trained staff who has been approved to work with henipavirus-infected AGMs at ABSL-4.

2.2 General

1. Well-characterized virus stocks of HeV or NiV; tested for lethality in NHP pilot studies and seed stock for mycoplasma and endotoxin content and fully sequenced genome.
2. Young adult to adult (~3 to 10 years of age) AGMs (*Chlorocebus aethiops*), male or female ~3 to 9 kg.
3. Animal medical record (AMR) for each AGM used in the study.
4. Cage with squeeze mechanism to house AGMs with dimensions based on animal size recommended in the National Research Council's *Guide for the Care and Use of Laboratory Animals* eighth edition [19] or equivalent.
5. NHP biscuits/chow.
6. Fruit and vegetables.
7. Environmental enrichment such as hides and toys.
8. Down draft table or procedure table of adequate size to place an anesthetized AGM for procedures.
9. Versi-Dry lab soaker or equivalent absorbent bench pads.
10. Digital rectal thermometer, other devices to measure temperature such as Star-Oddi data loggers or telemetry system.
11. Scale and tub for recording weights.
12. Clippers—to shave fur.
13. Forceps.
14. Rubbing alcohol or equivalent disinfectant.
15. Gauze.
16. Anesthetic, such as Ketamine (5–20 mg/kg) or Telazol (2–6 mg/kg).
17. Container to secure sharps while moving to a cage from the procedure table.
18. Sharps containers.
19. Clinical observation and humane endpoint considerations (Table 1).

2.3 Inoculation of AGMs with Henipaviruses

1. Hank's Balanced Salt Solution (1×) supplemented up to 2% Certified Heat-inactivated Fetal Bovine Serum (2% FBS-HBSS).
2. 15 and 50 mL conical tubes.
3. Disposable 3 or 10 mL "Luer lock" syringes.

Table 1
Considerations for clinical observations and scores

Observations/euthanasia score criteria for Henipavirus infected AGMs	
Appetite	Based on food and enrichment intake
Waste	Amount/quality of urine and feces output
Appearance	Depression Grooming Nasal exudate Weakness Recumbency Unresponsiveness
Respiration	Cough Respiration rate Exertion upon respiration
Neurologic	Balance Tremors Ataxia Seizures Paralysis

4. Laryngoscope.
5. Gavage tube.
6. LMA® MAD (Teleflex); atomizer capable of producing mist of particles of 30–100 μm in size.

2.4 Vaccination, Treatment, and Sampling of AGMs

1. Vaccine or therapeutic.
2. 1 mL up to 20 mL "Luer lock" syringes.
3. Disposable 25-gauge needles and 21-gauge intravenous needles.
4. Vacutainer one-use blood collection needle holders.
5. 22- or 21-gauge blood collection needles.
6. Vacutainer blood collection tubes appropriate for the desired analyses:
   (a) K_2-EDTA—for viral load, immunoglobulin (Ig)/neutralizing antibodies, cytokines/chemokines, and hematology.
   (b) Serum Separator—for viral load, Ig/neutralizing antibodies, cytokines/chemokines, and blood chemistries.
   (c) Sodium Heparin—for peripheral blood mononuclear cell (PBMC) preparation.
   (d) Sodium Citrate—for coagulopathy profiles.
7. Disposable "break-away" cotton tipped swabs.

2.5 Euthanasia of AGMs at Humane and Scientific Endpoints

1. Disposable 5 mL "Luer lock" syringes.
2. 20-gauge intravenous needles.
3. American Veterinary Medical Association (AVMA), or equivalent, approved euthanasia solution; typically, a pentobarbital sodium solution such as Euthasol.

3 Methods

3.1 Vaccination

Depending on the vaccine vector being evaluated, the dosing regimen will be a prime only or prime-boost strategy where AGMs are vaccinated and sampled for replication of the vaccine vector (if applicable), detection of cell-mediated immune response, and detection of humoral immune response. The vaccination antigenicity assessment phase typically lasts for 21–56 days after vaccination and before exposure of the AGMs to henipaviruses.

1. Assess the AGMs from the cage-side for general health and behavior to determine if they are healthy enough for anesthesia and procedures.
2. Set up the procedure table and scale/tub with absorbent bench pads to work with the AGMs.
3. Use the squeeze mechanism of the NHP cage to pull the first AGM to the front of the cage and control the AGM so that the triceps or thigh are available for intramuscular (i.m.) injection of anesthetic (e.g., Ketamine [5–20 mg/kg] or Telazol [2–6 mg/kg]) using a 25-gauge needle and syringe.
4. Once the AGM appears sedated, verify that the animal is completely sedated and remove the animal from the cage, weigh the animal, and then place the animal on the procedure table. Examine the animal for overall health by observing the eyes, mucus membranes, fur, skin, and hydration status through skin turgor test as well as recording the rectal temperature. Assess the baseline respiration quality by holding the thorax between the examiner's hands to feel for crackles upon inspiration. Additionally, baseline X-ray or CT scans can be performed.
5. Disinfect the inguinal region or other region allowing access to a vein for phlebotomy. Depending on the size of the AGM use a 21-gauge (>4 kg) or 22-gauge (<4 kg) needle for blood collection. For inguinal bleeds, penetrate the skin with bleeding needle (needle is seated in a needle holder/hub) toward the femoral vein. Once the needle is under the skin, place the desired blood tube type into the needle holder and push the top of the tube onto the blood collection needle and insert the needle into the femoral vein. Once the desired amount of

blood is collected in each of the different tubes required for analysis, remove the needle and place pressure on the venipuncture site with the thumb and a piece of gauze to assist in clotting. Dispose the needle in a sharps container. At this point, the mucus membranes can be swabbed if needed.

6. Inject the vaccine formulation i.m. using a 25-gauge needle and syringe into as many locations as desired; typically one or two injection sites in either the caudal thigh muscles or deltoid.
7. Assess the venipuncture site to assure clotting has occurred and then place AGM back into the cage on their side facing the front of the cage so they can be monitored as they come out of anesthesia.
8. Fill out the AMR with the health of the animal, weight, temperature, type and amount of anesthetic used, details of the vaccination given. and time of recovery from the anesthetic. Remain in the room until all AGMs have recovered from the anesthetic.
9. If multiple doses of vaccines are to be given as part of the vaccine regimen, repeat **steps 1–8** on subsequent days of vaccination.
10. Repeat **steps 1–8**, except for the vaccination step (**step 6**), on the sampling days for humoral and/or the cellular immune response analysis.
11. On the day post-vaccination where the vaccination regimen is considered complete, proceed with exposure of the AGMs to the henipavirus, as described below in Subheading 3.2.

3.2 Henipavirus Exposure in AGMs

Henipaviruses are lethal in AGMs by the intratracheal (i.t.) [16, 20, 21], aerosol [22, 23], and intranasal (i.n.) [24] exposure routes; however, i.t. or i.t. plus i.n. exposure are the routes published for a majority of vaccine and therapeutic studies to date [20, 21, 25–28]. Small particle and intermediate size aerosol exposure models using NiV have been described but have yet to have countermeasure efficacy assessed against these challenge routes [22, 29]. Additionally, the i.n. route model was recently described using an atomizer for delivery of a mist with 30–100 μm sized particles i.n. [24]; however, this route also has yet to be tested against vaccine and therapeutics. Currently, the i.t. and i.t./i.n. exposure dose for NiV (*see* **Note 1**) used for countermeasure efficacy studies is 5×10^5 plaque forming units (PFU) and represents a very high "bar" to overcome as this dose of exposure is less likely during a natural exposure. These methods will cover the i.t./i.n. exposure dose that has been used to evaluate vaccines and therapeutics and currently is reported in the literature.

1. For the i.t./i.n. henipavirus exposure, thaw the chosen henipavirus stock and dilute the virus in 2% FBS-HBSS starting with at least 0.5 mL of virus stock (*see* **Note 2**). For the i.t. challenge preparation, dilute the virus stock to 50,000 PFU/mL and place on ice to keep cool until use. For the i.n. challenge preparation, dilute the virus stock to 500,000 PFU/mL and place on ice to keep cool until use.
2. Assess the AGMs from the cage-side for general health, respiration rate/exertion, and behavior to determine if they are healthy enough for anesthesia and procedures.
3. Set up the procedure table and scale/tub with absorbent bench pads to work with the AGMs.
4. Use the squeeze mechanism of the NHP cage to pull the first AGM to the front of the cage and control the AGM so that the triceps or caudal thigh muscles are available for i.m. injection of anesthetic (e.g., Ketamine [5–20 mg/kg] or Telazol [2–6 mg/kg]) using a 25-gauge needle and syringe.
5. Once the AGM appears sedated, verify that the animal is completely sedated and remove the animal from the cage, weigh the animal, and then place the animal on the procedure table. Examine the animal for overall health by observing the eyes, mucus membranes, fur, skin, and hydration status through a skin turgor test as well as recording the rectal temperature. Assess the respiration quality by holding the thorax between the examiner's hands to feel for crackles upon inspiration. Additionally, baseline X-ray or CT scans can be performed.
6. Disinfect the inguinal region or other region allowing access to a vein for phlebotomy. Depending on the size of the AGM, use a 21-gauge (>4 kg) or 22-gauge (<4 kg) needle for blood collection. For inguinal bleeds, penetrate the skin with bleeding needle (needle is seated in a needle holder/hub) toward the femoral vein. Once the needle is under the skin, place the desired blood tube type into the needle holder and push the top of the tube onto the blood collection needle and insert the needle into the femoral vein. Once the desired amount of blood is collected in each of the different tubes required for analysis, remove the needle and place pressure on the venipuncture site with the thumb and a piece of gauze to assist in clotting. Dispose the needle in a sharps container. At this point, the mucus membranes can be swabbed if needed.
7. For i.t. portion of henipavirus challenge: sit the AGM upright and have a second person keep the mouth open using gauze hooked around canines. Use a laryngoscope to locate the opening of the trachea and insert the gavage tube attached to a syringe filled with 5 mL (250,000 PFU) of the i.t. virus

preparation and then depress syringe plunger to instill into the trachea. For i.n. portion of henipavirus challenge: lay the AGM dorsally and have a second person keep the head angled for i.n. instillation of the i.n. virus preparation. Instill 0.250 mL (250,000 PFU) per nostril using a pipette.

8. After the inoculation, assess the venipuncture site again to assure clotting has occurred and then place AGM back into the cage on their side facing the front of the cage so they can be monitored as they come out of anesthesia.
9. Fill out the AMR with the health of the animal, weight, temperature, type and amount of anesthetic used, details of the inoculation, and time of recovery from the anesthetic. Remain in the room until all AGMs have recovered from the anesthetic.
10. Repeat **steps 1–9**, minus the virus inoculation step (**step 7**), on desired sampling days.
11. If evaluating a post-exposure treatment continue with treatments as described in Subheading 3.3 starting at the chosen time point post-henipavirus exposure.

3.3 Post-Exposure Treatment

The treatment dosage and regimen will be adjusted for the candidate therapeutic to be assessed. As far as treatment regimen, pre-infection treatment can be evaluated; however, there are pre-clinical data in the literature that have shown monoclonal antibody (mAb) treatments beginning 1, 3, or 5 days post-henipavirus infection. Although pre-infection or time of infection treatment regimens should not be excluded from consideration, starting treatments at day 3 post-henipavirus infection should be considered as the current benchmark to meet.

1. Assess the AGMs from the cage-side for general health, respiratory rate/exertion and behavior to determine if they are healthy enough for anesthesia and procedures.
2. Set up the procedure table and scale/tub with absorbent bench pads to work with the AGMs.
3. Use the squeeze mechanism of the NHP cage to pull the first AGM to the front of the cage and control the AGM so that the triceps or caudal thigh muscles are available for i.m. injection of anesthetic (e.g., Ketamine [5–20 mg/kg] or Telazol [2–6 mg/kg]) using a 25-gauge needle and syringe.
4. Once the AGM appears sedated, verify that the animal is completely sedated and remove the animal from the cage, weigh the animal, and then place the animal on the procedure table. Examine the animal for overall health by observing the eyes, mucus membranes, fur, skin, and hydration status through a skin turgor test as well as recording the rectal temperature. Assess the respiration quality by holding the thorax

between the examiner's hands to feel for crackles upon inspiration. Additionally, baseline X-ray or CT scans can be performed.

5. If a blood sample is desired on the treatment day, disinfect the inguinal region or other region allowing access to a vein for phlebotomy. Depending on the size of the AGM, use a 21-gauge (>4 kg) or 22-gauge (<4 kg) needle for blood collection. For inguinal bleeds, penetrate the skin with bleeding needle (needle is seated in a needle holder/hub) toward the femoral vein. Once the needle is under the skin, place the desired blood tube type into the needle holder and push the top of the tube onto the blood collection needle and insert the needle into the femoral vein. Once the desired amount of blood is collected in each of the different tubes required for analysis, remove the needle and place pressure on the venipuncture site with the thumb and a piece of gauze to assist in clotting. Dispose the needle in a sharps container. At this point, the mucus membranes can be swabbed if needed.
6. For intravenous (i.v.) treatment: disinfect the inguinal region or saphenous vein region. Use a 21-gauge intravenous needle and syringe to deliver the treatment into the femoral or saphenous vein. Once under the skin insert the needle into the femoral vein (*see* **Note 3**) and pull back on the plunger until blood is drawn into syringe; at this point slowly depress the plunger releasing the treatment into the femoral vein. Remove the needle, place in a sharps container, and apply pressure to the venipuncture site with the thumb and a piece of gauze to assist in clotting. Alternatively, AGMs could have a vascular access port (VAP) or a catheter connected to an ambulatory infusion system for intravenous delivery of treatment. For oral treatment: sit the AGM upright and have a second person keep the mouth open using gauze hooked around canines. Use a laryngoscope to locate the opening of the esophagus and insert the gavage tube attached to a syringe filled with the treatment and then depress syringe plunger to release the treatment.
7. If i.v. treatment is used, assess the venipuncture site again and place the AGM back into the cage on their side facing the front of the cage.
8. Fill out the AMR with the health of the animal, weight, temperature, type and amount of anesthetic used, details of the treatment given, and time of recovery from the anesthetic. Remain in the room until all AGMs have recovered from the anesthetic.
9. Repeat all steps on additional treatment days, minus the treatment step on sampling days only (**step** 7).

3.4 Clinical Samples, Clinical Observations, Humane Endpoint Scoring, and Euthanasia

Infection of AGMs with henipaviruses leads to signs of disease such as depression, lethargy, fever, loss of appetite, labored breathing, tremors, ataxia, and limb paresis. Clinical pathology of AGMs infected with henipaviruses includes thrombocytopenia, lymphopenia, increase in blood urea nitrogen (BUN), and hypoalbuminemia, while the gross pathology includes lung congestion, hemorrhage and necrosis in all lung lobes, and enlarged spleen. Each of these signs of disease/pathology can be used to assess the efficacy of vaccine/treatment. Techniques for analyzing these signs/pathologies are described below.

1. On sampling days EDTA-plasma tubes and serum tubes can be collected for hematology and serum biochemistry, respectively. Remove 100 μL of whole blood from the EDTA-plasma tube and examine the blood using a hematology analyzer; the total number of lymphocytes, granulocytes, or neutrophils, and platelets are of the most interest. Remove 100 μL of serum from serum separator tube and examine the serum using a biochemistry analyzer; alanine aminotransferase (ALT), aspartate aminotransferase (AST), albumin, total protein (TP), BUN, and C-reactive protein (CRP) are the parameters that are of the most interest. (*see* **Note 4**).
2. After the henipavirus infection phase in a vaccine/treatment efficacy study (up to the study endpoint), clinical observations should be documented (see Table 1) during daily checks or during sampling/treatment days while the AGM is on the procedure table. These observations can be used to compare the control and vaccine/treatment cohorts' disease progression.
3. When AGMs are infected with henipaviruses via the i.n./i.t. route and there is no vaccine or therapeutic used to curtail the disease, the infection is up to 100% lethal depending on virus used in the study (*see* **Note 1**). Considering that HeV and NiV cause lethality, it is necessary to ensure that the AGMs infected with henipaviruses do not unnecessarily suffer but also allow the disease course to advance to a point where the animal serves as a proper control when testing a vaccine/treatment. To prevent suffering beyond the study criteria, humane endpoints should be set for each study based on respiration, appetite, activity/appearance, and neurological signs as shown in Table 1. Humane endpoint criteria (*see* **Note 5**) can be investigator and study specific; however, the decision on what is acceptable is made by the IACUC of the institution involved in AGM henipavirus studies. Scoring AGMs for these criteria should, at a minimum, begin day 1 post-henipavirus infection with certain scores/categories requiring additional monitoring to intervene with euthanasia in a timely manner (*see* **Note 5**).

4. When an AGM reaches a clinical score requiring euthanasia or study endpoint has been reached, set up the procedure table and scale/tub with absorbent bench pads to work with the AGMs.
5. Use the squeeze mechanism of the NHP cage to pull the first AGM to the front of the cage and control the AGM so that the triceps or caudal thigh muscles are available for i.m. injection of anesthetic (e.g., Ketamine [5–20 mg/kg] or Telazol [2–6 mg/kg]) using a 25-gauge needle and syringe.
6. Once the AGM appears sedated, verify they are completely sedated and remove them from the cage, weigh them, and then place them on the procedure table. Exam them for overall health by observing the eyes, mucus membranes, fur, skin, and hydration status through a skin turgor test as well as measuring their temperature.
7. Disinfect the inguinal region or other region allowing access to a vein for phlebotomy. Depending on the size of the AGM, use a 21-gauge (>4 kg) or 22-gauge (<4 kg) needle for blood collection. For inguinal bleeds, penetrate the skin with bleeding needle (needle is seated in a needle holder/hub) toward the femoral vein. Once the needle is under the skin, place the desired blood tube type into the needle holder and push the top of the tube onto the blood collection needle and insert the needle into the femoral vein. Once the desired amount of blood is collected in each of the different tubes required for analysis, remove the needle and place pressure on the venipuncture site with the thumb and a piece of gauze to assist in clotting. Dispose the needle in a sharps container. At this point, the mucus membranes can be swabbed if needed.
8. Deliver a pentobarbital sodium-based euthanasia solution (<4 kg use 1.5 mL; >4 kg 2.0 mL) via intracardiac stick using a 20-gauge needle and 5 mL syringe. Insert needle in between the ribs near the left nipple, targeting the heart, and pull back on the plunger until blood is drawn into the syringe; at this point depress the plunger injecting pentobarbital sodium solution into the heart and circulatory system.
9. In general, when the humane endpoint or the study endpoint (*see* **Note 6**) is reached, AGMs are typically necropsied with gross pathology observed and noted. Additionally, hematoxylin and eosin (H & E) staining for cytopathology and immunohistochemistry (IHC) staining for virus antigen should be performed on formalin-fixed tissues (*see* **Note 7**); tissue can also be used for detection of viral RNA by in situ hybridization (ISH). Tissues taken at necropsy can also be used to assess the infectious virus load when evaluating the effectiveness of a vaccine/treatment.

4 Notes

1. Henipavirus lethality in AGMs using either the i.t. (HeV) or the combined i.n./i.t. (NiV) challenge route has shown some variability depending on the virus used for the challenge. For HeV, the lethality found in the literature is ~73% [20, 30–32], while the NiV strains Malaysia and Bangladesh have been reported to be ~80% [16, 21, 22, 25, 27, 28] and 100% [26, 27, 30, 33], respectively. As the AGM model is considered the "gold standard" animal model, the Bangladesh strain has now become the "gold standard" strain chosen for countermeasure studies as the Bangladesh AGM model has been shown to be more pathogenic than the Malaysia AGM model [27], which is similar to what has been observed between the two strains in human outbreaks [34–36]. It is recommended to consult a biostatistician to ensure that there is enough power in the groups set for any vaccine or treatment study with NHPs.
2. Most henipavirus stocks will need to be diluted around 100–1000-fold to reach 500,000 PFU/mL, so an initial tenfold dilution is made by placing 0.5 mL of virus stock into 4.5 mL of 2%FBS-HBSS. Pulse vortex the tube of virus stock three times so that all liquid goes up the sides of the tube and then remove the 0.5 mL. This assures a more homogenous mixture of virus is pulled rather than pulling a smaller volume (e.g., 0.005 mL and placing it into 4.995 mL for 5000-fold dilution). Pulse vortex at each dilution step using at least 2 mL for tenfold dilutions.
3. If the treatment regimen requires multiple injections via the femoral vein, it is possible that scar tissue will build up so it is best practice to alternate left and right femoral veins for bleeding and treating on the same day and potentially on successive days of treatment. Alternatively, the saphenous vein can also be used to reduce build-up of scar tissue.
4. With the smaller numbers used for AGM cohorts, it is important that all hematology and clinical chemistry values are compared to the day of challenge which represents the baseline for each individual AGM. Ranges for hematology and blood chemistry that represent advanced disease: greater than 30–35% change in hematology total cell/platelet numbers and greater than 10- to 20-fold changes in liver enzymes, 30% reduction in albumin and TP, and changes in CRP levels over 20-fold.
5. Table 1 is a representation of henipavirus disease signs and humane endpoint considerations in AGMs. At a minimum, investigators need an established score for humane intervention along with the disease course resulting from henipavirus infection for the positive control animals to ensure the vaccine/

treatment has been assessed against the disease. These scores and clinical signs can be adjusted based on experience with the model.

6. The study endpoint may vary but has traditionally been around 28 days post-virus exposure due to space-usage constraints in the BSL4 labs. With NiV and HeV infection though the potential exists for recrudescence in neural tissues after recovery from an initial infection. To date, 65 and 92 days post-NiV exposure in AGMs are the most extended study endpoints [29, 33]; however, this would be difficult as a model for study length at most BSL4s considering the multi-user/multi-virus nature of studies run in these limited space laboratories. Careful consideration and planning would be needed when setting up a study design to observe recrudescence in the AGM model.
7. Formalin-fixed tissues can be removed from the ABSL4 based on an institution's validated inactivation procedure.

References

1. Selvey LA, Wells RM, McCormack JG, Ansford AJ, Murray K, Rogers RJ et al (1995) Infection of humans and horses by a newly described morbillivirus. Med J Aust 162(12):642–645
2. Chua KB, Goh KJ, Wong KT, Kamarulzaman A, Tan PS, Ksiazek TG et al (1999) Fatal encephalitis due to Nipah virus among pig-farmers in Malaysia. Lancet 354(9186):1257–1259. Epub 1999/10/16. https://doi.org/10.1016/S0140-6736(99)04299-3 [pii]
3. Mathieu C, Horvat B (2015) Henipavirus pathogenesis and antiviral approaches. Expert Rev Anti-Infect Ther 13(3):343–354. https://doi.org/10.1586/14787210.2015.1001838
4. Clayton BA, Wang LF, Marsh GA (2012) Henipaviruses: an updated review focusing on the pteropid reservoir and features of transmission. Zoonoses Public Health 60(1):69–83. Epub 2012/06/20. https://doi.org/10.1111/j.1863-2378.2012.01501.x
5. Halpin K, Young PL, Field HE, Mackenzie JS (2000) Isolation of Hendra virus from pteropid bats: a natural reservoir of Hendra virus. J Gen Virol 81(Pt 8):1927–1932. Epub 2000/07/19
6. Weatherman S, Feldmann H, de Wit E (2018) Transmission of henipaviruses. Curr Opin Virol 28:7–11. https://doi.org/10.1016/j.coviro.2017.09.004. PubMed PMID: 29035743; PubMed Central PMCID: PMCPMC5835161
7. Food, Drug Administration HHS (2002) New drug and biological drug products; evidence needed to demonstrate effectiveness of new drugs when human efficacy studies are not ethical or feasible. Final rule. Fed Regist 67(105): 37988–37998
8. Dhondt KP, Mathieu C, Chalons M, Reynaud JM, Vallve A, Raoul H et al (2013) Type I interferon signaling protects mice from lethal henipavirus infection. J Infect Dis 207(1): 142–151. Epub 2012/10/24. https://doi.org/10.1093/infdis/jis653 [pii]
9. Williamson MM, Hooper PT, Selleck PW, Westbury HA, Slocombe RF (2000) Experimental Hendra virus infectionin pregnant guinea-pigs and fruit bats (Pteropus poliocephalus). J Comp Pathol 122(2–3):201–207. https://doi.org/10.1053/jcpa.1999.0364
10. Middleton DJ, Westbury HA, Morrissy CJ, van der Heide BM, Russell GM, Braun MA et al (2002) Experimental Nipah virus infection in pigs and cats. J Comp Pathol 126(2–3): 124–136. Epub 2002/04/12. https://doi.org/10.1053/jcpa.2001.0532 S0021997501905328 [pii]
11. Tanimura N, Imada T, Kashiwazaki Y, Shahirudin S, Sharifah SH, Aziz AJ (2004) Monoclonal antibody-based immunohistochemical diagnosis of Malaysian Nipah virus infection in pigs. J Comp Pathol 131(2–3): 199–206. Epub 2004/07/28. https://doi.org/10.1016/j.jcpa.2004.03.006 S0021997504000477 [pii]
12. McEachern JA, Bingham J, Crameri G, Green DJ, Hancock TJ, Middleton D et al (2008) A recombinant subunit vaccine formulation

protects against lethal Nipah virus challenge in cats. Vaccine 26(31):3842–3852. Epub 2008/06/17. doi: S0264-410X(08)00572-0 [pii] https://doi.org/10.1016/j.vaccine.2008.05.016

13. Wong KT, Grosjean I, Brisson C, Blanquier B, Fevre-Montange M, Bernard A et al (2003) A golden hamster model for human acute Nipah virus infection. Am J Pathol 163(5): 2127–2137. Epub 2003/10/28. https://doi.org/10.1016/S0002-9440(10)63569-9 [pii]
14. Bossart KN, Zhu Z, Middleton D, Klippel J, Crameri G, Bingham J et al (2009) A neutralizing human monoclonal antibody protects against lethal disease in a new ferret model of acute Nipah virus infection. PLoS Pathog 5(10):e1000642. Epub 2009/11/06. https://doi.org/10.1371/journal.ppat.1000642
15. Marianneau P, Guillaume V, Wong T, Badmanathan M, Looi RY, Murri S et al (2010) Experimental infection of squirrel monkeys with Nipah virus. Emerg Infect Dis 16(3):507–510. Epub 2010/03/06. https://doi.org/10.3201/eid1603.091346
16. Geisbert TW, Daddario-DiCaprio KM, Hickey AC, Smith MA, Chan YP, Wang LF et al (2010) Development of an acute and highly pathogenic nonhuman primate model of Nipah virus infection. PLoS One 5(5):e10690. Epub 2010/05/27. https://doi.org/10.1371/journal.pone.0010690
17. Rockx B, Brining D, Kramer J, Callison J, Ebihara H, Mansfield K et al (2011) Clinical outcome of henipavirus infection in hamsters is determined by the route and dose of infection. J Virol 85(15):7658–7671. Epub 2011/05/20. https://doi.org/10.1128/JVI.00473-11 [pii]
18. Satterfield BA, Cross RW, Fenton KA, Agans KN, Basler CF, Geisbert TW et al (2015) The immunomodulating V and W proteins of Nipah virus determine disease course. Nat Commun 6:7483
19. Barthold SW, Bayne KA, Davis MA (2011) Guide for the care and use of laboratory animals. National Academy Press, Washington, DC
20. Bossart KN, Geisbert TW, Feldmann H, Zhu Z, Feldmann F, Geisbert JB et al (2011) A neutralizing human monoclonal antibody protects African green monkeys from Hendra virus challenge. Sci Transl Med 3(105):105ra3. Epub 2011/10/21. doi: 3/105/105ra103 [pii]. https://doi.org/10.1126/scitranslmed.3002901
21. Bossart KN, Rockx B, Feldmann F, Brining D, Scott D, LaCasse R et al (2012) A Hendra virus G glycoprotein subunit vaccine protects African green monkeys from Nipah virus challenge. Sci Transl Med 4(146):146ra07
22. Cong Y, Lentz MR, Lara A, Alexander I, Bartos C, Bohannon JK et al (2017) Loss in lung volume and changes in the immune response demonstrate disease progression in African green monkeys infected by small-particle aerosol and intratracheal exposure to Nipah virus. PLoS Negl Trop Dis 11(4): e0005532
23. Prasad AN, Agans KN, Sivasubramani SK, Geisbert JB, Borisevich V, Mire CE et al (2020) A lethal aerosol exposure model of Nipah virus strain Bangladesh in African Green monkeys. J Infect Dis 221(Suppl 4): S431–S435. https://doi.org/10.1093/infdis/jiz469
24. Geisbert JB, Borisevich V, Prasad AN, Agans KN, Foster SL, Deer DJ et al (2020) An intranasal exposure model of lethal Nipah virus infection in African green monkeys. J Infect Dis 221(Suppl 4):S414–S418. https://doi.org/10.1093/infdis/jiz391. PubMed PMID: 31665362; PubMed Central PMCID: PMCPMC7213566
25. Geisbert TW, Mire CE, Geisbert JB, Chan YP, Agans KN, Feldmann F et al (2014) Therapeutic treatment of Nipah virus infection in nonhuman primates with a neutralizing human monoclonal antibody. Sci Transl Med 6(242): 242ra82. Epub 2014/06/27. doi: 6/242/242ra82 [pii]. https://doi.org/10.1126/scitranslmed.3008929
26. Mire CE, Geisbert JB, Agans KN, Versteeg KM, Deer DJ, Satterfield BA et al (2019) Use of single-injection recombinant vesicular stomatitis virus vaccine to protect nonhuman primates against lethal Nipah virus disease. Emerg Infect Dis 25(6):1144–1152. https://doi.org/10.3201/eid2506.181620. PubMed PMID: 31107231; PubMed Central PMCID: PMCPMC6537706
27. Mire CE, Satterfield BA, Geisbert JB, Agans KN, Borisevich V, Yan L et al (2016) Pathogenic differences between Nipah virus Bangladesh and Malaysia strains in primates: implications for antibody therapy. Sci Rep 6: 30916
28. Prescott J, DeBuysscher BL, Feldmann F, Gardner DJ, Haddock E, Martellaro C et al (2015) Single-dose live-attenuated vesicular stomatitis virus-based vaccine protects African green monkeys from Nipah virus disease. Vaccine 33(24):2823–2829
29. Lee JH, Hammoud DA, Cong Y, Huzella LM, Castro MA, Solomon J et al (2020) The use of large-particle aerosol exposure to Nipah virus

to mimic human neurological disease manifestations in the African Green monkey. J Infect Dis 221(Suppl 4):S419–SS30. https://doi.org/10.1093/infdis/jiz502. PubMed PMID: 31687756; PubMed Central PMCID: PMCPMC7368178

30. Geisbert TW, Bobb K, Borisevich V, Geisbert JB, Agans KN, Cross RW et al (2021) A single dose investigational subunit vaccine for human use against Nipah virus and Hendra virus. npj Vaccines 6(1):23. https://doi.org/10.1038/s41541-021-00284-w. PubMed PMID: 33558494; PubMed Central PMCID: PMCPMC7870971

31. Mire CE, Geisbert JB, Agans KN, Feng YR, Fenton KA, Bossart KN et al (2014) A recombinant Hendra virus G glycoprotein subunit vaccine protects nonhuman primates against Hendra virus challenge. J Virol 88(9): 4624–4631. https://doi.org/10.1128/JVI.00005-14. PubMed PMID: 24522928; PubMed Central PMCID: PMCPMC3993805

32. Rockx B, Bossart KN, Feldmann F, Geisbert JB, Hickey AC, Brining D et al (2010) A novel model of lethal Hendra virus infection in African green monkeys and the effectiveness of ribavirin treatment. J Virol 84(19): 9831–9839. Epub 2010/07/28. doi: JVI.01163-10 [pii]. https://doi.org/10.1128/JVI.01163-10

33. Lo MK, Feldmann F, Gary JM, Jordan R, Bannister R, Cronin J et al (2019) Remdesivir (GS-5734) protects African green monkeys from Nipah virus challenge. Sci Transl Med 11(494). https://doi.org/10.1126/scitranslmed.aau9242. PubMed PMID: 31142680; PubMed Central PMCID: PMCPMC6732787

34. Chua KB, Bellini WJ, Rota PA, Harcourt BH, Tamin A, Lam SK et al (2000) Nipah virus: a recently emergent deadly paramyxovirus. Science 288(5470):1432–1435. Epub 2000/05/29. doi: 8529 [pii]

35. Lo MK, Lowe L, Hummel KB, Sazzad HM, Gurley ES, Hossain MJ et al (2012) Characterization of Nipah virus from outbreaks in Bangladesh, 2008–2010. Emerg Infect Dis 18(2):248–255. Epub 2012/02/07. https://doi.org/10.3201/eid1802.111492

36. Uppal PK (2000) Emergence of Nipah virus in Malaysia. Ann N Y Acad Sci 916:354–357. Epub 2001/02/24

Chapter 13

Nipah Virus Aerosol Challenge of Three Distinct Particle Sizes in Nonhuman Primates

Matthew G. Lackemeyer, J. Kyle Bohannon, and Michael R. Holbrook

Abstract

Aerosol and inhalational studies of high-consequence pathogens allow researchers to study the disease course and effects of biologicals transmitted through aerosol in a laboratory-controlled environment. Inhalational studies involving Nipah virus with small (1–3 μm), intermediate (6–8 μm), and large particles (10–14 μm) were explored in African green nonhuman primates to determine if the subsequent disease course more closely recapitulated what is observed in Nipah virus human disease. The aerosol procedures outlined describe the different equipment/techniques used to generate the three particle sizes and control the site of particle deposition within this animal model.

Key words Aerosol, Small particle, Intermediate particle, Large particle, Plethysmography, Inhalation, Aerobiology, Class III BSC, Biosampler, Nipah virus, African green monkey

1 Introduction

Aerosol transmission of biologicals has emerged as a focal point of interest for many researchers in recent years due to newly emerging, naturally airborne diseases (e.g., SARS-CoV, MERS, influenza, and tuberculosis) and potential for biological warfare or terrorist attack, with aerosolization being the most probable route of exposure [1, 2]. In fact, aerosolization of a pathogen is thought to be more of a concern than direct contact or fomite transmission due to the potential for easy dissemination and pandemic threat potential [3]. Advancements in aerobiology methods, technology, and equipment over the last two decades have allowed exploration into various aerosol particle sizes [4–8]. A modest amount of biological research involving aerosolized pathogens has been modeled in nonhuman primates but most of that work focused on small particle aerosols (1–3 μm), which target the alveolar region of the lower respiratory tract, and subsequent disease course [9–19]. Intermediate sized particles (6–8 μm), targeting the tracheobronchial region and large particles (10–14 μm), targeting the

Alexander N. Freiberg and Barry Rockx (eds.), *Nipah Virus: Methods and Protocols*, Methods in Molecular Biology, vol. 2682, https://doi.org/10.1007/978-1-0716-3283-3_13,

nasopharyngeal region, have not been as extensively studied and the disease course may be more indicative of what is observed in human disease [4, 19]. Few studies have explored a range of aerosol particle sizes and have shown a correlation with particle size directly affecting the median lethal dose with a slight alteration in disease presentation [4, 20, 21]. Thus, the ability to create aerosols and separate infectious particles based on aerodynamic size gives the researcher more control over the deposition site and region of interest within the respiratory tract.

Nipah virus is a highly pathogenic paramyxovirus known to cause severe respiratory and neurological disease in humans through animal–human contact, human–human contact, consumption of contaminated material, or inhalation through droplet transmission [22–25]. An African green (grivet) monkey animal model has been explored as a suitable nonhuman primate model to evaluate the effects of Nipah virus, with evidence of neuropathy after infection mimicking what is observed in human disease [26, 27]. The disease presentation in African Green monkeys exposed to aerosolized Nipah virus varies depending on estimated inhaled dose, aerodynamic particle size, and deposition site [24, 25, unpublished data]. The techniques and methods used to generate these differing particle sizes require multiple generators, applicable biosamplers, and addition of glycerol for creation of intermediate and larger particles. These processes and procedures are outlined.

2 Materials

Nipah virus is considered a biosafety level 4 (BSL-4) agent and should be handled in accordance with the guidelines stipulated in the "Biosafety in Microbiological and Biomedical Laboratories" (BMBL) (https://www.cdc.gov/labs/BMBL.html).

2.1 Aerosol Equipment

1. Class III Biosafety Cabinet (Class III BSC).
2. Autoclave.
3. Automated aerosol management platform containing flow controllers, connections, and temperature and relative humidity probe.
4. A 16-L head-only aerosol exposure chamber.
5. Laptop station controlling the automated management platform.
6. Laboratory house air and vacuum sources connected inside the Class III BSC.
7. 3 or 6-jet small particle generator.
8. Centered flow tangential aerosol intermediate/large particle generator.

9. Non-human primate (NHP) supine positioning ramp.
10. Stainless steel delivery and exhaust lines.
11. Aerodynamic particle sizer.
12. Biosamplers (swirling impaction mechanism or gelatin membrane filter).
13. Syringe pump.
14. ½″ rubber tubing connecting HEPA filters via a plastic Tee fitting.
15. HEPA filters for exhaust ports.
16. External siphon vacuum controller.
17. Pneumotach plethysmography mask.
18. Plethysmography control station.

2.2 Aerosol Consumables

1. Wet ice and ice bucket for samples and virus starting concentration.
2. Spray bottle filled with appropriate disinfectant (5% quaternary ammonium).
3. 10/50 mL conical tubes for sample preparation and collection.
4. 250 mL bottle containing virus starting concentration.
5. 60 mL syringe and delivery line attaching to the syringe pump and cannula needles.
6. Virus stock, media diluent (Dulbecco's modified eagle medium (DMEM) with 2% fetal bovine serum (FBS) or DMEM with 4% bovine serum albumin (BSA), glycerol (5–15%), and virus starting concentration.
7. Gelatin membrane filter.
8. Dental dam to create a seal around the NHP neck while in the head-only chamber.
9. Autoclave bags for generated waste.

3 Methods

3.1 Class III BSC Preparation

1. Visually and physically verify the Class III biosafety cabinet (BSC) is operational prior to experimentation (Fig. 1; *see* **Note 1**).
2. Inspect the Class III BSC looking for cracks on the view panels, worn gaskets and O-rings, damage to synthetic rubber gloves, dry rot, and a breach in containment (*see* **Notes 2** and **3**).
3. Check to ensure the integrated dunk tank is filled to the appropriate level with the proper concentration of dual quaternary ammonium.

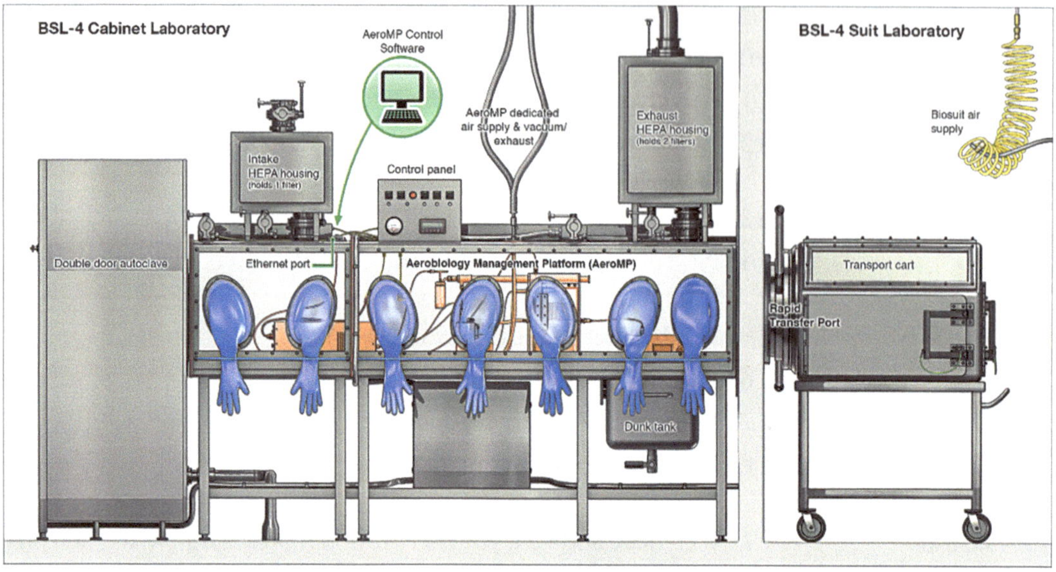

Fig. 1 A hermetically sealed stainless-steel Class III BSC containing aerosol equipment (peach color). The Class III BSC is always maintained under negative pressure (*see* **Note 1**). Synthetic rubber gloves (blue) allow the researcher to penetrate and manipulate the equipment while maintaining an enclosed environment. An interlocked double door autoclave is attached to the Class III BSC and requires a full 2-h sterilization cycle to unlock the inner autoclave door. A single HEPA filter is located at the inlet air intake, and a double HEPA filter is located at the exhaust air outlet so all air entering/leaving the Class III BSC is filtered. A dunk tank containing a 5% dual quaternary ammonium disinfectant solution allows for materials to pass in/out of the Class III BSC without disrupting functionality of the unit. A rapid transfer port (RTP) door provides easy access from the Class III BSC to the high containment side of the laboratory, where the viral solution and nonhuman primates reside. A control panel provides an audible and visual alarm in case there is a breach in the Class III BSC [28, 29]

4. Ensure the autoclave attached to the Class III BSC is cycled and functional to receive biological waste after experimentation (*see* **Note 4**).
5. Set up aerobiology equipment within the Class III BSC and test functionality of particle generators, automated aerosol system, biological aerosol impingers, and aerodynamic particle sizer instrument (Figs. 2 and 3).
6. Place signs indicating the current contamination status of the Class III BSC and contact information of the researcher.

3.2 Aerosol Equipment Assembly and Nipah Virus Preparation of a Nonhuman Primate Head-Only Exposure Chamber

1. Assemble a 16-L head-only NHP exposure chamber with stainless steel delivery and exhaust lines, relative humidity and temperature sensor, pressure sensor and stabilization NHP ramp (Figs. 2 and 3; *see* **Note 5**).
2. Determine the exposure configuration (push, pull, push/pull) and connect the house air/vacuum sources contained within the Class III BSC to the automated aerosol management platform (*see* **Note 6**).

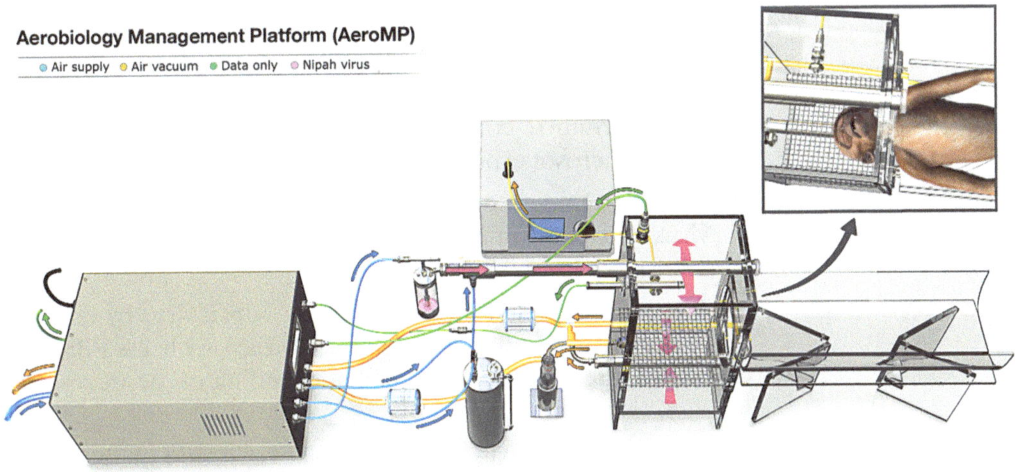

Fig. 2 Schematic of the aerosol equipment setup for a small particle aerosol challenge. Compressed air (blue hoses) is pushed into the system as a primary and secondary generation source. Particles are generated in the nebulizer, conditioned, mixed, and passed through to the inlet of the head only aerosol exposure chamber. Simultaneously, a vacuum source (yellow hoses) pulls the generated viral material through the chamber and into an exhaust HEPA filter system, biosampler collection impinger, and aerodynamic particle sizer. Negative pressure (green hose) is maintained during the aerosol exposure [28, 29]

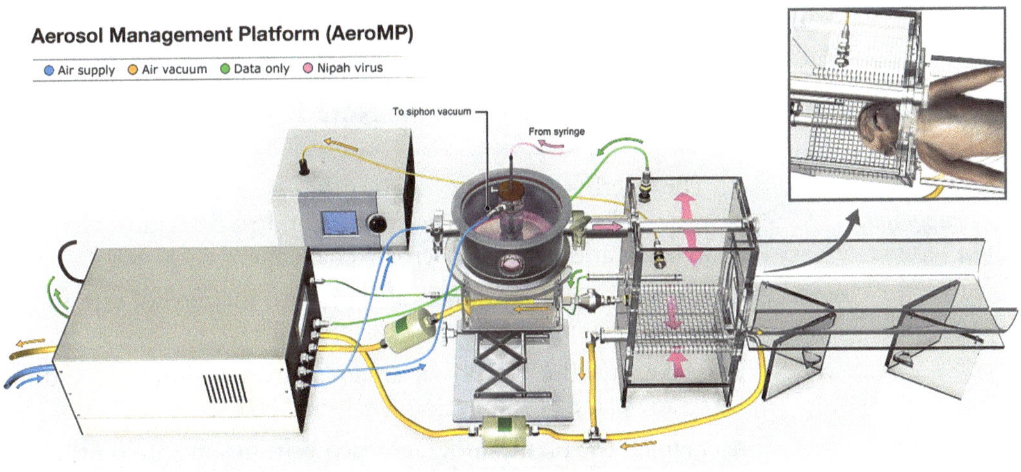

Fig. 3 Schematic of the aerosol equipment setup for an intermediate/large particle aerosol challenge. Compressed air (blue hoses) is pushed into the system as a primary and secondary generation source. Particles are generated in the aerosol generator, conditioned, mixed, and passed through to the inlet of the head only aerosol exposure chamber. Simultaneously, a vacuum source (yellow hoses) pulls the generated viral material through the chamber and into an exhaust HEPA filter system, biosampler collection impinger, and aerodynamic particle sizer. Negative pressure (green hose) is maintained during the aerosol exposure [6]

3. Attach an aerosol generator, biosampler, and aerodynamic particle sizer to the head-only chamber (*see* **Note 7**).
4. Launch the automated aerosol software and input the pre-determined criteria for a small, intermediate, and large particle aerosol exposure (*see* **Note 8**).
5. At room temperature, thaw the proper volume of Nipah stock virus and pool/mix the contents of individual vials into one 15 mL conical tube (*see* **Note 9**).
6. Prepare the starting concentration of Nipah virus by diluting a pre-calculated stock volume into DMEM with 2% FBS and a percentage of glycerol (variable depending on desired particle size) (*see* **Note 10**).
7. Additionally, prepare the biosampler collection medium using DMEM with 4% BSA (*see* **Note 11**).
8. Fill the appropriate aerosol generator with the starting concentration of Nipah virus needed to achieve the desired target dose (*see* **Note 12**).
9. Coat and prime the aerosol exposure chamber with a pre-run or viral coat of starting concentration for ~10 min.
10. After ~10 min, turn off the generator and replace starting concentration material with fresh virus if using small particle generator, since this type of generator recirculates the material. If using medium/large particle generator, pause the syringe pump until ready since this generator continuously dispenses new virus to the system (*see* **Note 13**).

3.3 Plethysmography Section

1. The plethysmography acquisition data for each NHP are required to estimate inhaled dose and to determine the exposure duration for each aerosol challenge.
2. Obtain a minute volume value prior to the aerosol exposure by using a pneumotach mask (*see* **Note 14**).
3. Make sure the NHP is at an adequate sedation level and in a steady plane of respiration (*see* **Note 15**).
4. Launch the plethysmography acquisition software on the local laptop.
5. Place the NHP in the supine position and place the pneumotach mask over the snout of the animal (*see* **Note 16**; Fig. 4).
6. Calibrate the software to the appropriate peak inspiratory and expiratory flows then record the NHP minute ventilation for a determined time period (*see* **Note 17**).
7. Remove the pneumotach mask from the NHP snout and save the minute ventilation data on the local laptop.

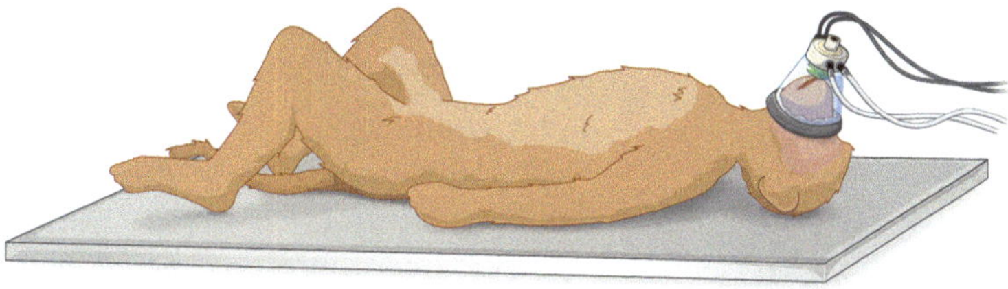

Fig. 4 Anesthetized NHP in the supine position undergoing plethysmography acquisition via a pneumotach mask. The pneumotach mask is placed over the snout of the NHP to record NHP respiratory parameters. A dental dam creates a tight seal around the NHP's snout to ensure accurate measurements. Once the pneumotach mask is calibrated by the corresponding plethysmography software, respiratory recording may commence. Once respiratory measurements have been recorded, the mask may be removed. The software will calculate breaths per minute (BPM), tidal volume (TV), and minute volume (MV) for the aerosol challenge [30]

8. Calculate the minute ventilation average from the recorded respiratory data (*see* **Note 18**).
9. The minute ventilation value is used to determine the aerosol challenge duration (*see* **Note 19**).
10. Additionally, this data is used for the calculation of the estimated inhaled exposure dose at the completion of the experiment using the titer data from the biosampler.

3.4 NHP Nipah Virus Head-Only Aerosol Exposure Using a Small Particle Generator

1. Use a 3- or 6-jet recirculating nebulizer connected to a conditioning tube leading to the inlet of head-only chamber (Fig. 2) (*see* **Note 20**).
2. Fill the generator with an appropriate amount of starting concentration Nipah virus material (*see* **Note 21**).
3. Attach a biosampler to the head-only exposure chamber filled with DMEM and 4% BSA (*see* **Note 22**).
4. Verify whether the NHP is at an adequate depth of anesthesia and pass the NHP through the rapid transfer port (RTP) door of the Class III BSC (*see* **Note 23**).
5. Place the NHP in the supine position on the exposure ramp and gently pass the NHP's head through the rubber/dental dam attached to the head portal of the exposure chamber (*see* **Note 24**).
6. Enter the aerosol information, parameters, and challenge time into the automated aerosol exposure system software (*see* **Note 25**).
7. Ensure the particle size is of the desired target size for each challenge run using the aerodynamic particle sizer (*see* **Note 26**).

8. Expose the NHP to the small particle Nipah virus for the calculated challenge time.
9. After completion of the aerosol challenge, remove the NHP's head from the exposure chamber and back through the rubber/dental dam. Be sure to wipe the animal's face with an appropriate disinfectant to reduce contamination (*see* **Note 27**).
10. Purge the aerosol chamber with an air wash for ~5 min to remove residual particles from the previous exposure. This will create an environment that is "clean" for subsequent aerosol exposures.
11. Pass the NHP back through the RTP door to be returned to its home cage located in high containment.
12. Prior to the next NHP and challenge run, remove the biosampler contents and place in the pre-labeled sample tube. Store these samples on wet ice. Additionally, discard the used challenge material from the small particle generator and replace with fresh material (the next run).
13. Repeat the process from **step 2** of this section until all NHPs have been challenged (*see* **Note 28**).
14. Upon completion of all challenges, pass the accumulated biosampler runs back through the RTP door into high containment for biological assaying (*see* **Note 29**).
15. All trash and sterilizable equipment are passed into the double-doors autoclave for a complete 2-h sterilization cycle (121 °C).
16. Breakdown and dissemble all equipment and decontaminate the NHP head-only exposure chamber, conditioning tubes, inlets, outlets, aerodynamic particle sizer, and all associated contents within the Class III BSC (*see* **Note 30**).

3.5 NHP Nipah Virus Head-Only Aerosol Exposure Using an Intermediate/Large Particle Generator

1. Use a spinning disc aerosol generator connected to a shortened conditioning tube leading to the inlet of head-only chamber (Fig. 3; *see* **Note 31**).
2. Fill the syringe pump with an appropriate amount of starting concentration Nipah virus material (*see* **Note 32**).
3. Attach a biosampler to the head-only exposure chamber filled with DMEM and 4% BSA (*see* **Note 33**).
4. Verify the NHP is at an adequate depth of anesthesia and pass the NHP through the RTP door of the Class III BSC (*see* **Note 23**).
5. Place the NHP in the supine position on the exposure ramp and gently pass the NHP's head through the rubber/dental dam attached to the head portal of the exposure chamber (*see* **Note 24**).

6. Enter the aerosol information, parameters, and challenge time into the automated aerosol exposure system software (*see* **Note 25**).
7. Ensure the particle size is of the desired target size for each challenge run using the aerodynamic particle sizer (*see* **Notes 26** and **34**).
8. Expose the NHP to the intermediate or large particle Nipah virus for the calculated challenge time.
9. After completion of the aerosol challenge, remove the NHP's head from the exposure chamber and back through the rubber/dental dam. Be sure to wipe the animal's face with an appropriate disinfectant to reduce contamination (*see* **Note 27**).
10. Purge the aerosol chamber with an air wash for ~5 min to remove residual particles from the previous exposure. This will create an environment that is "clean" for subsequent aerosol exposures.
11. Pass the NHP back through the RTP door to be returned to its home cage located in high containment.
12. Prior to the next NHP and challenge run, remove the biosampler contents and place in the pre-labeled sample tube. Store these samples on wet ice. The challenge material from the intermediate/large particle generator is single use and does not require replacement prior to next aerosol run (the syringe pump is paused).
13. Repeat the process from **step 2** of this section until all NHPs have been challenged (*see* **Note 28**).
14. Upon completion of all challenges, pass the accumulated biosampler runs back through the RTP door into high containment for exposure validation by biological assay (*see* **Note 29**).
15. All trash and sterilizable equipment are passed into the double-doors autoclave for a complete 2-h sterilization cycle (121 °C).
16. Breakdown and dissemble all equipment and decontaminate the NHP head-only exposure chamber, conditioning tubes, inlets, outlets, aerodynamic particle sizer, and all associated contents within the Class III BSC (*see* **Note 30**).

4 Notes

1. The Class III BSC operates under negative pressure (250 Pa or −1.0 in. water gauge (wg) recommended; a minimum value of 125 Pa or −0.5 in. wg required). Verify the Class III BSC HEPA filtration system has been certified annually. Ensure the

functionality of the audible and visual alarms on the unit. Class II BSCs may be used; however, they are not fully enclosed and require a different set of safety precautions (Class II BSC information not shown).

2. Worn gaskets and O-rings can compromise the integrity of the units and allow a breach in containment when working with biological agents.

3. Synthetic rubber gloves and O-rings are often a focal point for weak spots. Ensure to inspect both for tears, rips, and dry rot. Replace synthetic rubber gloves and O-rings regularly and, if possible, when the Class III BSC is not contaminated with biological agent. If the Class III BSC is contaminated and a synthetic rubber gloves requires changing, disinfect the integrated glove with a dual quaternary ammonium, remove O-rings leaving the integrated synthetic rubber glove attached and gently move the cuff of the compromised glove off the gloveport but keep the glove attached to the Class III BSC. Over top of the compromised glove, replace with a new synthetic rubber glove and hold the new glove into place with O-rings. Gently, pull the compromised glove inward while maintaining biocontainment. The audible alarm will sound if there is a breach and done incorrectly. The compromised glove will be decontaminated and discarded after the procedure.

4. Autoclaves are operated on cycled and integrated door system, with only one door opened at a time. Opening the inner autoclave door, or contaminated side door, requires a 2-h sterilization cycle at 121 °C to release and open the outer autoclave door, or non-contaminated side.

5. Inspect the 16-L chamber for leaks or cracks and keep the chamber pressure negative during aerosolization.

6. Most small particle aerosolization experiments use the push/pull configuration. The intermediate and large particle aerosolization experiments use the pull configuration.

7. The small particle generator used is a 3- or 6-jet nebulizer, which nebulizes the solution and recycles the medium/viral starting concentration contained within the precious fluids jar. The intermediate/large particle generator used is a syringe-fed spinning disc particle distributor, which uses a single pass droplet viral solution to create particles. The aerodynamic particle sizer attaches to the 16-L chamber and gives a real-time time-of-flight aerodynamic size of the generated particles.

8. Parameters and flow rates are determined during aerosol characterization, which takes place over several experiments not involving NHPs prior to an aerosol animal exposure. These characterization tests provide the necessary data needed to achieve a desired particle size and target dose.

9. Stock virus vials kept at −80 °C and must be thawed/pooled prior to any dilutions to ensure a homogenous mixture.
10. All dilutions are performed under sterile conditions in a high-containment environment within a Class II BSC. The more glycerol used, the larger the particles and no more than 20% glycerol used. A high-glycerol concentration can impact the functionality of the aerosol equipment.
11. BSA is chosen downstream in the impingers over FBS as media additive due to better titer results during characterization. BSA is not recommended upstream as part of the starting concentration due to the starting concentration (challenge material) entering the NHP respiratory system and the potential for negative or misleading interactions.
12. Generator type will be based on desired particle size.
13. Nipah virus starting concentration and biosampler contents should remain on wet ice pre/post aerosolization.
14. The pneumotach mask is calibrated by the plethysmography acquisition software on the local laptop by connecting the pneumotach mask to a known vacuum flow. The calibration is performed prior to collecting NHP respiration parameters.
15. Veterinary staff observes the NHP under anesthesia to determine if the NHP is not exhibiting labored breathing and is in steady state anesthesia. Tiletamine/zolazepam is the preferred anesthetic to achieve steady state anesthesia for aerosol and plethysmography procedures due to the minimal effects on the cardiovascular system and respiratory rate [31].
16. The calibrated pneumotach mask has dental dam at the base of the mask to ensure an air-tight seal is formed over the snout of the NHP.
17. Once respiratory waveforms are observed on the laptop, a further calibration needs to be performed within the plethysmography software. Due to the sensitivity of the pneumotach mask, this calibration removes background "noise" from the respiration signal and allows for "good" breaths to be recorded. A recording period is pre-determined by the end user, and the respiratory parameters are recorded for the NHP.
18. Open the saved file from the previously collected NHP respiratory data. Average the data from the recoded data to obtain an average minute ventilation.
19. The minute ventilation value determines the duration of the challenge to achieve the target dose. The preferred duration of an aerosol exposure is 10–30 min to achieve an adequate dosing strategy with a uniform aerosol concentration within the aerosol exposure chamber.

20. A recirculating nebulizer is the generator used for small particles (ranging from 1 to 3 μm). No glycerol is added to the starting concentration.
21. The generator will be filled with fresh Nipah virus starting concentration for every run of the challenge. Each run tube of virus must be kept on wet ice when not in use. ~10 mL of virus solution will be enough for a 30-min aerosolization with a flow rate of 7.5 L per minute.
22. The preferred biosampler for this application uses a 3-orifice swirling mechanism which preserves pathogen integrity and viability. Prior and post-storage conditions require the media to be kept on wet ice.
23. Adequate depth of anesthesia is defined as unresponsive to external stimuli with muscular tone and stable respiratory and heart rates. Verify the NHP's vital signs with a portable subject monitor.
24. The rubber/dental dam creates a seal around the NHP's neck during the exposure thus ensuring the system always remains sealed during the process.
25. Information and parameters obtained from several pre-characterization studies using only Nipah virus without NHPs. Challenge times are determined by the plethysmography rates and target dose just prior to the exposure.
26. The aerodynamic particle sizer uses 5 L per min of vacuum to operate and will potentially affect the flow rates unless adjusted by the aerosol system. The automated aerosol system does monitor the flow rate and adjusts accordingly.
27. The appropriate disinfectant wipe for NHPs exposed to Nipah virus is 1–2% chlorhexidine solution.
28. A typical challenge run takes ~10–30 min to complete.
29. Typical biological assays following an aerosol exposure include viral plaque assay and RT-PCR.
30. Paraformaldehyde gas validated with biological indicators is the preferred method of decontamination for high-consequence pathogens at this facility.
31. A single use spinning disc generator is used for intermediate particles (6–8 μm) and large particles (10–14 μm). Glycerol is added to the starting concentration depending on the desired particle size. The more glycerol, the more viscous the solution and the larger the generated particles. Additionally, the speed of the spinning disc determines the size range with the faster the disc creating smaller-sized particles.

32. The spinning disc generator uses a syringe pump at a flow rate of 1 mL/min. The syringe is filled with the viral starting concentration for aerosolization.
33. The preferred biosampler of for this application uses a gelatin impaction filter minimizing particle movements and angled turns. Prior and post-storage conditions require the media to be kept on wet ice.
34. The aerodynamic particle sizer is directly connected to the head-only chamber to minimize the distance the intermediate/large particles travel.

Acknowledgments

The authors thank Jiro Wada and Fabian de Kok-Mercado for their medical illustrations and expertise, and Jeremy Boydston for his critical review of the content.

This work was funded in part through Battelle Memorial Institute's prime contract with the US National Institute of Allergy and Infectious Diseases (NIAID) under Contract No. HHSN272200700016I. The content of this publication does not necessarily reflect the views or policies of the US Department of Health and Human Services (DHHS) or of the institutions and companies affiliated with the authors.

References

1. Roy CJ, Reed DS (2012) Infectious disease aerobiology: miasma incarnate. Front Cell Infect Microbiol 2:163
2. Roy C, Pitt L (2006) Infectious disease aerobiology: aerosol challenge methods. Taylor & Francis Group, Boca Raton, pp 61–75
3. Roy CJ, Reed DS (2010) Aerobiology and inhalation exposure to biological select agents and toxins. Vet Pathol 47(5):779–789
4. Dabisch PA, Xu Z, Boydston JA, Solomon J, Bohannon JK, Yeager JJ, Taylor JR, Reeder RJ, Sayre P, Seidel J, Mollura DJ, Hevey MC, Jahrling PB, Lackemeyer MG (2017) Quantification of regional aerosol deposition patterns as a function of aerodynamic particle size in rhesus macaques using PET/CT imaging. Inhal Toxicol 11:506–515
5. Lackemeyer MG, de Kok-Mercado F, Wada J, Kindrachuk J, Wahl-Jensen V, Kuhn JH, Jahrling PB (2013) ABSL-4 aerobiology biosafety and technology at the NIH/NIAID integrated research Facility at Fort Detrick. Viruses 1: 137–150
6. Bohannon JK, Lackemeyer MG, Kuhn JH, Wada J, Bollinger L, Jahrling PB, Johnson RF (2015) Generation and characterization of large-particle aerosols using a center flow tangential aerosol generator with a non-human-primate, head-only aerosol chamber. Inhal Toxicol 27(5):247–253
7. Hartings JM, Roy CJ (2004) The automated bioaerosol exposure system: preclinical platform development and a respiratory dosimetry application with nonhuman primates. J Pharmacol Toxicol Methods 49(1):39–55
8. Bohannon JK, Honko AN, Reeder RJ, Cooper K, Byrum R, Bollinger L, Kuhn JH, Wada J, Qin J, Jahrling PB, Lackemeyer MG (2016) Comparison of respiratory inductive plethysmography versus head-out plethysmography for anesthetized nonhuman primates in an animal biosafety level 4 facility. Inhal Toxicol 14:670–676
9. Geisbert TW, Daddario-Dicaprio KM, Geisbert JB, Reed DS, Feldmann F, Grolla A, Stroher U, Fritz EA, Hensley LE, Jones SM (2008) Vesicular stomatitis virus-based

vaccines protect nonhuman primates against aerosol challenge with Ebola and Marburg viruses. Vaccine 26:6894–6900

10. Pratt WD, Wang D, Nichols DK, Luo M, Woraratanadharm J, Dye JM, Holman DH, Dong JY (2010) Protection of nonhuman primates against two species of Ebola virus infection with a single complex adenovirus vector. Clin Vaccine Immunol 17:572–581
11. Reed DS, Lind CM, Sullivan LJ, Pratt WD, Parker MD (2004) Aerosol infection of cynomolgus macaques with enzootic strains of Venezuelan equine encephalitis viruses. J Infect Dis 189:1013–1017
12. Reed DS, Lind CM, Lackemeyer MG, Sullivan LJ, Pratt WD, Parker MD (2005) Genetically engineered, live, attenuated vaccines protect nonhuman primates against aerosol challenge with a virulent IE strain of Venezuelan equine encephalitis virus. Vaccine 23:3139–3147
13. Glynn AR, Alves DA, Frick O, Erwin-Cohen R, Porter A, Norris S, Waag D, Nalca A (2016) Comparison of experimental respiratory tularemia in three nonhuman primate species. Comp Immunol Microbiol Infect Dis 39:13–24
14. Tree JA, Hall G, Pearson G, Rayner E, Graham VA, Steeds K, Bewley KR, Hatch GJ, Dennis M, Taylor I, Roberts AD, SGP F, Vipond J (2015) Sequence of pathogenic events in cynomolgus macaques infected with aerosolized Monkeypox virus. J Virol 89(8): 4335–4344
15. Reed DS, Bethel LM, Powell DS, Caroline AL, Hartman AL (2014) Differences in aerosolization of Rift Valley fever virus resulting from choice of inhalation exposure chamber: implications for animal challenge studies. Pathog Dis 71(2):227–233
16. Reed DS, Lackemeyer MG, Garza NL, Sullivan LJ, Nichols DK (2011) Aerosol exposure to Zaire ebolavirus in three nonhuman primate species: differences in disease course and clinical pathology. Microbes Infect 11:930–936
17. Johnson RF, Hammoud DA, Lackemeyer MG, Yellayi S, Solomon J, Bohannon JK, Janosko KB, Jett C, Cooper K, Blaney JE, Jahrling PB (2015) Small particle aerosol inoculation of cowpox Brighton Red in rhesus monkeys results in a severe respiratory disease. Virology 481:124–135
18. Alves DA, Glynn AR, Steele KE, Lackemeyer MG, Garza NL, Buck JG, Mech C, Reed DS (2010) Aerosol exposure to the Angola strain of Marburg virus causes lethal viral hemorrhagic fever in cynomolgus macaques. Vet Pathol 5:831–851
19. Hinds WC (1999) Particle size statistics. In: Aerosol technology: properties, behavior, and measurement of airborne particles, 2nd edn. Wiley, New York, pp 75–110
20. Druett HA, Henderson DW, Packman L, Peacock L, Peacock S (1953) Studies on respiratory infection. I. The influence of particle size on respiratory infection with anthrax spores. J Hyg (Lond) 51:359–371
21. Day WC, Berendt RF (1972) Experimental tularemia in Macaca mulatta: relationship of aerosol particle size to the infectivity of airborne Pasteurella tularensis. Infect Immun 5: 77–82
22. Chua KB, Bellini WJ, Rota PA, Harcourt BH, Tamin A, Lam SK, Ksiazek TG, Rollin PE, Zaki SR, Shieh W, Goldsmith CS, Gubler DJ, Roehrig JT, Eaton B, Gould AR, Olson J, Field H, Daniels P, Ling AE, Peters CJ, Anderson LJ, Mahy BW (2000) Nipah virus: a recently emergent deadly paramyxovirus. Science 288:1432–1435
23. Paton NI, Leo YS, Zaki SR, Auchus AP, Lee KE, Ling AE, Chew SK, Ang B, Rollin PE, Umapathi T, Sng I, Lee CC, Lim E, Ksiazek TG (1999) Outbreak of Nipah-virus infection among abattoir workers in Singapore. Lancet 354:1253–1256
24. Cong Y, Lentz MR, Lara A, Alexander I, Bartos C, Bohannon JK, Hammoud D, Huzella L, Jahrling PB, Janosko K, Jett C, Kollins E, Lackemeyer M, Mollura D, Ragland D, Rojas O, Solomon J, Xu Z, Munster V, Holbrook MR (2017) Loss in lung volume and changes in the immune response demonstrate disease progression in African green monkeys infected by small-particle aerosol and intratracheal exposure to Nipah virus. PLoS Negl Trop Dis 11(4): e0005532
25. Hammoud DA, Lentz MR, Lara A, Bohannon JK, Feurstein I, Huzella L, Jahrling PB, Lackemeyer M, Laux J, Rojas O, Sayre P, Solomon J, Cong Y, Munster V, Holbrook M (2018) Aerosol exposure to intermediate size Nipah virus particles induces neurological disease in African green monkeys. PLoS Negl Trop Dis 12:e0006978
26. Geisbert TW, Daddario-DiCaprio KM, Hickey AC, Smith MA, Chan YP, Wang LF, Mattapallil JJ, Geisbert JB, Bossart KN, Broder CC (2010) Development of an acute and highly pathogenic nonhuman primate model of Nipah virus infection. PLoS One 5(5):e10690
27. Johnston SC, Briese T, Bell TM, Pratt WD, Shamblin JD, Esham HL, Donnelly GC, Johnson JC, Hensley LE, Lipkin WI, Honko AN (2015) Detailed analysis of the African green

monkey model of Nipah virus disease. PLoS One 10(2):e0117817

28. Bohannon JK, Janosko K, Holbrook MR, Barr J, Pusl D, Bollinger L, Coe L, Hensley LE, Jahrling PB, Wada J, Kuhn JH, Lackemeyer MG (2016) Safety precautions and operating procedures in an (A)BSL-4 laboratory: 3. Aerobiology. J Vis Exp 116:53600
29. Lackemeyer MG, Kok-Mercado F, Wada J, Bollinger L, Kindrachuk J, Wahl-Jensen V, Kuhn JH, Jahrling PB (2014) ABSL-4 aerobiology biosafety and technology at the NIH/-NIAID integrated research facility at Fort Detrick. Viruses 6(1):137–150
30. Bohannon JK, Honko AN, Reeder RJ, Cooper K, Byrum R, Bollinger L, Kuhn JH, Wada J, Qin J, Jahrling PB, Lackemeyer MG (2016) Comparison of respiratory inductive plethysmography versus head-out plethysmography for anesthetized nonhuman primates in an animal biosafety level 4 facility. Inhal Toxicol 28(14):670–676
31. Besch TK, Ruble DL, Gibbs PH, Pitt MLM (1996) Steady-state minute volume determination by body-only plethysmography in juvenile rhesus monkeys. Lab Anim Sci 46(5):539–544

Chapter 14

Generation and Characterization of a Humanized Lung Xenograft Mouse Model for Studying Henipavirus Pathogenesis

Gustavo Valbuena, Barry Rockx, and Olivier Escaffre

Abstract

The development of humanized mouse models has recently opened new avenues in the field of infectious diseases. These models allow research on many human viruses that were once difficult to study, because finding suitable animal models of infection can be challenging, cost prohibitive, and often do not entirely recapitulate all parameters of the disease. Here, we describe the procedure of human immune system reconstitution (humanization) of NOD.Cg-Prkdc^{scid} Il2rg^{tm1Wjl}/SzJ (NSG) mice by the bone marrow, liver, and thymus (BLT) reconstitution method as well as the process of human lung engraftment. We then describe how to infect these human lung grafts with the paramyxovirus Nipah virus (NiV) that can cause lethal respiratory disease in humans, and for which there is only limited understanding of pathogenesis to acute lung injury.

Key words NSG mice, BLT reconstitution, Humanized mouse model, Human lung xenograft, Henipavirus, Immune response

1 Introduction

Severely immune-incompetent NOD.Cg-Prkdc^{scid} Il2rg^{tm1Wjl}/SzJ mice, also known as NOD/SCID/gamma or NSG mice, have been extensively used to study human diseases and virus pathogenesis [1–6], and offer multiple advantages using animal models that often do not entirely mimic disease of interest. NSG mice can support human tissue engraftment, such as a fetal lung graft sutured on the muscle fascia in the dorsal subcutaneous space, and maintain its microenvironment enabling evaluation of lung response and damage following, for example, Nipah virus (NiV) infection [7]. Generation of improved NSG mouse models allows to study more complex virus–human graft interactions by having a nearly complete functional human immune system through a process of engraftment of human CD34+ hematopoietic stem cells and tissues using the bone marrow, liver, and thymus (BLT) method

Alexander N. Freiberg and Barry Rockx (eds.), *Nipah Virus: Methods and Protocols*, Methods in Molecular Biology, vol. 2682, https://doi.org/10.1007/978-1-0716-3283-3_14, © Springer Science+Business Media, LLC, part of Springer Nature 2023

[8–16]. These improved NSG mice are known as humanized BLT mice, and after undergoing additional tissue engraftment, (e.g., fetal human lung), it becomes possible to evaluate the contribution of the immune system and the lung tissue in pathogenesis of respiratory viruses including NiV [17]. Here we describe a protocol for the preparation and surgery of NSG mice for human immune system reconstitution by the BLT method as well as for the engraftment of additional human lung tissues. We also detail how to verify immune system reconstitution post-surgery as well as describe how to infect these lung grafts with NiV and perform immunostaining for virus antigen and immune cells.

2 Material

2.1 Processing of Tissues for Grafting onto NSG Mice

1. Obtain human fetal tissues from an authorized source under institutional guidelines and in compliance with appropriate local and national laws, ethical principles, and regulations.
2. Isolation/wash buffer: Dulbecco's PBS (without Ca or Mg) containing 1 × Gibco's antibiotic–antimycotic mixture, 10 mM HEPES, 2% BGS, and 2 mM EDTA. Keep on ice.
3. Diprotin A solution: 15 mM in PBS: it will be used to resuspend hematopoietic stem cells (HSCs) so animals will receive 200 μL (which is 4.5 μmol).
4. Sterile forceps and scissors.
5. Sterile arm with blade for McIllwain Tissue Chopper.
6. DNAse.
7. 10% Bleach solution.
8. Controlled-rate cell freezing system.
9. Serum-based freezing medium: Mix 90% warm Bovine growth serum (BGS) with 10% DMSO by adding the DMSO to the serum very slowly as you swirl the medium. It needs to be brought to 4 °C because cells do not tolerate DMSO higher than 0.5% at higher temperatures.
10. OKT3 monoclonal antibody diluted to 2 mg/mL solutions in sterile PBS containing 2% BGS. Produce 0.5 mL aliquots.
11. McIllwain Tissue Chopper.
12. Dounce homogenizer with A and B pestles.

2.2 Tissue Grafting onto NSG Mice and Care of NSG Mice

1. Parenteral Antibiotics: Azithromycin dose per mouse is 300 μg/0.2 mL, Levofloxacin is 300 μg/0.2 mL (*see* **Note 1**).
2. Post-surgical drinking water with antibiotics (to be used for 2 weeks after surgery). Adjust water to pH 3.0 with

concentrated HCl, autoclave, and sterilely transfer to bottles. Then add the following combination of antibiotics.

- Azithromycin: 100 mg/mL after reconstitution.
- Levofloxacin: Levaquin injection 500 mg in 20 mL.

3. Maintenance drinking water after 2 weeks of water with antibiotics above will consist of only acidified water.
4. Mice will be kept on food with bactrim or bactrim+carprofen (rimadyl). One possible source is BioServ (*see* **Note 2**).
5. Pre-surgical analgesia: slow release formulation of buprenorphine. Use at 1 mg/kg.
6. Post-surgical analgesia: diet (e.g., BioServ) containing Bactrim and Rimadyl. Alternatively, buprenorphine, p.o. (0.14 mg/ 300 mL drinking water) (*see* **Note 3**).
7. Certified irradiator for use with animals (cesium or X-ray source).
8. Isoflurane vaporized for use with rodents.
9. Numbered ear tags for mice.
10. Depilatory cream.
11. Ophthalmic ointment.
12. Blood collection buffer: PBS containing 3 mg/mL EDTA and 1 U/mL heparin.

2.3 NiV Infection of NSG Mice

Inoculation of NiV in recipient mice is performed under a biosafety cabinet (BSC) class 2 type A2. All equipment and veterinary instruments used to prepare virus inoculum, inject virus, and handle animals during the infection process or necropsy are sterile. Some are directly provided sterile by the manufacturers. Sterilization of instruments can be otherwise achieved by autoclaving at a temperature of 121 °C for at least 30 min by using saturated steam under at least 15 psi of pressure.

1. 5% MicroChem.
2. 70% ethanol.
3. Phosphate-buffered saline (PBS).
4. 15 mL conical tubes.
5. 200 μL pipettes.
6. 200 μL tips.
7. 1 mL syringes.
8. 27-gauge × 1″ needles.
9. Waste pan.
10. Sharp container.
11. Ice.

12. Anesthesia apparatus for the anesthesia procedures includes gas mixer, vaporizer, induction chamber, nose cones, tubing, and isoflurane or other approved anesthetics by your institution. Forceps are required to handle the animals. The induction chamber and nose cone need to be thoroughly decontaminated as they are under the BSC in direct contact with the animals. The hose only need to be surface decontaminated.

2.4 Euthanasia and Necropsy of NSG Mice

1. Euthanasia and necropsy of animals are performed in an animal procedure room that is equipped with a downdraft table.
2. The same anesthesia apparatus is used for euthanasia.
3. Operating scissors.
4. Forceps.
5. 5 mL syringes.
6. 23-gauge × 1″ needles.
7. Repetitive dispensing pipette such as Stepper™ series dispensing pipettes.

2.5 Processing of Human Lung Grafts

1. 10% neural-buffered formalin. The formalin fixative solution can be prepared from mixing one part of a saturated (37%) formaldehyde solution to nine parts of deionized water. Neutral pH is then obtained by adding sodium phosphate (4 g/L of NaH2PO4 and 6.5 g/L Na2HPO4).
2. 50 mL leak-proof containers.
3. Operating scissors.
4. Forceps.
5. 1 mL pipettes.
6. 1 mL tips.
7. Clear safe-lock 2 mL microcentrifuge tubes.
8. Phosphate-buffered saline (PBS).
9. Acid-guanidinium-phenol reagent such as TRI Reagent® or TRIzol®.
10. Sterile stainless steel beads, 5 mm.
11. Tissue homogenization equipment such as TissueLyser® with two 48 samples adapters.
12. Benchtop centrifuge.

3 Method

Use procedures approved by your institution to work with human tissues and fluids. All equipment and instruments are sterile. Some are directly provided sterile by the manufacturers. Sterilization of instruments can be otherwise achieved by autoclaving at a temperature of 121 °C for at least 30 min by using saturated steam under at least 15 psi of pressure.

All procedures with cells, tissues, and animals must be performed in a sterile environment. We recommend using a cage-changing station with laminar flow and opening on both sides to facilitate work standing up with one surgeon on each side. Procedures with mice must be approved by your local Institutional Animal Care and Use Committee. Surgical tables for mice should be temperature controlled at 37°C.

Animals can be engrafted with only human lung if the focus of interest is in analyzing the interaction between human target tissues and NiV, as we have done in the past [7]. If that is the case, begin with Subheading 3.5, disregard Subheading 3.8, and ignore specific steps related to HSCs grafting in other sections. If there is interest in producing a fully humanized model with human leucocytes, all sections and steps are relevant.

3.1 Preparation of OKT3 Antibody Solution

1. The antibody is injected I.P. (8 mg/kg: ~200 μg/mouse; each aliquot is sufficient for 10 mice) or incubated with cells in suspension on ice for at least 30 min at a concentration of at least 1 μg/1 million white blood cells (WBCs).
2. If tissues are to be frozen before implantation, prepare 15 mL of serum-based freezing medium with 250 μL of OKT3 (final concentration is 33.33 μg/mL). Transfer from 15 mL tube to one 5 mL tube to make dispensing easy without contaminating.
3. If tissues will be implanted fresh, prepare similarly but using wash buffer instead. For the day of surgery, prepare the rest of the same OKT3 aliquot (250 μL) in 15 mL of PBS with 2% BGS and Diprotin A (15 mM).

3.2 Processing of Human Thymus

1. Wash the thymus in ice-cold isolation/wash buffer by filling a tube, gently mixing, and carefully decanting. Repeat five times; this is to minimize microbial contamination, which would be present mainly on the surface.
2. Place the entire thymus inside a petri dish with ice-cold isolation/wash buffer on top of an ice-cold metal block. Trim and discard any tissues outside the capsule.
3. Cut small pieces for implantation (about 1.5 mm^3) and count the total number of pieces.
4. Transfer fragments to 0.5 mL cryotubes preloaded with 0.3 mL of medium with OKT3 so that each one has 11–12 thymus fragments (keep them ice-cold); each one of these tubes will be sufficient for 10 mice (1–2 additional fragments

in case of difficulties with surgical implantation). The final tube may have fewer fragments; label accordingly.

5. Freeze to −80°C according to protocol used for cells with your device of preference. We follow the protocol described by Yoyokama et al. [18].
6. The day of grafting surgery, thaw thymus rapidly and keep on ice [18].
7. Wash once by centrifuging at 200×g × 1 min and change medium to isolation/wash buffer. Transfer to 6-well plate and add 0.5 mL of buffer containing OKT3 antibody for the contents of one tube (multiply by number of tubes to be used).

3.3 Processing of Human Liver

1. Wash the liver in ice-cold isolation/wash buffer by filling the tube, gently mixing, and carefully decanting. Repeat five times.
2. Place the entire liver inside a petri dish with ice-cold isolation/wash buffer on top of an ice-cold metallic block or another ice-cold surface.
3. Cut small pieces for implantation (about 2 mm^3). Produce at least as many fragments as thymus fragments.
4. Process these fragments in a similar way as the thymus (*see* Subheading 3.2).
5. Process the rest of the liver with a McIllwain Tissue Chopper to 0.3 mm^3 fragments.
6. Centrifuge at 70×g × 3 min and save supernatant.
7. Transfer pelleted fragments to a Dounce homogenizer and process with pestle A only. Transfer to a 15-mL conical tube, centrifuge as above, save supernatant, and process remaining tissue fragments, if needed.
8. Pool with saved supernatants and filter through a 70-μm filter mounted on a 50-mL conical tube.
9. Pellet cells at 400×g × 8 min and aspirate supernatant.
10. Resuspend in a volume of OKT3 solution equivalent to number of thymus tubes ×0.5 mL and distribute among an equal number of 1.5 mL cryotubes kept ice-cold; label as HSCs (hematopoietic stem cells).
11. Incubate at 4°C for at least 30–45 min; mix gently every 6–8 min.
12. Take an aliquot to count cells (note number to know how many cells will be given to each mouse).
13. Freeze according to the standard protocol [18].
14. Also, thaw HSCs rapidly (according to the same protocol used for cells [18]) and keep on ice. Add an equal volume of wash buffer and then wash twice with ice-cold PBS-2% BGS; pellet at

$200 \times g \times 8$ min. If viscous, resuspend pellets in 1 mL of PBS-2% BGS containing 20 μg/mL DNAse and incubate at room temperature for 30 min.

15. Pellet cells from each tube at $200 \times g \times 10$ min and resuspend in 1.1 mL of OKT3-PBS 2% BGS containing Diprotin A (15 mM) to give 200 μL to each one of 5 mice per tube, and keep on ice.

3.4 Processing of Human Bone

1. Clean all long bones and vertebral bodies from adjacent tissues.
2. Wash bones in ice-cold isolation/wash buffer by filling the tube, gently mixing, and carefully decanting. Repeat 3–5 times.
3. Separate cortical bone from bone marrow by cutting bones open with bone cutters and scrapping off the bone marrow. Cut the bone marrow in small fragments for kidney implantation (produce at least as many fragments as thymus fragments).
4. Process following the same procedures as the thymus (*see* Subheading 3.2).
5. The day of surgery, thaw and wash tissues in a similar manner as the thymus (*see* Subheading 3.2), transfer to a well of the same 6-well plate containing the washed fragments of thymus and liver.

3.5 Processing of Human Lung

1. Dissect out the central areas containing large vessels and bronchi. Cut into thin fragments that expose the parenchyma (about $0.5 \times 0.5 \times 0.3$ cm). If needed for other experiments, separately dissect central airways.
2. Suspend in serum-based freezing medium with OKT3 antibody solution and keep on ice for 1 h to allow medium to penetrate tissues before freezing following the same procedure as in Subheading 3.2.
3. The day of surgery, thaw and wash tissues in a similar manner as the thymus, transfer to a well of the same 6-well plate containing the washed fragments of thymus, liver, and bone.

3.6 Pre-surgical Procedures

If animals are to be grafted with HSCs in addition to human lung, they must be irradiated 24–48 h before grafting procedures.

1. Anesthetize recipient mice with Isofluorane (vaporizer at ~2.5%).
2. Inject slow-release formulation of buprenorphine, s.c., in the ventral aspect of the abdomen.
3. Inject 0.2 mL of antibiotic parenteral solution subcutaneously in a separate site of the abdomen.
4. Tag mice with numbered tags.

5. Shave an area bounded cranial-caudal by the neck and iliac crest and dorsal-ventral by the spine and lower third of thorax and abdominal wall (both sides).
6. Add depilatory cream with sterile cotton swabs, leave for 30 s and then clean with gauze and 70% ethanol.
7. Once mice are awake and active again, irradiate at a dose of 200 cGy.
8. Return mice to animal facility.

3.7 Surgical Grafting of Tissues onto NSG Mice

1. Anesthetize mice as above and place ophthalmic ointment on eyes.
2. Inject 0.2 mL of antibiotic parenteral solution subcutaneously.
3. Place mouse in ventral recumbent position.
4. Prepare surgical site by disinfection of the skin. Disinfect with gauzes dipped in iodine (hold with sterile forceps); apply swab with 70% ethanol to clean the iodine and dry with sterile gauze.
5. Make a 2.5-cm linear incision on the mouse skin along the midline and produce a subcutaneous pocket by blunt dissection.
6. Make a 4–7-mm incision in the abdominal wall over the midline. This location will allow to access either kidney with the same skin incision.
7. Elevate the right kidney through the incision in the abdominal wall by pulling with ring forceps (set separation of forceps to about 3–4 mm) while at the same time depressing the adjacent abdominal wall under the kidney using forceps. The kidney should be grabbed from the area around the hilum and not from the middle because this will fracture the kidney.
8. Dry the renal capsule with sterile gauze, sterile cotton swab or just by letting it be exposed to room air.
9. While the renal capsule dries, grab one small fragment of human bone marrow, one of liver, and one of thymus, and place them next to the kidney so you are ready to implant them after incising the capsule.
10. Use a small and sharp hook to make a small incision on the kidney capsule.
11. Grab the edge of the incision with small blunt forceps and pull capsule up.
12. Implant the thymus first followed by liver and bone marrow fragments using another pair of blunt forceps between the open renal capsule and the renal cortical parenchyma.
13. Return kidney to its anatomical position. You can either increase the size of the wall incision or use ring forceps to

guide the kidney back inside while holding the abdominal wall with forceps in order to avoid contact with the graft area so that the implant is not displaced as the kidney returns inside the cavity.

14. Inject all HSCs (resuspended in 200 μL of PBS containing diprotin A, 15 mM), 100 μL i.v., 50 μL in the liver, and 50 μL i.m. (*see* **Note 4**).
15. Suture the incision in the abdominal wall with at least two 4–0 or 5–0 absorbable sutures.
16. Suture one small fragment of human fetal lung to the muscle mass adjacent to the lumbar spine on each side.
17. Close skin incision with staples. Apply supplemental tissue adhesive (e.g., VetBond) to the suture line and the surgical staples.
18. If procedure is long and/or there is bleeding, administer 1 cc of warm saline or PBS, s.c.
19. Place mouse in a box on top of a heated pad. Observe until mobile.
20. Provide oral antibiotics in the water for 2 weeks post-operatively and diet containing bactrim and rimadyl.
21. Label cage with surgical procedure and initials of the surgeon. Follow institutional rules for record-keeping.
22. One week after injection of HSCs, inject (i.p. or i.v.) 200 μg of OKT3 monoclonal antibody.
23. Continue diet with only bactrim-containing pellets.

3.8 Analysis of HSC Grafting

1. Eight weeks after irradiation and xenotransplantation, anesthetize recipient mice with Isofluorane (vaporizer at ~2.5%).
2. Place a sterile glass Pasteur pipette at the medial canthus of the eye and thrust it past the eyeball to pass through the slightly resistant membrane of the retro-orbital sinus.
3. Collect 0.1–0.3 mL blood from humanized mice into 0.5 mL of blood collection buffer. Mix well but gently.
4. Withdraw the pipette and apply pressure with a piece of gauze on the eyeball for about 30 s to stop bleeding.
5. Process blood sample to perform staining and flow cytometry analysis for mouse CD45 and human CD3, CD45, and CD20 in order to determine the level of chimerism of each mouse. The specific staining and cytometric analysis procedure are beyond the scope of this protocol. They can be consulted from sources such as Current Protocols in Cytometry. The levels of reconstitution with human leukocytes are variable

within the same cohort of animals, generally ranging from 10% to 70% [17].

3.9 NiV Infection

NiV is a risk group 4 agent, and all experiments conducted with this virus are carried out at biosafety level 4. Obey federal and state laws and your institution policies, regulations and rules regarding proper handling, inactivation methods, and disposal of the agent. Follow all waste disposal regulations when disposing non-infectious waste materials as well. The housing, care, handling, and euthanasia of animals must be conforming to standards specified in "The Guide for the Care and Use of Laboratory Animals," Animal Welfare Regulations, and the institution ethics and IACUC committees. Personnel must be trained and signed off for each procedure.

1. Of the 12-week post-engraftment, animals are transferred to an animal biosafety level 4 (ABSL4) facility for challenge with NiV.
2. Surface decontaminate all equipment needed and cage prior placing them in the BSC. Prepare the virus inoculum on ice. Carefully open the cage and transfer the recipient mice with the use of forceps in the anesthesia induction chamber sitting on a heat pad. Anesthesia is performed using a vaporizer releasing 5 L/min 100% O_2 and 2% of isoflurane. Visual monitoring of optimal/deep anesthesia signs includes breath rate of the animal dropping to 55–65 breaths per minute, with no gasping, and no response to pinching leg extremities. Do not proceed to infection if still at a light anesthesia stage as indicated by breath rate above 70 breaths per min.
3. Infection of the recipient mice. NiV master stock was provided by the Special Pathogens Branch (Centers for Disease Control and Prevention, Atlanta, GA, USA).
   (a) Intravenous (i.v.) inoculation of NiV: Remove one mouse at a time from the induction chamber and place the mouse flat on another heat pad while still maintaining anesthesia with the help of a nose cone connected to the anesthesia machine. Hold the tail straight and inoculate 100 μL (10^5TCID$_{50}$) of NiV in a buffered saline solution into the lateral tail vein using a 1-mL syringe and 27-gauge × 1″ needle. Dispose the syringe and needle into the sharp container in the BSC when done.
   (b) Intragraft (i.g.) inoculation of NiV: Remove one mouse at a time from the induction chamber and place the mouse flat on a heat pad. This procedure does not require to maintain anesthesia unless more than two grafts per subject need to be infected. Localize the grafts under the skin, secure one at a time with forceps, and directly inoculate 50 μL (10^5TCID$_{50}$) of NiV in a buffered saline solution

through the skin into each graft using a 1 mL syringe and 27-gauge × 1″ needle. Dispose the syringe and needle into a sharp container placed under the BSC.

(c) Intraperitoneal (i.p.) inoculation of NiV: Remove one mouse at a time from the induction chamber and use the one-handed mouse restraint technique to proceed to infection. Firmly grasp the mouse by the scruff, paying attention not to pull the skin around the neck too tightly that the animal cannot breathe. While holding the mouse vertically, use a 1-mL syringe with 27-gauge × 1″ needle inserted into a repetitive fluid dispensing pipette, to inject 100 μL ($10^5 TCID_{50}$) of NiV in a buffered saline solution into the abdominal cavity penetrating the peritoneum of the mouse. Dispose the syringe and needle into a sharp container under the BSC.

(d) Intranasal (i.n.) inoculation: While holding the mouse vertically, use a pipette with a 200-μL tip size, and place a drop of NiV in a buffered saline solution by each nostril of the animal. Watch for the inoculum to be inhaled and repeat as necessary until 50 μL ($10^5 TCID_{50}$) per nostril has been administered.

4. Once NiV inoculation is completed, each mouse will be placed into its original cage and observed until it recovers from anesthesia. Animals are then monitored daily for weight loss and clinical signs of disease, including ataxia, scruffy coat, hunched posture, lethargy, irregular breathing, seizure, and paralysis. Animals are humanely sacrificed at predetermined time points for the purpose of the study.

3.10 Euthanasia and Necropsy of Animals

Termination of animals is performed in the animal procedure room. Disinfect surfaces of the work area with MicroChem and then ethanol. The procedure is performed with mice on bench pads.

1. Using forceps, animals are first placed into the induction chamber for isoflurane anesthesia overdose (5 L/min 100% O_2 and 5% of isoflurane). Visual signs of a too deep anesthesia/overdose are animal gasping with breath rate under 50 breaths/min. One animal at a time is then placed on its back, and while still under deep/overdose isoflurane anesthesia using the nose cone accessory, proceed to terminal bleed via cardiac puncture with a 5-mL syringe and 23-gauge × 1″ needle. Place the needle, bevel up, into the chest to puncture the heart. Apply slight back pressure with the syringe to collect as much blood as possible.
2. The animal is finally place on its stomach for cervical dislocation. Firmly grasp the base of the tail with one hand. Using the other hand, place a closed scissor against the neck at the base of

the skull. Simultaneously push forward with the scissor restraining the head and pull backward with the hand holding the tail. Confirm death by checking for respiratory arrest or cardiac arrest after performing chest opening using scissors and forceps.

3.11 Graft Sampling and Processing

1. Once animals are euthanized, use scissors and forceps to make an incision immediately above each graft. Gently dissect the surrounding connective tissues and harvest the graft.
2. Section the graft into three equal pieces.
   (a) Place one piece in a leak-proof container with fresh 10% neutral-buffered formalin for the purpose of histochemistry/immunohistochemistry. Use 10 parts formalin to one part tissue ratio (vol/wt) and store at room temperature. Total sample size must be smaller than 1 cm^3. Transfer the tissue after a minimum of 24 h into a clean container with fresh 10% formalin. Tissue can be further processed after an additional 48 h of fixation. All subsequent steps following formalin fixation are performed at biosafety level 2.
   (b) Place one piece in a sterile 2-mL microcentrifuge tube for the purpose of either virus titration or virus genome isolation. Do not use more than 5 mg tissue per tube. Add 500 μL of sterile PBS (infectious virus titration) or 1 mL of acid-guanidinium-phenol reagent (virus genome extraction), and one sterile 5-mm stainless steel bead per tube (*see* **Note 5**). Load the tube into the tissue lyser and run for 5 min at 25–50 Hz to disrupt the tissue and homogenize the lysate. Centrifuge the lysate at $6000 \times g \times 4$ min at 4 °C and save the clarified PBS- or phenol-based supernatant to respectively titer infectious virus and to recover virus genome. Virus titration is done at biosafety level 4 by either plaque assay [19] or $TCID_{50}$ [20]. All subsequent steps following lysis of tissue in acid-guanidinium-phenol reagent are performed at biosafety level 2. Virus genome purification can be performed by either the acid-guanidinium-phenol-chloroform extraction [21, 22] or the spin column-based nucleic acid purification [23] method.

4 Notes

1. Doses for post-surgical drinking water with antibiotics were calculated based on average daily consumption of 6 mL of water. In addition, we house 5 mice per cage and the water bottles contain 250–300 mL of water.

2. Medicated diets are formulated based on an intake of 5 g/mouse/day. Thus, for a cage with 5 mice, you will need $25g \times 7$ days $= 175$ g of food for 1 week.
3. The diet with bactrim + rimadyl will be used for only 1 week. After that, use only the diet with bactrim.
4. The number of HSCs is not precise. It depends on the gestational age of the fetus and individual factors that cannot be controlled. In our experience, we have obtained excellent human HSC grafting by following the protocol without attention to the specific number of cells.
5. Use chilled PBS and precooled tissuelyser adapters to avoid heating up samples.

References

1. Agliano A, Martin-Padura I, Mancuso P et al (2008) Human acute leukemia cells injected in NOD/LtSz-scid/IL-2Rgamma null mice generate a faster and more efficient disease compared to other NOD/scid-related strains. Int J Cancer 123:2222–2227
2. Arnold L, Tyagi RK, Meija P et al (2011) Further improvements of the P. falciparum humanized mouse model. PLoS One 6:e18045. 3069031
3. Foreman O, Kavirayani AM, Griffey SM, Reader R, Shultz LD (2011) Opportunistic bacterial infections in breeding colonies of the NSG mouse strain. Vet Pathol 48:495–499. 3101569
4. Racki WJ, Covassin L, Brehm M et al (2010) NOD-scid IL2rgamma(null) mouse model of human skin transplantation and allograft rejection. Transplantation 89:527–536. 2901915
5. Sanchez PV, Perry RL, Sarry JE et al (2009) A robust xenotransplantation model for acute myeloid leukemia. Leukemia 23:2109–2117. 3659827
6. Zhang L, Meissner E, Chen J, Su L (2010) Current humanized mouse models for studying human immunology and HIV-1 immunopathogenesis. Sci China Life Sci 53:195–203. 4224686
7. Valbuena G, Halliday H, Borisevich V, Goez Y, Rockx B (2014) A human lung xenograft mouse model of Nipah virus infection. PLoS Pathog 10:e1004063. 3974875
8. Berges BK, Rowan MR (2011) The utility of the new generation of humanized mice to study HIV-1 infection: transmission, prevention, pathogenesis, and treatment. Retrovirology 8:65. 3170263
9. Bird BH, Spengler JR, Chakrabarti AK et al (2016) Humanized mouse model of Ebola virus disease mimics the immune responses in human disease. J Infect Dis 213:703–711. 4747627
10. Calderon VE, Valbuena G, Goez Y et al (2013) A humanized mouse model of tuberculosis. PLoS One 8:e63331. 3656943
11. Lee J, Brehm MA, Greiner D, Shultz LD, Kornfeld H (2013) Engrafted human cells generate adaptive immune responses to Mycobacterium bovis BCG infection in humanized mice. BMC Immunol 14:53. 3924189
12. Morton JJ, Bird G, Refaeli Y, Jimeno A (2016) Humanized mouse xenograft models: narrowing the tumor-microenvironment gap. Cancer Res 76:6153
13. Nusbaum RJ, Calderon VE, Huante MB et al (2016) Pulmonary tuberculosis in humanized mice infected with HIV-1. Sci Rep 6:21522. 4808832
14. Smith DJ, Lin LJ, Moon H et al (2016) Propagating humanized BLT mice for the study of human immunology and immunotherapy. Stem Cells Dev 25:1863
15. Spengler JR, Lavender KJ, Martellaro C et al (2016) Ebola virus replication and disease without immunopathology in mice expressing transgenes to support human myeloid and lymphoid cell engraftment. J Infect Dis 214:S308
16. Stoddart CA, Maidji E, Galkina SA et al (2011) Superior human leukocyte reconstitution and susceptibility to vaginal HIV transmission in humanized NOD-scid IL-2Rgamma(-/-) (NSG) BLT mice. Virology 417:154–160. 3152643
17. Escaffre O, Saito TB, Juelich TL et al (2017) Contribution of human lung parenchyma and

leukocyte influx to oxidative stress and immune system-mediated pathology following Nipah virus infection. J Virol 91:e00275-17. 5651721

18. Yokoyama WM, Thompson ML, Ehrhardt RO (2012) Cryopreservation and thawing of cells. Curr Protoc Immunol Appendix 3:3G
19. Cooper PD (1961) The plaque assay of animal viruses. Adv Virus Res 8:319–378
20. Reed LJMH (1938) A simple method of estimating fifty per cent endpoints. Am J Hyg 27: 493–497
21. Chomczynski P, Sacchi N (1987) Single-step method of RNA isolation by acid guanidinium thiocyanate-phenol-chloroform extraction. Anal Biochem 162:156–159
22. Chomczynski P, Sacchi N (2006) The single-step method of RNA isolation by acid guanidinium thiocyanate-phenol-chloroform extraction: twenty-something years on. Nat Protoc 1:581–585
23. Boom R, Sol CJ, Salimans MM, Jansen CL, Wertheim-van Dillen PM, van der Noordaa J (1990) Rapid and simple method for purification of nucleic acids. J Clin Microbiol 28:495–503. 269651

Chapter 15

Ferret Models for Henipavirus Infection

Barry Rockx and Chad E. Mire

Abstract

Henipaviruses are emerging zoonotic viruses that can cause outbreaks of severe respiratory and neurological disease in humans and animals such as horses. The mechanism by which these viruses can cause disease remain largely unknown and to date there are no therapeutics or vaccines approved for use in humans. Nipah virus is listed on the World Health Organization R & D Blueprint list of epidemic threats. In order to advance the availability of effective therapeutics and vaccines and medicines that can be used to save lives and avert large scale crises, animal models are required which recapitulate the disease progression in humans. Ferrets are highly susceptible to infection with henipaviruses and develop both severe respiratory and neurological disease. Therefore, the ferret model is highly suitable for studies into both the pathogenesis of henipaviruses, as well as pre-clinical evaluation of intervention strategies.

Key words Henipavirus, Ferret, Vaccination, Treatment

1 Introduction

Hendra (HeV) and Nipah (NiV) viruses are emerging zoonotic viruses within the genus henipavirus, family of *Paramyxoviridae*, that can cause severe acute respiratory and neurological disease in humans with an average case-fatality rate of 57% [1]. Transmission of henipaviruses primarily occurs through direct contact with infected animals (swine, horse), consumption of contaminated date palm sap, and direct contact with human cases [2–5]. To date, no vaccines or therapeutics have been approved for use in humans. Although no licensed vaccine or therapeutic is available for human use, several candidates are currently in development, including a human monoclonal antibody, recombinant protein vaccines, and several vectored vaccine candidates including vesicular stomatitis virus, rabies virus, and chimpanzee adenovirus [6–10].

Understanding the pathogenesis of henipaviruses in relevant animal models, which recapitulate the disease seen in humans, is important for the evaluation of the efficacy of vaccine and therapeutic candidates. This is particularly true for highly virulent

Alexander N. Freiberg and Barry Rockx (eds.), *Nipah Virus: Methods and Protocols*, Methods in Molecular Biology, vol. 2682, https://doi.org/10.1007/978-1-0716-3283-3_15,

viruses, for which human efficacy trials are not feasible or ethical, such as for henipaviruses. The United States Food and Drug Administration (FDA) has established an "Animal Rule," (described in the FDA Code of Federal Regulations CFR 21314.600), which states that a product can be licensed through substantial evidence of effectiveness shown in one or more well-characterized animal models that are expected to react with a response predictive for humans [11].

Several animal models of experimental infection have been proposed to study henipavirus infection in vivo [12]. Experimental infections in cats [13], guinea pigs, and mice do not develop the full spectrum of pathological features observed in the human disease, whereas Syrian hamsters, ferrets, and African green monkeys (AGM) develop both severe respiratory and neurological disease [13–19]. While hamsters do recapitulate both respiratory and neurological diseases, their use in evaluating responses to vaccines and therapeutics is limited due to a lack of reagents. Alternatively, non-human primates, specifically AGM, are considered the gold standard for evaluating intervention strategies; however, their use is limited by ethical and financial constraints. Ferrets are widely used as experimental models of infection for a variety of respiratory viruses including influenza, due to the recapitulation of key pathological features observed in human infections [20]. In case of experimental henipavirus infection in ferrets, the animals develop severe respiratory and neurological disease. The ferret model has not only been used to study the clinical and pathological aspects of henipavirus infection but also to study other relevant aspects such as virus shedding, transmission studies, and efficacy testing of vaccines and therapeutics [6, 16, 21–23]. The use of ferrets as experimental models of infection has increased following the availability of the ferret transcriptome which has facilitated host gene expression analysis in this animal model [24, 25].

Here, we describe a ferret model to consider for therapeutic or vaccine studies and how to conduct these henipavirus countermeasure evaluation studies.

2 Materials

2.1 Requirements to Work with Henipaviruses in Ferrets

1. Laboratory space for work at animal biosafety level 4 (ABSL4) approval to work with henipaviruses in ferrets from the U.S. Centers for Disease Control and Prevention (CDC) or equivalent.
2. Approval to work with henipaviruses in ferrets from the U.S. Centers for Disease Control and Prevention (CDC) or equivalent.

3. Approval from the Institution/University, or equivalent, to work with henipaviruses in ferrets at ABSL4.
4. Institutional Animal Care and Use Committee (IACUC), or equivalent, approval to work with ferrets at ABSL4.
5. Staff that has been trained and approved to work with henipavirus infected ferrets at ABSL4.

2.2 General

1. Virus stocks of NiV or HeV.
2. Ferrets (*Mustela putorius furo*), male or female, 0.750–1.000 kg (18–22 weeks in age).
3. Animal medical record (AMR) for each individual ferret under study.
4. Cage to socially house ferrets with dimensions recommended in the National Research Council's *Guide for the Care and Use of Laboratory Animals* eighth edition [26] or equivalent.
5. Ferret chow.
6. Environmental enrichment such as hides and chew toys.
7. Down draft table or biosafety cabinet (BSC) for procedures.
8. Versi-Dry lab soaker, or equivalent absorbent bench pads.
9. Lab animal identification (ID) information chip and temperature monitor.
10. Bio Medics Data Systems (BMDS) lab animal ID chip reader; or equivalent.
11. Scale for weights.
12. Gauze.
13. Rubbing alcohol or equivalent disinfectant.
14. Anesthetic, such as KAX [Ketamine (35–50 mg/Kg); Acepromazine (0.75 mg/Kg); Xylazine (5 mg/Kg)] or isoflurane at continuous flow up to 5% by volume.
15. Sharps containers.
16. Stainless steel mesh hand glove.
17. Leather hand glove to go over stainless steel mesh glove.
18. Clippers; to shave fur.
19. Forceps.
20. Clinical observation sheet (Table 1).
21. Clinical score sheet (Table 2).

2.3 Inoculation of Ferrets

1. Hank's Balanced Salt Solution (1×) supplemented up to 2% Certified Heat-inactivated Fetal Bovine Serum (2% FBS-HBSS).
2. 15 mL and 50 mL conical tubes.

Table 1
Clinical Observations Sheet for Henipavirus in Ferrets

IACUC Protocol #		Virus
Ferret ID#: Gender:		
Day	Day 0; [Actual date]	Day 1; [Actual date] Add more columns as needed
Weight		
Chip Temperature		
Depression		
Weakness		
Hunched Posture		
Unresponsive		
Dyspnea		
Nasal Exudate		
Ocular Exudate		
Head and Neck Edema		
Ventral Neck rash		
Tremors		
Paresis		

Back of the page used for specific comments about observations

3. Disposable 1 mL "Luer lock" syringes.
4. Disposable 25 gauge needles.

2.4 Vaccination, Treatment, Sampling of Ferrets

1. Vaccine or therapeutic.
2. 1 mL up to 5 mL "Luer lock" syringes.
3. Disposable 25 gauge needles and 23 gauge intravenous needles.
4. Mini-collect blood collection tubes appropriate for the desired analyses and volume:

   K_2-EDTA: for viral load/immunoglobulin (Ig) analysis/hematology.

   Serum Separator: for viral load/Ig analysis/blood chemistries

   Lithium Heparin: for peripheral blood mononuclear cell (PBMC) preparation/Ig analysis/plasma analysis.
5. Disposable "break-away" cotton tipped swabs.

Table 2
Clinical score sheet for henipavirus in ferrets

Parameter	Degree of parameter	Possible Score
Appearance	Normal	0#
	Reduced grooming	1
	Dull/rough coat and/or ocular dishcharge	2
	Absence of grooming, piloerection, hunched up	3
Skin	Normal	0
	Facial edma or cutaneous petechial hemorrhage	4
	Cutaneous ecchymosis	6
Behavior	Normal, Playing, Active, comes to cage front upon approach	0
	Mild lethargy, does not approach cage front without stimulation	2
	Lethargic, only active when stimulated	4
	Very weak, little to no response when stimulated*	9
Respiration	Normal	0
	Sneezing	1
	Increased or decreased respiration rate or coughing	3
	Occluding nasal discharge	6
	Overt respiratory distress/open mouth breathing*	9
Neurological Signs	Normal	0
	Ear or facial myoclonus	1
	Tremors	3
	Single limb paresis or ataxia	4
	Multi-limb paresis or seizures*	9
Total		#
Observer		
Time		

Bold* No matter the total score any ferret showing these clinical signs should be humanely euthanized
The maximum score for each category is up to the investigator and/or defined by their institutional policies
Date, time, and animal ID# should be on the score sheets as well

2.5 Euthanasia of Ferrets at Humane and Scientific Endpoints

1. Disposable 1 mL and 5 mL "Luer lock" syringes.
2. 23–25 gauge intravenous needles.
3. American Veterinary Medical Association (AVMA), or equivalent, approved euthanasia solution; typically, a pentobarbital sodium solution.

3 Methods

3.1 Vaccination

Depending on the vaccine platform, the vaccine regimen will be a prime only or prime-boost strategy where the ferrets are vaccinated and sampled for replication of the vaccine vector, detection of cell-mediated immune response, and detection of humoral immune response. This phase will typically last 21–56-day post-vaccination before exposure of the ferrets to henipaviruses.

1. Assess the ferrets for general health and behavior to see if they are fit for anesthesia and procedures.
2. Set up the procedure table and scale/tub with absorbent bench pads to work with the ferrets.
3. Place stainless steel mesh glove on hand and place leather glove over top of the stainless steel mesh glove.
4. Open the cage and coax a ferret to your leather gloved hand and remove it from the cage. Use the BMDS chip reader to ID and measure the temp of the ferret to get a reading pre-anesthesia. Using a partner, immobilize the ferret so that the thigh is available for i.m. injection of anesthetic (KAX) using a 25-gauge needle and syringe; place needle and syringe in sharps container. Alternatively, the ferret can be placed in an anesthesia box with isoflurane under continuous flow at 5% volume. If using isoflurane, a nose cone for continuous flow is placed over the ferret's nose during the procedures.
5. Once the ferret is sedated, it can be handled for weighing and placed on the procedure table. Assess overall health by observing the eyes, mucus membranes, fur, skin, and hydration status.
6. Place the ferret in dorsal recumbency and disinfect the ventral neck region for phlebotomy. Use a 23-gauge needle attached to a 3 mL "luer lock" syringe for blood collection. This is a "blind stick" where one inserts the needle just lateral of the manubrium and cranial to the first rib at a 45-degree angle toward the opposite hind limb. Once under the skin, insert the needle into the cranial vena cava and pull back on the syringe and collect the desired amount of blood (no more than 20% total blood volume per 2 week period). After collecting the desired amount of blood, deposit blood in each of the different tubes needed for downstream analysis and remove the needle and place pressure on the venipuncture site with the thumb and a piece of gauze to assist in clotting. Place syringe and needle into sharps container. Swab the mucus membranes if desired.
7. Inject the vaccine to be tested using a 25-gauge needle and syringe into as many sites as desired; typically one injection site in either the upper back or front leg muscle is used.
8. Check the venipuncture site and place ferret in the front of the cage.
9. Record information in the AMR with the health of the animal, weight, temperature, type and amount of anesthetic used, details of the vaccination given, and time of recovery from the anesthetic. Remain in the room until all ferrets have recovered from the anesthetic.
10. If multiple vaccination doses are to be given, repeat **steps 1–9** on subsequent vaccination days.

11. Repeat **steps 1–8**, except for the vaccination step (**step 6**), on desired sampling days where the humoral and/or the cellular immune response to vaccination will be assayed.
12. On the day post-vaccination where the vaccination regimen is considered complete, proceed with exposure of the ferrets to the henipavirus, as described below in Subheading 3.2.

3.2 Henipavirus Inoculation

Henipaviruses are lethal in ferrets through intransal (i.n.) exposure routes with the typical lethal dose of 5000 plaque forming units (PFU) or tissue culture infectious dose 50 ($TCID_{50}$). A thorough 50% lethal dose (LD_{50}) study for older ferrets has yet to be conducted though a study found the LD_{50} in 6-week-old ferrets to be 5–22 $TCID_{50}$. Based on these small cohorts for LD_{50}, the dose of 5000 PFU represents a stringent challenge to overcome henipavirus infection. Medical countermeasures that can provide protection against the stringent challenge are more likely to move on toward advanced development and further testing in the AGM model.

1. Thaw the chosen henipavirus stock and dilute the virus in 2% FBS-HBSS starting with at least 0.5 mL of virus stock (*see* **Note 1**). Dilute preparation to 10,000 PFU/mL and place on ice to keep cool until use.
2. Observe the ferrets cage-side for general health and whether or not they are fit for anesthesia and procedures.
3. Set up the procedure table and scale/tub with absorbent bench pads to work with the ferrets.
4. Place stainless steel mesh glove on hand and place leather glove over top of the stainless steel mesh glove.
5. Open the cage and coax a ferret to your leather gloved hand and remove it from the cage. Use the BMDS chip reader to ID and measure the temp of the ferret to get a reading pre-anesthesia. Using a partner, immobilize the ferret so that the thigh is available for i.m. injection of anesthetic (KAX) using a 25-gauge needle and syringe; place needle and syringe in sharps container. Alternatively, the ferret can be placed in an anesthesia box with isoflurane under continuous flow at 5% volume. If using isoflurane, a nose cone for continuous flow is placed over the ferret's nose during the procedures.
6. Once the ferret is sedated, it can be handled for weighing and placed on the procedure table. Assess overall health by observing the eyes, mucus membranes, fur, skin, and hydration status.
7. Place the ferret in dorsal recumbency and disinfect the ventral neck region for phlebotomy. Use a 23-gauge needle attached to a 3 mL "luer lock" syringe for blood collection. This is a "blind stick" where one inserts the needle just lateral of the

manubrium and cranial to the first rib at a 45-degree angle toward the opposite hind limb. Once under the skin, insert the needle into the cranial vena cava and pull back on the syringe and collect the desired amount of blood (up to 20% total blood volume per 2-week period). After collecting the desired amount of blood, deposit blood in each of the different tubes needed for downstream analysis and remove the needle and place pressure on the venipuncture site with the thumb and a piece of gauze to assist in clotting. Place syringe and needle into sharps container. Swab the mucus membranes if desired.

8. Slowly instill 0.5 mL (5000 PFU) of the diluted henipavirus preparation using a 1 mL syringe into both nostrils of the ferret (0.250 mL per nostril).
9. Assess the venipuncture site again and place the NHP back into the cage on their side facing the front of the cage.
10. 10 Check the venipuncture site and place ferret in the front of the cage.
11. Record information in the AMR with the health of the animal, weight, temperature, type and amount of anesthetic used, details of the vaccination given, and time of recovery from the anesthetic. Remain in the room until all ferrets have recovered from the anesthetic.
12. Repeat **steps 1–10**, minus the virus inoculation step (**step** 7), on desired sampling days.
13. If conducting an evaluation of post-exposure treatment continue with treatments as described in Subheading 3.3 starting at the appropriate time point post-henipavirus inoculation.

3.3 Post-exposure Treatment

The treatment regimen and dosage will vary depending on the candidate therapeutic used, while pre-infection treatment can be tested there is precedence for monoclonal antibody (mAb) treatments to begin 1 or 3 days post-henipavirus infection. We will cover intraperitoneal (i.p.) treatment route below; however, oral dosing is also a possibility depending on the treatment selected (*see* **Note 2**)

1. Assess the ferrets for general health and behavior to see if they are fit for anesthesia and procedures.
2. Set up the procedure table and scale/tub with absorbent bench pads to work with the ferrets.
3. Place stainless steel mesh glove on hand and leather glove over top of the stainless steel mesh glove.
4. Open the cage and coax a ferret to your leather gloved hand and remove it from the cage. Use the BMDS chip reader to ID and measure the temp of the ferret to get a reading pre-anesthesia. Using a partner, immobilize the ferret so that

the thigh is available for i.m. injection of anesthetic (KAX) using a 25-gauge needle and syringe; place needle and syringe in sharps container. Alternatively, the ferret can be placed in an anesthesia box with isoflurane under continuous flow at 5% volume. If using isoflurane, a nose cone for continuous flow is placed over the ferret's nose during the procedures.

5. Once the ferret is sedated, it can be handled for weighing and placed on the procedure table. Assess overall health by observing the eyes, mucus membranes, fur, skin, and hydration status.
6. If bleeding on a treatment day, place the ferret in dorsal recumbency and disinfect the ventral neck region for phlebotomy. Use a 23-gauge needle attached to a 3 mL "luer lock" syringe for blood collection. This is a "blind stick" where one inserts the needle just lateral of the manubrium and cranial to the first rib at a 45-degree angle toward the opposite hind limb. Once under the skin, insert the needle into the cranial vena cava and pull back on the syringe and collect the desired amount of blood (up to 20% total blood volume over 2 week period). After collecting the desired amount of blood, deposit blood in each of the different tubes needed for downstream analysis and remove the needle and place pressure on the venipuncture site with the thumb and a piece of gauze to assist in clotting. Place syringe and needle into sharps container. Swab the mucus membranes if desired.
7. For i.p. treatment: shave and disinfect the lower abdomen. Use a 23-gauge intravenous needle and syringe to deliver the treatment into the peritoneal cavity using forceps to "tent" lower abdominal skin. Once under the skin and in the peritoneal cavity pull back on the plunger to ensure you have not pierced any organs; at this point slowly depress the plunger releasing the treatment into the peritoneal cavity. Remove the needle and place needle and syringe in sharps container.
8. Fill out the AMR with the health of the animal, weight, temperature, type and amount of anesthetic used, and time of recovery from the anesthetic. Remain in the room until all NHPs have recovered from the anesthetic.
9. Repeat all steps on additional treatment days, minus the treatment step on sampling days only (*see* **Step** 7).

3.4 Clinical Samples, Clinical Observations, Humane Endpoint Scoring, and Euthanasia

Infection of ferrets with henipaviruses leads to signs of disease such as depression, lethargy, sneezing, ocular and nasal discharge, fever, loss of appetite, labored breathing, rash on the ventral neck, edema of the head and neck, tremors, and limb paresis. Clinical pathology of ferrets infected with henipaviruses includes thrombocytopenia, lymphopenia, increase in blood urea nitrogen (BUN), and hypoalbuminemia, while the gross pathology includes lung congestion, hemorrhage and necrosis in all lung lobes, and enlarged spleen. Each of these signs of disease/pathology can be used to assess the efficacy of vaccine/treatment. Techniques for analyzing these signs/pathology are described below.

1. On sampling days EDTA-plasma tubes and serum tubes can be collected for hematology and serum biochemistry, respectively. Remove 100 μL of whole blood from EDTA-plasma tube and run it on a hematology machine. Separate the serum from the whole blood in the serum blood tube and then remove 100 μL of serum from serum tube and run it in a biochemistry panel disc.
2. After the henipavirus infection phase in a vaccine/treatment efficacy study (up to the study endpoint), clinical observations should be documented (see Table 1 as an example) during daily checks or while on the procedure table. These observations are critical data for comparing the control and vaccine/treatment cohort's disease progression.
3. When ferrets are infected with henipaviruses via the i.n. route and there is no intervention, the infection results in 100% lethality. Considering that these henipaviruses cause lethality, it is necessary to ensure that the ferrets in henipavirus studies do not suffer unnecessarily but also serve as a proper control when testing a vaccine/treatment. To prevent unnecessary suffering, humane endpoint criteria should be set for each study based on appearance, skin, behavior, respiration, and neurological signs as shown in Table 2. Humane endpoint criteria (*see* **Note 3**) can be investigator and study specific; however, the decision on what is acceptable is made by the IACUC of the institution involved in ferret henipavirus studies. Ferrets are scored for these criteria daily, at a minimum, beginning day 1 post-henipavirus infection with certain scores/categories requiring additional monitoring to intervene with euthanasia in a timely manner (*see* **Note 4**).
4. At the study endpoint or when a clinical score requires euthanasia, prepare the procedure table and scale/tub with Versi-dry®absorbent bench pads to place ferrets on.
5. Place stainless steel mesh glove on hand and leather glove over top of the stainless steel mesh glove.
6. Open the cage and coax the ferret to your leather gloved hand and remove it from the cage. Use the BMDS chip reader to ID and measure the temp of the ferret to get a reading pre-anesthesia. Using a partner, immobilize the ferret so that the thigh is available for i.m. injection of anesthetic (KAX) using a 25-gauge needle and syringe; place needle and syringe in sharps container. Alternatively, the ferret can be placed in an

anesthesia box with isoflurane under continuous flow at 5% volume. If using isoflurane, a nose cone for continuous flow is placed over the ferret's nose during the procedures.

7. Once the ferret is sedated, it can be handled for weighing and placed on the procedure table. Assess overall health by observing the eyes, mucus membranes, fur, skin, and hydration status.
8. Place the ferret in dorsal recumbency and disinfect the ventral neck region for phlebotomy. Use a 23-gauge needle attached to a 3 mL "luer lock" syringe for blood collection. This is a "blind stick" where one inserts the needle just lateral of the manubrium and cranial to the first rib at a 45-degree angle toward the opposite hind limb. Once under the skin, insert the needle into the cranial vena cava and pull back on the syringe and collect the desired amount of blood. After collecting the desired amount of blood, deposit blood in each of the different tubes needed for downstream analysis and remove the needle and place pressure on the venipuncture site with the thumb and a piece of gauze to assist in clotting. Place syringe and needle into sharps container. Swab the mucus membranes if desired.
9. Once a blood sample has been taken, deliver pentobarbital sodium solution (0.5 mL) via intracardiac stick using a 23-gauge needle and a 3-mL syringe. Insert needle between the 3–5 ribs up from the diaphragm and pull back on the plunger until blood is drawn into the syringe; at this point depress the plunger injecting pentobarbital sodium solution into the heart and circulatory system.
10. Depending on the study design, when the humane endpoint or the study endpoint is reached, ferrets are typically necropsied with gross pathology observed and noted with further analysis through hematoxylin and eosin (H & E) staining for cytopathology and immunohistochemistry (IHC) staining for virus antigen. Tissues taken at necropsy can also be used to assess the infectious virus load when evaluating the effectiveness of a vaccine/treatment.

4 Notes

1. Most henipavirus stocks will need to be diluted around 10,000-fold to reach 10,000 PFU/mL, so an initial tenfold dilution is made by placing 0.5 mL of virus stock into 4.5 mL of 2% FBS-HBSS. Pulse vortex the tube of virus stock three times so that all liquid goes up the sides of the tube and then remove the 0.5 mL. This assures the user pulls in a more homogenous mixture of virus than pulling a smaller volume (e.g., 0.001 mL and placing it into 4.999 mL for 5000 fold dilution). Pulse vortex at each dilution step using at least 2 mL for tenfold dilutions.

2. While intravenous (i.v.) treatment is possible with ferrets mAb treatment studies in the henipavirus ferret model have shown that treatment through the i.p. route is sufficient to mitigate henipavirus disease. If choosing oral delivery for treatment of ferrets, the preferred method is through syringe delivery versus gavage.
3. Table 2 is a representation of henipavirus disease signs in ferrets typically observed and scored. At a minimum, investigators need an established score for humane intervention along with the disease course resulting from henipavirus infection for the control animals to ensure the vaccine/treatment has been assessed against the disease. This score can be adjusted based on experience with the model.
4. The clinical scores in Table 2 provide a humane endpoint for the ferrets on study, although the disease course of henipaviruses can be slightly variable in this outbred ferret model. Additionally, due to the lethality of the henipaviruses and the acute onset of clinical signs, there is the possibility of an unintended death even when the intent was to intervene with euthanasia.

References

1. Escaffre O, Borisevich V, Rockx B (2013) Pathogenesis of Hendra and Nipah virus infection in humans. J Infect Dev Ctries 7:308–311
2. Chew MH, Arguin PM, Shay DK, Goh KT, Rollin PE, Shieh WJ, Zaki SR, Rota PA, Ling AE, Ksiazek TG, Chew SK, Anderson LJ (2000) Risk factors for Nipah virus infection among abattoir workers in Singapore. J Infect Dis 181:1760–1763
3. Luby SP, Gurley ES, Hossain MJ (2009) Transmission of human infection with Nipah virus. Clin Infect Dis 49:1743–1748
4. Luby SP, Rahman M, Hossain MJ, Blum LS, Husain MM, Gurley E, Khan R, Ahmed BN, Rahman S, Nahar N, Kenah E, Comer JA, Ksiazek TG (2006) Foodborne transmission of Nipah virus, Bangladesh. Emerg Infect Dis 12:1888–1894
5. O'Sullivan JD, Allworth AM, Paterson DL, Snow TM, Boots R, Gleeson LJ, Gould AR, Hyatt AD, Bradfield J (1997) Fatal encephalitis due to novel paramyxovirus transmitted from horses. Lancet 349:93–95
6. Bossart KN, Zhu Z, Middleton D, Klippel J, Crameri G, Bingham J, McEachern JA, Green D, Hancock TJ, Chan YP, Hickey AC, Dimitrov DS, Wang LF, Broder CC (2009) A neutralizing human monoclonal antibody protects against lethal disease in a new ferret model of acute nipah virus infection. PLoS Pathog 5: e1000642
7. Kurup D, Wirblich C, Feldmann H, Marzi A, Schnell MJ (2015) Rhabdovirus-based vaccine platforms against henipaviruses. J Virol 89: 144–154
8. Lo MK, Bird BH, Chattopadhyay A, Drew CP, Martin BE, Coleman JD, Rose JK, Nichol ST, Spiropoulou CF (2014) Single-dose replication-defective VSV-based Nipah virus vaccines provide protection from lethal challenge in Syrian hamsters. Antivir Res 101:26–29
9. McEachern JA, Bingham J, Crameri G, Green DJ, Hancock TJ, Middleton D, Feng YR, Broder CC, Wang LF, Bossart KN (2008) A recombinant subunit vaccine formulation protects against lethal Nipah virus challenge in cats. Vaccine 26:3842–3852
10. van Doremalen N, Lambe T, Sebastian S, Bushmaker T, Fischer R, Feldmann F, Haddock E, Letko M, Avanzato VA, Rissanen I, LaCasse R, Scott D, Bowden TA, Gilbert S, Munster V (2019) A single-dose ChAdOx1-vectored vaccine provides complete protection against Nipah Bangladesh and Malaysia in Syrian golden hamsters. PLoS Negl Trop Dis 13:e0007462
11. Food, Drug Administration HHS (2002) New drug and biological drug products; evidence

needed to demonstrate effectiveness of new drugs when human efficacy studies are not ethical or feasible. Final rule. Fed Regist 67: 37988–37998
12. Rockx B (2014) Recent developments in experimental animal models of Henipavirus infection. Pathog Dis doi. https://doi.org/10.1111/2049-632X.12149
13. Middleton DJ, Westbury HA, Morrissy CJ, van der Heide BM, Russell GM, Braun MA, Hyatt AD (2002) Experimental Nipah virus infection in pigs and cats. J Comp Pathol 126:124–136
14. Dhondt KP, Mathieu C, Chalons M, Reynaud JM, Vallve A, Raoul H, Horvat B (2013) Type I interferon signaling protects mice from lethal henipavirus infection. J Infect Dis 207:142–151
15. Geisbert TW, Daddario-DiCaprio KM, Hickey AC, Smith MA, Chan YP, Wang LF, Mattapallil JJ, Geisbert JB, Bossart KN, Broder CC (2010) Development of an acute and highly pathogenic nonhuman primate model of Nipah virus infection. PLoS One 5:e10690
16. Pallister J, Middleton D, Wang LF, Klein R, Haining J, Robinson R, Yamada M, White J, Payne J, Feng YR, Chan YP, Broder CC (2011) A recombinant Hendra virus G glycoprotein-based subunit vaccine protects ferrets from lethal Hendra virus challenge. Vaccine 29: 5623–5630
17. Rockx B, Bossart KN, Feldmann F, Geisbert JB, Hickey AC, Brining D, Callison J, Safronetz D, Marzi A, Kercher L, Long D, Broder CC, Feldmann H, Geisbert TW (2010) A novel model of lethal Hendra virus infection in African green monkeys and the effectiveness of ribavirin treatment. J Virol 84: 9831–9839
18. Williamson MM, Hooper PT, Selleck PW, Westbury HA, Slocombe RF (2000) Experimental hendra virus infectionin pregnant Guinea-pigs and fruit bats (Pteropus poliocephalus). J Comp Pathol 122:201–207
19. Wong KT, Grosjean I, Brisson C, Blanquier B, Fevre-Montange M, Bernard A, Loth P, Georges-Courbot MC, Chevallier M, Akaoka H, Marianneau P, Lam SK, Wild TF, Deubel V (2003) A golden hamster model for human acute Nipah virus infection. Am J Pathol 163:2127–2137
20. Smith H, Sweet C (1988) Lessons for human influenza from pathogenicity studies with ferrets. Rev Infect Dis 10:56–75
21. Clayton BA, Middleton D, Bergfeld J, Haining J, Arkinstall R, Wang L, Marsh GA (2012) Transmission routes for nipah virus from Malaysia and Bangladesh. Emerg Infect Dis 18:1983
22. Mire CE, Versteeg KM, Cross RW, Agans KN, Fenton KA, Whitt MA, Geisbert TW (2013) Single injection recombinant vesicular stomatitis virus vaccines protect ferrets against lethal Nipah virus disease. Virol J 10:353
23. Pallister JA, Klein R, Arkinstall R, Haining J, Long F, White JR, Payne J, Feng YR, Wang LF, Broder CC, Middleton D (2013) Vaccination of ferrets with a recombinant G glycoprotein subunit vaccine provides protection against Nipah virus disease for over 12 months. Virol J 10:237
24. Leon AJ, Banner D, Xu L, Ran L, Peng Z, Yi K, Chen C, Xu F, Huang J, Zhao Z, Lin Z, Huang SH, Fang Y, Kelvin AA, Ross TM, Farooqui A, Kelvin DJ (2013) Sequencing, annotation, and characterization of the influenza ferret infectome. J Virol 87:1957–1966
25. Leon AJ, Borisevich V, Boroumand N, Seymour R, Nusbaum R, Escaffre O, Xu L, Kelvin DJ, Rockx B (2018) Host gene expression profiles in ferrets infected with genetically distinct henipavirus strains. PLoS Negl Trop Dis 12:e0006343
26. Barthold SW, Bayne KA, Davis MA (2011) Guide for the care and use of laboratory animals. National Academy Press, Washington

Chapter 16

Syrian Golden Hamster Model for Nipah Virus Infection

Terry Juelich, Jennifer Smith, and Alexander N. Freiberg

Abstract

Small rodent animal models that recapitulate the symptomology and pathology of the human disease caused by Nipah virus (NiV) are crucial not only to study virus-induced disease but also a critical component for the development of vaccine and therapeutic candidates. The Syrian golden hamster is the most commonly used small animal model for NiV and develops clinical symptoms and pathologies that closely resemble NiV disease in humans. In this chapter, we describe standard techniques used to infect hamsters and conduct evaluation of therapeutics and vaccine candidates.

Key words Nipah virus, Syrian golden hamster, Small animal model, Pathogenicity, Antiviral, Vaccine

1 Introduction

Nipah virus (NiV) and Hendra virus (HeV) are emerging and highly pathogenic zoonotic bat-borne paramyxoviruses (genus henipavirus, HNV). In humans, they cause severe encephalitis and respiratory disease with high fatality rates [1, 2]. While outbreaks are relatively rare and confined in Southeast and Southern Asia (Malaysia, Singapore, Bangladesh, India, and Philippines for NiV, and Australia for HeV), the extreme virulence, documented person-to-person transmission, and lack of approved vaccines or therapeutics have led the World Health Organization to label NiV a priority pathogen for the development of medical countermeasures [3].

Our understanding of HNV-induced disease primarily originates from pathogenicity studies of experimentally infected animals and only to a minor extent from end-stage histopathology findings from fatal human cases [4]. The animal challenge models that most accurately recapitulate pathology and symptomology of human disease are the Syrian golden hamster, ferrets, and African Green monkeys (AGM) [5–8].

While AGMs are considered the most relevant animal model for NiV disease, the advantage of the hamster model is their small size,

Alexander N. Freiberg and Barry Rockx (eds.), *Nipah Virus: Methods and Protocols*, Methods in Molecular Biology, vol. 2682, https://doi.org/10.1007/978-1-0716-3283-3_16,

ease of handling, and economical housing. Pathogenicity studies in hamsters with both NiV and HeV have informed on the development of disease course and also allowed to evaluate the efficacy of vaccine candidates and antivirals [9, 10]. Non-protected animals typically develop labored breathing, severe respiratory distress, pulmonary infiltrates, as well as hemorrhagic lesions of the lungs [11]. Hamsters also develop neurological signs of disease, including lethargy, muscle twitching, imbalance, tremors, and limb paralysis [12]. Vasculitis and thrombosis are prominent in multiple organs including the lungs and brain but also the liver, kidneys, and heart, with rare detection of endothelial syncytial cells [13]. Infectious virus is detectable in multiple organs and urine but typically not in serum [5]. Viral antigens and RNA have been detected in the lungs, brain, liver, spleen, kidneys, and heart. Vascular and parenchymal lesions are most prominent in the brain. Here, neurons in the vicinity of vasculitis show eosinophilic inclusion bodies in the cytoplasm, which are often positive for viral RNA and antigen. Other parenchymal changes include ischemia and edema. In the lungs, the areas of parenchymal inflammation which are often associated with vasculitis can be observed. In affected lung tissues, inflammatory cells, such as macrophages, lymphocytes, and neutrophils, can be found. Disease progression in the hamster model appears to be dependent on the route of inoculation and challenge dose [5, 14]. While infection via the intranasal (IN) and intraperitoneal (IP) routes induces similar symptoms and pathologies, IP inoculation causes a more rapid disease course compared to the IN route. Regarding challenge doses, high doses induce a primarily respiratory syndrome, while lower doses induce both, respiratory and neurological symptoms [14]. In addition to the IP and IN routes, infection via the aerosol route resulted in both respiratory and neurological diseases, while feeding of hamsters with artificial date palm sap containing NiV resulted in predominantly neurological disease [15, 16].

Here, we describe standard procedures used for NiV infection in the hamster model to study viral pathogenicity, and to evaluate the efficacy of antivirals and vaccines.

2 Materials

NiV is a biosafety level 4 (BSL-4) agent and should be handled in accordance with the guidelines stipulated in the current edition of "Biosafety in Microbiological and Biomedical Laboratories" (BMBL) (https://www.cdc.gov/labs/BMBL.html).

Work with NiV in hamsters requires animal biosafety level 4 (ABSL-4) space approved by the U.S. Centers for Disease Control and Prevention (CDC) or equivalent as well as approval from the Institution or University, or equivalent, to work with NiV in hamsters at ABSL-4. Furthermore, approval from the Institutional Animal Care and Use Committee (IACUC) to work with hamsters at ABSL-4 is required.

2.1 General Materials and Supplies

1. NiV stock.
2. Hamsters (Mesocricetus auratus), female or male, 4–8 weeks of age (or 80–100 grams).
3. Microisolator cages to house hamsters with dimensions recommended in the National Research Council's *Guide for the Care and Use of Laboratory Animals* eighth edition [4] or equivalent.
4. Rodent food.
5. Class II biosafety cabinet (BSC) or downdraft table for procedures.
6. Forceps or salad tongs.
7. 2-L beaker.
8. Scale.
9. Appropriate anesthetic (for example isoflurane or Ketamine/Xylazine).
10. Anesthesia system with isoflurane vaporizer.
11. Oxygen.
12. Anesthesia induction chamber and nose-cone.
13. Bio Medics Data Systems (BMDS) lab animal identification (ID) chip reader; or equivalent.
14. Lab animal ID chip; temperature monitor if desired.
15. Sheets to record clinical observations and body weights.
16. Sheets summarizing clinical scoring.
17. Adsorbent bench pads.
18. Appropriate disinfectant (5% quaternary ammonium, 70% ethanol, etc.).
19. Gauze.
20. Sharps container.
21. Minimal Essential Media (MEM).
22. Sterile Dulbecco's phosphate-buffered saline (DPBS).
23. TRIzol® Reagent (Invitrogen).
24. 26-gauge 1 mL disposable syringes for intraperitoneal (IP) injection (BD syringe).
25. Stainless steel beads for tissue homogenization.
26. Tissuelyser.
27. Tabletop centrifuge.
28. Pipettes and pipette tips.

2.2 Specialized Supplies for Biosampling, Vaccination, or Therapeutic Administration

1. 1–5 mL syringes with 23-gauge or 25-gauge needles for cardiac puncture.
2. 0.3–0.5 mL syringes with 30-gauge or 31-gauge needles for intramuscular (IM) injection.
3. Standard Mylar-wrapped non-heparinized micro-hematocrit capillary tubes.
4. Plastic disposable transfer pipets.
5. Topical ophthalmic anesthetic (if wanted).
6. BNP triple antibiotic ophthalmic ointment.
7. Oral gavage needles—18-gauge or 20-gauge, 1.5—2 inches long, rigid or flexible, reusable or disposable, straight or curved may be used depending on preference.
8. 1 or 3 mL luer lock syringes for PO dosing needles, depending on dose volume to be administered.
9. Blood collection tubes for desired analyses of whole blood, plasma, and serum. Standard tubes would be Lithium Heparin (for plasma analysis, peripheral blood mononuclear cell preparation, and immunoglobulin analysis), K2EDTA (primarily used for hematology), and Serum Separator (for blood chemistry).
10. Sterile collection tubes prefilled with stainless steel beads and DPBS or TRIzol® for the collection and homogenization of tissues.
11. Specimen jars pre-filled with 10% buffered formalin for the fixation and storage of tissue specimens.
12. Vaccine or therapeutic.

3 Methods

3.1 Nipah Virus Inoculation

1. On the day of infection, thaw NiV stock at room temperature and prepare the challenge concentration by diluting a pre-calculated NiV stock volume into plain MEM or DPBS inside BSC. Keep on ice until use. (*see* **Note 1**).
2. Set up BSC or downdraft table with absorbent bench pads, anesthesia chamber, sharps container, and spray bottle with appropriate disinfectant.
3. Transfer the cage from rack to BSC or downdraft table (depending on laboratory set up). Open the cage, remove hamsters using large forceps or salad tongs, and transfer into 2-L beaker. Identify hamster ID (e.g., by BMDS chip reader).
4. Measure body temperature and body weight prior to infection (if required by protocol).

5. Anesthetize hamster. For inhaled anesthetics (e.g., isoflurane), anesthesia induction chambers or nose-cones are required. Adjust the oxygen flow-meter to approximately 0.5–1.0 L/min and adjust the isoflurane vaporizer to approximately 2–5% for induction. To maintain anesthesia, a continuous flow set to approximately 1–3% should be used. For injectable anesthetics, combined Ketamine/Xylazine via the IP route is preferred (Ketamine: 100–200 mg/kg; Xylazine: 10 mg/kg).
6. Verify the sedation level (either inside BSC or on downdraft table—depending on laboratory set up) according to approved animal study protocol.
7. Inoculate animal with NiV. According to the experimental design, different viral doses and routes of administration can be used (e.g., IP, IN, and aerosol exposure). Detailed information about inoculation protocols can be found elsewhere.
8. After virus infection has been completed, place hamsters back into the microisolator cage and monitor animals to recover from anesthesia. Remain in the room until all hamsters have recovered from anesthesia.
9. Perform daily health checks as specified in the animal use protocol. Repeat **steps 3** and **4** and assess each hamster for the development of clinical signs of disease, such as ruffled fur, lethargy, paralysis, and orbital tightening. Record body weight, temperature, clinical scoring, and type and amount of anesthetic used in the study protocol.
10. If the efficacy of therapeutics will be evaluated, follow the procedures as outlined in Subheading 3.2.
11. According to the study protocol, once infected hamsters reach the humane endpoint or the endpoint of the study, they are euthanized. Biosampling, such as blood collection or necropsy, might need to be performed. Follow the procedures as outlined in Subheading 3.4. Record all procedures in the study protocol.

3.2 Evaluation of Therapeutics

To evaluate the efficacy of therapeutics (e.g., antiviral compounds or monoclonal antibodies), dosing can be performed prior to (prophylactic evaluation) or after (therapeutic evaluation) virus inoculation. Several factors of the candidate therapeutic are influencing the treatment dosage and regimen (*see* **Note 2**). Here, we will only cover administration via the IP and oral gavage (PO) routes.

1. On the day of administration, have candidate therapeutic prepared and ready to use according to study protocol. Pre-fill syringe(s) if possible and store at the recommended temperature.

2. Set up BSC or downdraft table with absorbent bench pads, sharps container, and spray bottle with appropriate disinfectant.
3. Transfer the cage from the rack to BSC or downdraft table (depending on laboratory set up). Open the cage, remove hamsters using large forceps, and transfer into a 2-L beaker. Identify hamster ID (e.g., by BMDS chip reader).
4. Measure body temperature and body weight prior to infection (if required by protocol).
5. Transfer hamster into the anesthesia induction chamber.
6. Anesthetize hamster using either inhaled or injectable anesthetics.
7. Verify sedation level (either inside BSC or on downdraft table—depending on laboratory set up) according to the approved animal study protocol.
8. For treatment via the IP route: Disinfect the lower abdomen by using alcohol wipes. Use a 21-gauge 1 mL disposable syringe to deliver the candidate therapeutic. Once the needle has penetrated the skin and is in the peritoneal cavity, slowly pull back on the plunger to ensure that no organs have been pierced. To administer the candidate therapeutic, slowly depress the plunger. Remove the needle from the animal and discard it with the syringe in the sharps container.
9. For treatment via the PO route:
   (a) Load the syringe with therapeutic and attach the gavage needle. Push therapeutic into gavage needle so that administered dose is accurate.
   (b) Once the hamster is anesthetized, grasp it loosely by the scruff. Hold the hamster in an upright position so that the hind legs are dangling, the neck/throat are straight, and the hamster is facing you.
   (c) Measure the length of the gavage needle needed to reach from the mouth to the stomach on the outside of the hamster.
   (d) Introduce the oral gavage needle to the side of the teeth and run along the roof of the mouth. Once the needle reaches the back of the throat gently tilt the head back and push the needle down the esophagus. There should be no resistance. If resistance is felt, remove the needle and start again. Slowly and gently depress the plunger to administer the therapeutic. The maximum volume that can be administered is 0.3 mL.
   (e) Gently remove the gavage needle and return hamster to the cage. Observe for signs of distress. If the animal shows

immediate signs of respiratory distress, inadvertent dosing into the lungs has occurred and the hamster should be humanely euthanized.

(f) Monitor until all hamsters have recovered from anesthesia.

10. For the control groups, equivalent volumes of vehicle solution or 1X DPBS are typically used for each route of inoculation.
11. After the administration of candidate therapeutic has been completed, place hamsters back into the microisolator cage and monitor animals to recover from anesthesia. Remain in the room until all hamsters have recovered from anesthesia.
12. Perform daily health checks as specified in the animal use protocol and record body weight, temperature, clinical scoring, type, and amount of anesthetic and therapeutic used in the study protocol.
13. Repeat **steps 1–9** on all dosing days as specified in the study protocol.

3.3 Evaluation of Vaccines

To evaluate the efficacy of vaccine candidates, the specifics of the vaccine candidate will determine the vaccine strategy (prime only or prime-boost). Typically, the vaccination phase will last between 21 and 56 days prior to challenge with NiV. During this time, as well as after infection, blood will typically be collected from immunized hamsters to assess humoral and cell-mediated immune responses, as well as viremia. Here, we will only cover administration via the IM route. While the procedures in handling hamsters are nearly identical, immunizations are typically performed at ABSL-2, prior to moving immunized animals to ABSL-4 for challenge with NiV and to evaluate protective efficacy.

1. On the day of administration, have candidate vaccine prepared and ready to use according to the study protocol. Pre-fill syringe(s) if possible and store at the recommended temperature.
2. Set up BSC or downdraft table with absorbent bench pads, anesthesia chamber, sharps container, and spray bottle with appropriate disinfectant.
3. Transfer the cage from the rack to BSC or downdraft table (depending on laboratory set up). Open cage, remove hamsters using large forceps, and transfer into 2 L beaker. Identify hamster ID (e.g., by BMDS chip reader).
4. Measure body temperature and body weight prior to immunization (if required by protocol).
5. Transfer hamster into the anesthesia induction chamber.

6. Anesthetize hamster using either inhaled or injectable anesthetics.
7. Verify the sedation level (either inside BSC or on the downdraft table—depending on laboratory set up) according to approved animal study protocol.
8. Injection of the vaccine candidate will depend on the study protocol but typically one IM injection is given into each in the hind limb with typically 50 μL volume per leg. The same needle and syringe can typically be used for multiple animals within the same vaccine group. Once immunization has been completed, discard the needle and syringe in the sharps container.
9. After the administration of vaccine candidate has been completed, place hamsters back into the microisolator cage and monitor animals to recover from anesthesia. Remain in the room until all hamsters have recovered from anesthesia.
10. Perform daily health checks as specified in the animal use protocol and record body weight, temperature, clinical scoring, type and amount of anesthetic used in the study protocol.
11. Repeat **steps 1–9** on all immunization days as specified in the study protocol.
12. On desired sampling days to access humoral and/or cellular immune responses, repeat **steps 1–9** (without the vaccination step) and follow the procedures as outlined in Subheading 3.4. Record all procedures in the study protocol.
13. Once the vaccination regimen has been completed, transfer immunized hamsters into the BSL4, acclimate, and then follow procedures for NiV challenge as outlined in Subheading 3.1.

3.4 Biosampling, Euthanasia, and Necropsy

The development of clinical signs of disease, as well as clinical pathology and viral load in blood and tissues can be utilized to describe henipavirus-induced disease and to assess the efficacy of a vaccine or therapeutic treatment. Techniques used for biosampling, euthanasia, and necropsy are described below:

1. *Retro-orbital bleeding:*
   (a) For blood collection, non-heparinized Mylar-wrapped micro-hematocrit capillary tubes can be used.
   (b) Anesthetize animals as outlined in Subheading 3.1, **steps 2** through **6**.
   (c) Position the anesthetized hamster on the table, laying on its side. A topical ophthalmic anesthetic, e.g. proparacaine or tetracaine drops may be used.
   (d) Restrain the hamster with the facial skin pulled taut while gently grasping the skin at the back of the neck (the scruff). This results in a slight protrusion of the upward

facing eye. Be careful not to stretch the skin too tight, which can result in the compression of the thoracic cavity.

(e) Place the tip of the capillary tube at the lateral canthus and gently insert at an approximate 45° angle into the space between the globe and the lower eyelid.

(f) Gently twist the capillary tube between the thumb and forefinger until blood begins to flow or when the capillary tube reaches the bone at the back of the eye (orbit). Blood will enter the tube by capillary action. It may be helpful to retract the tube or loosen the grip on the scruff to facilitate blood flow.

(g) Following blood collection, remove the capillary tube and transfer the blood into a blood tube using a transfer pipet. To prevent further bleeding of the eye, place gauze over the eye and apply light pressure for approximately 30 s. BNP eye ointment may be applied to the eye at this time.

(h) If repeated bleeding is planned, it is recommended to alternate eyes to minimize the risk of damage. No more than 0.1 mL to 0.5 mL of blood should be collected via retro-orbital bleed at any one time.

(i) Once the procedure has been completed, place hamsters back into the microisolator cage and monitor animals until all hamsters have recovered from anesthesia.

(j) Process blood according to tube manufacturer instructions.

2. *Cardiac puncture:*

Cardiac puncture (or terminal bleed) is performed when an animal reaches euthanasia criteria as outlined per the study protocol or on surviving animals at the predefined end of the study.

(a) Prior to initiation of the cardiac puncture, the animal must be under deep anesthesia. Anesthetize animals as outlined in Subheading 3.1, **steps 2** through **6**.

(b) Once the animal is anesthetized, remove it from the chamber, and place the animal on its back with its nose and mouth in a nose cone that is attached to an isoflurane vaporizer.

(c) Blood is collected by introducing a 23-gauge or 25-gauge needle into the sagittal plane at the posterior extremity of the sternum and pushing forward. Gently and slowly pull the syringe plunger (up to 5 mL) to prevent the heart from collapsing.

(d) Following blood collection, transfer blood into the appropriate tubes for further analysis (e.g., blood chemistry or hematology) and process following established protocols (*see* **Note 3**). Dispose of needle and syringe in sharps container.

3. *Necropsy:*

   Depending on the study design, when the humane endpoint (*see* **Note 4**) or study endpoint is reached, hamsters are euthanized and typically necropsied. Gross pathology is performed, and tissues taken at necropsy can either be processed to analyze the histopathology of tissues, assess viral load, or determine cellular responses.

   (a) Remove hamsters from the cage and place them under deep terminal anesthesia. Recommended methods of euthanasia are asphyxiation using CO_2 or inhalant/injectable anesthetic followed by bilateral thoracotomy or exsanguination or cervical dislocation.

   (b) During necropsy, different organs (e.g., brain, lungs, heart, kidneys, liver, and spleen) can be taken. Tissues can then be processed for RNA isolation (homogenization in TRIzol®), analysis of viral load (homogenization in DPBS), or histopathological analysis (fixation in 10% formalin) following established protocols.

4 Notes

1. All dilutions of viral stocks are performed under sterile conditions in a high containment BSL4 environment within a Class II BSC.
2. Depending on the mechanism of action, dosing might need to be initiated prior to or after infection. Dosing might also need to be administered more than once daily and/or over several days post infection.
3. Depending on the study protocol, collected blood might need to be separated in multiple aliquots to allow for the analysis of blood chemistry and hematology, or determination of viral titers. For extraction of viral RNA, whole blood or serum would need to be mixed with TRIzol.
4. Euthanasia criteria of moribund animals will need to be determined by the investigator. Typical signs of the disease include the development of ruffled fur, lethargy, hunched posture, and rapid respiration. Euthanasia criteria are met if, in addition to the above-listed symptoms, animals are reluctant to move when stimulated, show paralysis, and agonal or distressed breathing or a 20% body weight loss.

References

1. Kenmoe S, Demanou M, Bigna JJ et al (2019) Case fatality rate and risk factors for Nipah virus encephalitis: a systematic review and meta-analysis. J Clin Virol 117:19–26
2. de Wit E, Munster VJ (2015) Animal models of disease shed light on Nipah virus pathogenesis and transmission. J Pathol 235(2):196–205
3. Prioritizing Diseases for Research and Development in Emergency Contexts; Available online: https://www.who.int/activities/prioritizing-diseases-for-research-and-development-in-emergency-contexts
4. Escaffre O, Borisevich V, Rockx B (2013) Pathogenesis of Hendra and Nipah virus infection in humans. J Infect Dev Ctries 7(4): 308–311
5. Wong KT, Grosjean I, Brisson C et al (2003) A golden hamster model for human acute Nipah virus infection. Am J Pathol 163:2127–2137
6. Pallister J, Middleton D, Wang LF et al (2011) A recombinant Hendra virus G glycoprotein-based subunit vaccine protects ferrets from lethal Hendra virus challenge. Vaccine 29: 5623–5630
7. Geisbert TW, Daddario-DiCaprio KM, Hickey AC et al (2010) Development of an acute and highly pathogenic nonhuman primate model of Nipah virus infection. PLoS One 5:e10690
8. Rockx B, Bossart KN, Feldmann F et al (2010) A novel model of lethal Hendra virus infection in African green monkeys and the effectiveness of ribavirin treatment. J Virol 84:9831–9839
9. Pelissier R, Iampietro M, Horvat B (2019) Recent advances in the understanding of Nipah virus immunopathogenesis and anti-viral approaches. F1000Research 8(F1000 Faculty Rev):1763
10. Johnson K, Vu M, Freiberg AN (2021) Recent advances in combating Nipah virus. Faculty Rev 10:74
11. Rockx B (2014) Recent developments in experimental animal models of Henipavirus infection. Pathog Dis 71:199–206
12. Dhondt KP, Horvat B (2013) Henipavirus infections: lessons from animal models. Pathogens 2:264–287
13. Williamson MM, Torres-Velez FJ (2010) Henipavirus: a review of laboratory animal pathology. Vet Pathol 47:871–880
14. Rockx B, Brining D, Kramer J et al (2011) Clinical outcome of henipavirus infection in hamsters is determined by the route and dose of infection. J Virol 85:7658–7671
15. Escaffre O, Hill T, Ikegami T et al (2018) Experimental infection of Syrian hamsters with aerosolized Nipah virus. J Infect Dis 218(10):1602–1610
16. de Wit E, Prescott J, Falzarano D et al (2014) Foodborne transmission of nipah virus in Syrian hamsters. PLoS Pathog 10:e1004001

Part IV

Immune Assays for Henipaviruses

Chapter 17

Anti-Nipah Virus Enzyme-Linked Immunosorbent Assays with Non-human Primate and Hamster Serum

Elena Postnikova, Janie Liang, Shuiqing Yu, Yingyun Cai, Yu Cong, and Michael R. Holbrook

Abstract

Enzyme-linked Immunosorbent assays or ELISAs are a versatile method for detecting various immunological ligands of interest. As the name suggests, ELISAs rely on the interaction between a ligand and an antibody to produce results. In the study of infectious disease, ELISAs are commonly used to determine if a pathogen-specific immune response has occurred in a host organism. These assays can be performed in serosurveys as part of epidemiological investigations during, or following, an infectious disease outbreak. In the research environment, ELISAs are used to quantify the humoral immune response following infection or vaccination of a host organism. Data from these assays can be used to determine the type of immune response elicited (e.g. IgG1 vs IgG2) and the robustness of the response. Here, we describe ELISAs that were developed for the study of either hamsters or non-human primates vaccinated against Nipah virus infection, or infected with Nipah virus. The ELISAs described include assays for both IgG and IgM in the hamster and non-human primate models for Nipah virus-induced disease. An assay was also developed for the detection of IgA in bronchoalveolar lavage from non-human primates.

Key words Nipah virus, ELISA, Humoral response, IgG antibody, IgM antibody, IgA antibody

1 Introduction

Nipah virus (NiV) is a single-strand negative-sense RNA from the *Paramyxoviridae* family that is found primarily in Bangladesh and India [1]. ELISAs are an effective method for detecting the presence of immunological responses against NiV [1–3]. There are a variety of methods for performing an ELISA depending on the choices of ligands and antibodies. For this method, there are two types of ELISA that were used, the indirect ELISA and the sandwich/capture ELISA. For the indirect ELISA, the plates were coated with an irradiated cell lysate [3–7] containing whole NiV. Serum potentially containing the antibody of interest binds to the

Elena Postnikova and Janie Liang contributed equally with all other contributors.

Alexander N. Freiberg and Barry Rockx (eds.), *Nipah Virus: Methods and Protocols*, Methods in Molecular Biology, vol. 2682, https://doi.org/10.1007/978-1-0716-3283-3_17,

viral protein coated on the plate. Following the primary antibody, a secondary antibody with a conjugated horseradish peroxidase (HRP) is added. The secondary antibody is then detected with a colorimetric substrate and the optical density (OD) at 450 nm is quantified using a plate reader.

For the capture ELISA, the purpose is to detect the presence or absence of the antibody of interest. To achieve this objective, the plates are coated with a capture antibody that is designed to bind the antibody of interest in the serum and varies dependent upon the animal species under study, for example, Goat Anti-Monkey IgM antibody. Following the application of the capture antibody and the test serum, irradiated cell culture supernatant containing NiV is added. An anti-NiV antibody is used to bind the NiV G-protein and then an HRP-conjugated secondary antibody is used to detect the anti-NiV antibody. The plate is developed with a substrate and the optical density is measured on a plate reader.

2 Materials

Nipah virus is considered a biosafety level 4 (BSL-4) agent and should be handled in accordance with the guidelines stipulated in the "Biosafety in Microbiological and Biomedical Laboratories" (BMBL) (https://www.cdc.gov/labs/BMBL.html).

2.1 Nipah Virus Preparation

1. Nipah virus stock.
2. T225 Flasks.
3. VeroE6 cells.
4. 50-mL conical tubes.
5. Centrifuge.
6. Cell Scraper.
7. Virus Growth Medium (VGM): Dulbecco's Modified Eagle Medium (DMEM) with L-glutamine and 2% Fetal Bovine Serum (FBS) (*see* **Note 1**).
8. 1X Radioimmunoprecipitation assay (RIPA) Buffer: (*see* **Note 2**).
9. Protease inhibitor tablets.
10. 10X PBS.
11. Bicinchoninic acid (BCA) Assay Kit.

2.2 Plate Coating

1. 1X coating buffer: Dilute 5X coating buffer 1:5 in water [2].
2. Wash solution (PBST): 1X PBS containing 0.1% Tween-20 (v/v) [8] (*see* **Note 3**).

3. Blocking buffer: 1X PBST containing 3% Normal Chicken Serum and 2% Milk.
4. Non-sterile 96-well clear flat-bottom plates coated with Immulon 2 HB.
5. Nipah virus cell culture slurry lysate (see methods section for preparation procedure).
6. Capture antibody (*see* **Note 4**) [9, 10]:
   (a) IgM: Goat Anti-Monkey IgM Antibody (KPL,071–11-031) or Mouse Anti-Hamster IgM Antibody (BD Pharmington, 554031).
   (b) IgG1: Mouse Anti-Human IgG1 Fc Antibody (LSBio, LS-351375).
   (c) IgG2: Mouse Anti-Human IgG2 Fab Antibody (ThermoFisher, MA5–16715) or Mouse Anti-Hamster IgG2 Antibody (BD Pharmington, 624084).

2.3 ELISA Procedure

1. 3,3′,5,5′-Tetramethylbenzidine (TMB) substrate solution.
2. Stop solution for TMB substrate solution.
3. 96-well dilution block.
4. Nipah virus supernatant or slurry (see methods for preparation).
5. Non-Human Primate (NHP) or Hamster serum (test agent), Bronchioalveolar Lavage (BAL) (*see* **Note 5**).
6. Anti-Nipah Antibody (NiV G protein-specific rabbit polyclonal antiserum) [7].
7. Secondary Antibody (*see* **Note 6**):
   (a) IgM Capture ELISA: Goat Anti-Rabbit IgG HRP Antibody (Sigma, 6154).
   (b) IgG indirect ELISA: Rabbit-Anti-Monkey IgG HRP (Sigma, A2054) or Goat-Anti-Hamster IgG HRP (Abcam, ab6892).
   (c) IgA indirect ELISA: Goat-anti-Monkey IgA HRP (Novus Biological, NBP1-737251).
8. Wypalls.

3 Methods

3.1 Nipah Virus Procedure

1. Growing Nipah Virus.
   (a) Seed VeroE6 cells in T225 flasks so that the cell monolayer confluency on the day of use is at 70–80% confluency—

this should be done at least 24 h in advance to give cells time to adhere to the flasks.

(b) In the BSL-4, infect cells with the Nipah virus at a multiplicity of infection (MOI) of 0.01 and rock the flasks every 15 min for a total of 60 min.

(c) Add enough VGM to bring the total volume of the flask to 60 mL and incubate for 2–4 days until up to 50% cytopathic effects (CPE) are observed.

2. Harvesting Supernatant.

(a) Remove the supernatant and divide it into 50-mL conical tubes, keep the flasks for the preparation of the NiV cell culture slurry described in Subheading 3.2.

(b) Spin the supernatant in a centrifuge at 7500 × g for 10 min at 4 °C to clarify.

(c) Remove the supernatant and aliquot into 50-mL conical tubes at a volume no greater than 40 mL.

(d) Irradiate the supernatant using a dose of no less than 5 Mrad while maintaining the material on dry ice throughout the irradiation cycle.

(e) Store at −80 °C until use. Avoid freeze-thaw cycles.

(f) Use for subsequent ELISA procedure.

3.2 NiV Slurry Preparation

1. Lysis of Nipah virus-infected cells.

(a) Use cells retained from the previous procedure.

(b) Add 9–10 mL of 1X PBS per T225 flask and scrape cells off with a cell scraper.

(c) Transfer the cell slurry into a labeled, sterile 50-mL conical tube. Repeat the process until each 50-mL conical tube contains 40 mL of slurry (approximately 4X T225 flasks will fill a single 50-mL conical tube).

(d) After harvesting, spin down 50-mL conical tubes 224 × g for 5 min at 4 °C to pellet the cells and discard supernatants.

(e) Add 1–2 mL of 1X PBS into each 50-mL conical, and resuspend the cell pellets thoroughly using a serological pipette.

(f) Combine slurries (not more than 40 mL per 50-mL conical tube). Write down the number of T225 flasks combined per 50-mL conical tube.

(g) Spin down 50-mL conical tubes 224 × g for 5 min at 4 °C and discard supernatants.

(h) Lyse cells with RIPA buffer by adding 1X RIPA buffer and mix well by pipetting up and down repeatedly.

(i) Each T225 flask has approximately 1.5 × 10^7 cells, use 400–600 μL of 1X RIPA buffer per flask to lyse the cells completely. Let tubes sit on ice at 4 °C for 10–20 min.

(i) Freeze at −80 °C until ready to remove from BSL-4 for irradiation.

(j) Irradiate at 5 Mrad while maintaining the material on dry ice throughout the irradiation cycle prior to transferring material to BSL-2.

2. Homogenization and Sonication of irradiated cell slurries (BSL-2).

(a) Thaw-lysed irradiated NiV cell slurries at room temperature. Disrupt samples by using 15-mL PYREX Dounce Tissue Homogenizer.

(i) On ice, pour sample one by one into sterile homogenizer and make approximately 30 vertical movements with pestle A.

(ii) Transfer samples from the homogenizer to the corresponding 50-mL conical tubes.

(b) Sonicate the viral lysate on the Misonix Sonicator according to manufacturers' instructions (*see* **Note 7** for sonicator settings).

(c) Transfer sonicated NiV cell lysate into Eppendorf™ LoBind Microcentrifuge Tubes (2 mL) and spin down for 10,000 × g for 15 min at 4 °C.

(d) Combine supernatant in a new 50-mL conical tube. Label the tube and place on ice. Determine the protein concentration by using a BCA assay (Pierce) following manufacturer instructions.

(e) After determining the protein concentration, aliquot the cell lysate into 250–500 μL samples and store at −80 °C.

3.3 Indirect IgG ELISA Procedure

1. Coating Plates.

(a) Coat the plates with irradiated NiV cell slurry lysate (Subheading 3.2) diluted in 1X ELISA Coating Buffer (*see* **Notes 8, 9,** and **10**).

(b) Add 50 μL/well (final protein concentration–0.05 μg/well) of diluted irradiated NiV slurry lysate to the 96-well plates.

(c) Store plates at 4 °C and cover to prevent evaporation.

2. ELISA Procedure.
   (a) Wash plates 6X with PBST buffer with at least 200 μL per well of buffer. Soak once in PBST buffer for 1–2 min.
   (b) Dump liquid and tap on paper towel to dry, add 300 μL/well of Blocking Buffer, and incubate the plates at 37 °C for 2 h.
   (c) Meanwhile, heat inactivate all test sera at 56 °C for 1 h.
   (d) Make serial dilutions of sera in Serum Dilution Buffer in dilution blocks or 96 well plates using the following plate map (plate should be run in triplicate); include a positive and negative control:

	1	2	3	4	5	6	7	8	9	10	11	12
Dil.	100	200	400	800	1600	3200	6400	12,800	25,600	51,200	102,400	204,800
A	O	O	O	O	O	O	O	O	O	O	O	O
B	O	O	O	O	O	O	O	O	O	O	O	O
C	O	O	O	O	O	O	O	O	O	O	O	O
D	O	O	O	O	O	O	O	O	O	O	O	O
E	O	O	O	O	O	O	O	O	O	O	O	O
F	O	O	O	O	O	O	O	O	O	O	O	O
G	O	O	O	O	O	O	O	O	O	O	O	O
H	O	O	O	O	O	O	O	O	O	O	O	O

   (e) Remove the plates from the incubator, dump liquid and tap on paper towel to dry.
   (f) Add 40 μL/well of diluted sera to appropriate wells.
   (g) Incubate, covered to prevent evaporation, OVERNIGHT on a rocker at 4 °C.
   (h) The next day, dilute secondary antibody (*see* **Note 6**) in Blocking Buffer.
   (i) Remove plates from 4 °C and wash plates 6X with PBST buffer with at least 200 μL per well of buffer. Soak once in PBST buffer for 1–2 min.
   (j) Add 100 μL/well of diluted secondary antibody and incubate for 1 h at 37 °C.
   (k) Wash plates 6X with PBST buffer with at least 200 μL per well of buffer. Soak once in PBST buffer for 1–2 min.
   (l) Apply 100 μL/well of TMB Substrate Solution to each well (one to two plate(s) at a time). Incubate at room temperature for about 10 min.

(m) Add 100 μL/well of Stop Solution and incubate at room temperature for 10–30 min.

(n) Measure absorbance at 450 nm by Tecan plate reader.

(o) Analyze data.

3.4 Indirect IgA (NHP Only) ELISA Procedure

1. Coating Plates.
   (a) Coat the plates with irradiated NiV slurry lysate diluted in 1X ELISA Coating Buffer (*see* **Notes 8, 9**, and **10**).
   (b) Add 50 μL/well (final protein concentration – 0.05 μg/well) of diluted irradiated NiV slurry lysate to the 96-well plates.
   (c) Store plates at 4 °C overnight and cover to prevent evaporation.
2. ELISA Procedure.
   (a) Wash plates 6X with PBST buffer with at least 200 μL per well of buffer. Soak once in PBST buffer for 1–2 min.
   (b) Dump liquid and tap on paper towel to dry, add 300 μL/well of Blocking Buffer, and incubate the plates at 37 °C for 2 h.
   (c) Make serial dilutions of BAL in Serum Dilution Buffer in dilution blocks or 96-well plates using the following plate map (plate should be run in triplicate); include a positive and negative control if possible:

	1	2	3	4	5	6	7	8	9	10	11	12
Dil.	Und*	2	4	8	16	32	64	128	256	512	1024	2048
A	O	O	O	O	O	O	O	O	O	O	O	O
B	O	O	O	O	O	O	O	O	O	O	O	O
C	O	O	O	O	O	O	O	O	O	O	O	O
D	O	O	O	O	O	O	O	O	O	O	O	O
E	O	O	O	O	O	O	O	O	O	O	O	O
F	O	O	O	O	O	O	O	O	O	O	O	O
G	O	O	O	O	O	O	O	O	O	O	O	O
H	O	O	O	O	O	O	O	O	O	O	O	O

   (d) Remove the plates from the incubator, empty them by tapping against a paper towel.
   (e) Add 40 μL/well of diluted target analytes to appropriate wells.

(f) Incubate, covered to prevent evaporation, OVERNIGHT on a rocker at 4 °C.

(g) The next day dilute secondary antibody (*see* **Note 8**) in Blocking Buffer.

(h) Remove plates from 4 °C and wash plates 6X with PBST buffer with at least 200 μL per well of buffer. Soak once in PBST buffer for 1–2 min.

(i) Add 100 μL/well of diluted secondary antibody and incubate for 1 h at 37 °C.

(j) Wash plates 6X with PBST buffer with at least 200 μL per well of buffer. Soak once in PBST buffer for 1–2 min.

(k) Apply 100 μL/well of TMB Substrate Solution to each well (one–two plate(s) at a time). Incubate at room temperature for about 10 min.

(l) Add 100 μL/well of Stop Solution and incubate at room temperature for 10–30 min.

(m) Measure absorbance at 450 nm by Tecan plate reader.

(n) Analyze data.

3.5 IgM, IgG2, and IgG1 Capture ELISA Procedure

1. Plate Coating.

   (a) Dilute capture antibody in cold 1X ELISA Coating Buffer to bring concentration to 2 μg/ml (*see* **Note 4**).

   (b) Add 100 μl/well (final antibody concentration 0.2 μg/well) of diluted capture antibody to the 96-well plates.

   (c) Store plates at 4 °C overnight and cover to prevent evaporation.

2. ELISA Procedure.

   (a) Wash plates 6X with PBST buffer with at least 200 μL per well of buffer. Soak once in PBST buffer for 1–2 min.

   (b) Dump liquid and tap on paper towel to dry, add 300 μL/well of Blocking Buffer, and incubate the plates at 37 °C for 2 h.

   (c) Heat inactivate all sera at 56 °C for 1 h.

   (d) Make serial dilutions of sera (triplicate) in Serum Dilution Buffer in dilution blocks or 96-well plates using the following plate map (plate should be run in triplicate); include a positive and negative control:

	1	**2**	**3**	**4**	**5**	**6**	**7**	**8**	**9**	**10**	**11**	**12**
Dil.	100	200	400	800	1600	3200	6400	12,800	25,600	51,200	102,400	204,800
A	O	O	O	O	O	O	O	O	O	O	O	O
B	O	O	O	O	O	O	O	O	O	O	O	O
C	O	O	O	O	O	O	O	O	O	O	O	O
D	O	O	O	O	O	O	O	O	O	O	O	O
E	O	O	O	O	O	O	O	O	O	O	O	O
F	O	O	O	O	O	O	O	O	O	O	O	O
G	O	O	O	O	O	O	O	O	O	O	O	O
H	O	O	O	O	O	O	O	O	O	O	O	O

(e) Remove the plates from the incubator and empty them by tapping firmly against a paper towel.

(f) Add 40 μL/well of diluted target analytes to appropriate wells.

(g) Incubate, covered to prevent evaporation, overnight on a rocker at 4 °C.

(h) Dilute irradiated NiV supernatant in Blocking Buffer (*see* **Note 11**).

(i) Remove the plates from 4 °C and wash plates 6X with PBST buffer with at least 200 μL per well of the buffer. Soak once in PBST buffer for 1–2 min.

(j) Empty plates and tap them firmly against a paper towel. Add 50 μL/well of the diluted NiV supernatant to the plate and incubate for 1 h at 37 °C.

(k) Wash plates 6X with PBST buffer with at least 200 μL per well of buffer. Soak once in PBST buffer for 1–2 min.

(l) Dilute Rabbit-anti-NiV-G 1:4000 in Blocking Buffer (dilution may vary dependent upon the antibody used).

(m) Add 100 μL/well of the diluted anti-NiV-G Antibody to the plate and incubate for 1 h at 37 °C.

(n) Wash plates 6X with PBST buffer with at least 200 μL per well of buffer. Soak once in PBST buffer for 1–2 min.

(o) Dilute Goat Anti-Rabbit IgG (whole molecule) – HRP in Blocking Buffer (1:10,000)—1 μl of antibody per 10 ml of Blocking Buffer and apply 100 μL/well.

(p) Wash plates 6X with PBST buffer with at least 200 μL per well of buffer. Soak once in PBST buffer for 1–2 min.

(q) Apply 100 μL/well of TMB Substrate Solution to each well (one-two plate(s) at a time). Incubate at room temperature for about 10 min.

(r) Add 100 μL/well of Stop Solution and incubate at room temperature for 10–30 min.

(s) Measure absorbance at 450 nm using an appropriate plate reader.

(t) Analyze data.

4 Notes

1. For DMEM with L-glutamine and 2% FBS: add 10.2 mL of FBS to 500 mL of DMEM with L-glutamine.
2. Dilute 10X RIPA buffer in ultrapure water at a ratio of 1:10 and add 1–3 protease inhibitor tablets per 50 mL of buffer. Invert until fully dissolved and filter through a 0.2 μm filter.
3. For 1X PBST, mix 300 mL 10X PBS with 2697 mL distilled water and 3 mL of Tween-20.
4. Capture antibody dilution table (following instruction of vendor) [9]:

Serum Source	Antibody of interest	Capture Antibody/Conc.	Concentration
Hamster	IgM	Mouse anti-hamster IgM (0.5 mg/mL)	1:250
Hamster	IgG2	Mouse anti-hamster IgG2 (11.1 mg/mL)	1:5000
NHP	IgM	Goat anti-monkey IgM (1.0 mg/mL)	1:500
NHP	IgG1	Mouse anti-human IgG1 fc (0.5 mg/mL)	1:250
NHP	IgG2	Mouse anti-human IgG2 fab (1.0 mg/mL)	1:500

5. Human and NHP antibodies were tested against African Green Monkeys only.
6. Secondary antibody dilution table (following instruction of vendor):

Serum Source	Antibody of interest	Secondary Antibody	Concentration
Hamster	IgG	Goat Anti-Hamster IgG HRP	1:10,000
NHP	IgG	Rabbit Anti-Monkey IgG (whole molecule) HRP	1:45,000
NHP	IgA	Goat Anti-Monkey IgA HRP	1:10,000

7. Sonicator program using the cup:
   (a) 4 times—30 seconds of exposure time
   (b) Pulse on—30 sec exposure.
   (c) Pulse off—1 min.
8. All antigens and antibodies should be diluted in blocking buffer, only test samples are to be diluted in serum dilution buffer.
9. All buffers should be maintained at 4 °C. Plates must be placed at 4 °C at least 30 min prior to coating.
10. The NiV slurry lysate should be diluted to a final protein concentration of 1.0 μg/mL so that when 50 μL is added to each well, the protein concentration is 0.048 μg/well.
11. NiV supernatant should be diluted in blocking buffer to a concentration of approximately 10^6 pfu/well.

Acknowledgments

This work was funded in part through Battelle Memorial Institute's prime contract with the US National Institute of Allergy and Infectious Diseases (NIAID) under Contract No. HHSN272200700016I. The content of this publication does not necessarily reflect the views or policies of the US Department of Health and Human Services (DHHS) or of the institutions and companies affiliated with the authors.

References

1. Flint SJ et al (2015) Principles of virology, 4th edn. ASM Press, Washington, DC
2. Bausch DG et al (2000) Diagnosis and clinical virology of Lassa fever as evaluated by enzyme-linked immunosorbent assay, indirect fluorescent-antibody test, and virus isolation. J Clin Microbiol 38(7):2670–2677
3. Daniels P, Ksiazek T, Eaton BT (2001) Laboratory diagnosis of Nipah and Hendra virus infections. Microbes Infect 3(4):289–295
4. Cong Y et al (2009) Vaccination with a defined Francisella tularensis subsp. novicida pathogenicity Island mutant (DeltaiglB) induces protective immunity against homotypic and heterotypic challenge. Vaccine 27(41): 5554–5561
5. Pfaff E et al (1988) Analysis of neutralizing epitopes on foot-and-mouth disease virus. J Virol 62(6):2033–2040

6. Wacharapluesadee S et al (2005) Bat Nipah virus, Thailand. Emerg Infect Dis 11(12): 1949–1951
7. Yu F et al (2006) Serodiagnosis using recombinant nipah virus nucleocapsid protein expressed in Escherichia coli. J Clin Microbiol 44(9):3134–3138
8. Shirai J, Matsumura T (2007) Application of enzyme-linked immunosorbent assays for the diagnosis of emerging equine paramyxovirus infection. Acta Veterinaria 57(2–3):143–155
9. Chiang CF et al (2010) Use of monoclonal antibodies against Hendra and Nipah viruses in an antigen capture ELISA. Virol J 7:115
10. Ebersole JL et al (1990) Molecular approaches to leucotoxin as a virulence component in Actinobacillus actinomycetemcomitans. Arch Oral Biol 35(Suppl):69S–78S

Chapter 18

Assays for Detecting Henipavirus Antibodies

Lin-Fa Wang, Shailendra Mani, Chee Wah Tan, and Danielle E. Anderson

Abstract

While molecular detection has increasingly become the detection method of choice for infectious diseases, antibody detection remains an important approach for diagnosis and surveillance. For henipaviruses, antibody detection methods such as ELISA and Western blot played a key role in the initial discovery of bats as the natural reservoir host. Here, we will describe three additional antibody detection methods (LIPS, Luminex, and pseudovirus systems), which can be used in most BSL2 laboratories without the need for live virus and a high containment BSL4 facility.

Key words Henipavirus, Hendra, Nipah, Luciferase immunoprecipitation system (LIPS), Luminex, Pseudovirus

1 Introduction

The serological detection of pathogen-specific antibodies is used to play a key role in the diagnosis and surveillance of infectious diseases [1]. In the last few decades, with the rapid advance of molecular techniques, serology has almost become a "forgotten" tool that has been overshadowed by PCR and sequencing approaches. However, despite the lack of "revolutionary" advances of serological platforms in the same league as PCR for molecular detection, antibody detection still played a key role in several major outbreak investigations from epidemiological tracing [2, 3], reservoir identification [4] to assessment of zoonotic potential of emerging viruses [5]. For henipaviruses, serology played a key role in the identification of bats as the natural reservoir [4, 6] and for the mapping of high-risk bat species and geographical locations in different parts of the world [7–11].

The original antibody detection methods were ELISA-based, using whole virus antigens and the virus neutralization test (VNT) remains the "gold standard" [12]. Unfortunately, for henipaviruses, both platforms rely on the use of live viruses which can only be done in a biosafety level 4 (BSL4) facility, which is not

Alexander N. Freiberg and Barry Rockx (eds.), *Nipah Virus: Methods and Protocols*, Methods in Molecular Biology, vol. 2682, https://doi.org/10.1007/978-1-0716-3283-3_18,

available in most of the laboratories. Here, we describe three non-ELISA antibody detection methods which can be implemented in standard BSL2 laboratories and do not require the growth of live viruses, based on three different platforms, i.e., the luciferase immunoprecipitation system (LIPS) [13, 14], the Luminex bead-based liquid array system [15], and the pseudo virus system [16, 17] (*see* **Note 1**).

2 Materials

All reagents should be of AR grade. All solutions and buffers should be prepared using ultrapure water, autoclaved, or filter-sterilized where appropriate. Sterile tubes and filter tips should be used.

2.1 General

1. HEK 293T (Human Embryonic kidney cells) ATCC CRL-3216, COS-1 (*Cercopithecus aethiops* cells) ATCC CRL-1650.
2. Antibodies: Anti-human IgG PE conjugate (Stock- 0.5 mg/mL, eBioscience, Cat. No. 12-4998-82), Anti-human IgM PE conjugate (Stock- 0.5 mg/mL, Southern Biotech, Cat. No. 2020-09), and Anti-his antibody PE conjugate (Abcam, Cat. No. ab72467).
3. 100 mm tissue culture dish.
4. DMEM-Dulbecco's Modified Eagle Medium.
5. Fetal bovine serum.
6. Trypsin 0.25% EDTA.
7. Dulbecco's PBS (2.7 mM KCl, 1.5 mM KH_2PO_4, 136.9 mM NaCl, and 8.9 mM $Na_2HPO_4.7H_2O$).
8. Opti-MEM media.
9. Cell scraper.
10. FuGENE 6 transfection reagent.
11. Polyethylenimine (PEI) transfection reagent.
12. pREN-2, pcDNA3.1-C6his, pCAGGS vector.
13. Power supply, horizontal agarose gel electrophoresis tank, Mini-PROTEIN II SDS-PAGE system, and Mini Trans-Blot Module were all purchased from Bio-Rad (Hercules, CA).
14. Rocker and orbital shaker.

2.2 Gene Cloning

1. *BamH*I, *Xho*I, *Hind*III, *Nhe*I, and *Not*I restriction endonuclease.
2. OMEGA E.Z.N.A. gel extraction kit.
3. OMEGA E.Z.N.A. cycle-pure kit I.

4. OMEGA E.Z.N.A. plasmid DNA mini kit I.
5. OMEGA E.Z.N.A. endo-free plasmid DNA maxi kit.
6. Luria Broth (LB), Miller bacterial culture media.
7. LB Agar Miller.
8. Agarose biotechnology grade.
9. Kanamycin.
10. Glycerol biotechnology grade.
11. NEB 5-alpha competent *E. coli* (high efficiency).
12. Q5 High-fidelity PCR reagents, use as recommended by the supplier. It is essential to use high-fidelity DNA polymerases to reduce PCR-introduced error.
13. T4 DNA ligase and ligation buffer, use as recommended.

2.3 Luciferase Immunoprecipitation System (LIPS)

2.3.1 Primers

2.3.2 LIPS Assay

1. 96-well plate (white flat bottom).
2. 96-well culture plate (round bottom).
3. MultiScreen 96-well filter plate.
4. BIO-RAD microseal 'B' seal seals.
5. Multiscreen vacuum manifold separation system (Millipore-MSVMHTS00).
6. Renilla luciferase assay system.
7. Cold lysis buffer (50 mM Tris, pH 7.5, 100 mM NaCl, 5 mM $MgCl_2$, 1% Triton X-100, 50% glycerol, and protease inhibitors).
8. Buffer A (20 mM Tris, pH 7.5, 150 mM NaCl, 5 mM $MgCl_2$, and 1% Triton X-100).
9. Buffer B (Buffer A containing 100 μg/mL BSA).
10. CYTATION 5 imaging reader (BioTek).
11. Gen5 3.03 software.

2.4 Luminex

1. Trizma base.
2. Sodium chloride.
3. Triton-X100.
4. SDS.
5. Imidazole.

6. Protease inhibitor.
7. RIPA lysis buffer (10 mM Tris-Cl [pH 8.0], 1 mM EDTA. 1% Triton X-100, 0.1% sodium deoxycholate, 0.1% SDS, 140 mM NaCl, and 1 mM PMSF).
8. Cell lysis buffer (30 mM Tris, 300 mM NaCl, 1% Triton-X, 0.1% SDS, 10 mM βME, 25 mM Imidazole, pH 8.0).
9. Purification buffer 1 (30 mM Tris and 300 mM NaCl pH 8.0).
10. Purification buffer 2 (30 mM Tris, 300 mM NaCl, and 500 mM imidazole pH 8.0).
11. Ni Sepharose 6 Fast Flow.
12. AKTA start protein purification system.
13. UNICORN start control software.
14. Luminex MagPlex microsphere beads.
15. xMAP antibody coupling (AbC) Kit (Luminex-40-50016).
16. Luminex assay buffer (PBS supplemented with 1% Bovine serum albumin).
17. 96-well plate (round bottom).
18. BIO-RAD microseal 'B' seal seals.
19. 96-well plate (flat bottom).
20. Hercuvan lab system-microplate thermoshaker incubator.
21. Magnet plate separator.
22. Tecan hydrospeed plate washer with a magnetic platform.
23. MAGPIX Calibration kit (Luminex-MPXIVD-CAL-K25).
24. MAGPIX performance verification kit (Luminex-MPXIVD-PVER-K25).
25. MAGPIX NxTAG Enabled *Luminex* plate reader.
26. Luminex xPONENT for MAGPIX version 4.2 software.

2.5 Pseudovirus

1. Baby hamster kidney cells (BHK-21) ATCC CCL-10 and African green monkey kidney cells (Vero) ATCC CCL-81.
2. Defective vesicular stomatitis virus that expressing green fluorescent protein (GFP) (VSVΔG-GFP).
3. Plasmids: pCAGGS-NiV-F, pCAGGS-NiV-G.
4. Lipofectamine 3000.
5. CYTATION 5 imaging reader (BioTek).
6. 1 X Tris-acetate-EDTA (TAE) buffer (40 mM Tris, 20 mM Acetate, and 1 mM EDTA).

3 Methods

3.1 LIPS

3.1.1 Cloning of Target Gene

1. Amplify the open reading frame of NiV-N, NiV-M, NiV-F, and NiV-G genes from cDNA using forward and reverse primers listed in Table 1 (*see* **Note 2**).
2. Run 1% agarose gel to confirm the correct size of each DNA fragment.
3. Excise the correct DNA fragment for each gene by viewing on a UV gel illuminator and purify the DNA using the E.Z.N.A gel extraction kit according to the manufacturer's instructions.
4. Digest the amplicons and pREN-2 vector using *BamH*I and *Xho*I restriction enzymes in a 20 μL reaction at 37 °C for 1 h.
5. Purify the digested amplicons and pREN-2 vector DNA.
6. Ligate using T4 DNA ligase with an amplicon to a vector ratio of 3:1 at 4 °C for 16 h.
7. Add 1 μL of the ligation mix to 15 μL NEB 5-alpha competent *E. coli* and incubate on ice for 20 min.
8. Heat-shock the cells at 42 °C for 45 s in a water bath and immediately place on ice for 2 min.
9. Plate the cells on agar containing kanamycin as the selection marker. Incubate at 37 °C overnight.
10. Select the positive clones by colony PCR and extract the plasmid DNA for restriction enzyme analysis and sequencing.

3.1.2 Production of Recombinant Luc-Fusion Proteins

1. Seed COS-1 cells using DMEM supplemented with 10% FBS into 100 × 20 mm tissue culture dishes at 2×10^6 cells per plate and incubate at 37 °C for 24 h.
2. The COS-1 cells should be 80–95% confluent at the time of transfection. Allow the FuGENE 6 transfection reagent, which is stored at 4 °C, to warm up to room temperature.
3. Add 230 μL of Opti-MEM media to each tube. Add 15 μL of FuGENE 6 transfection reagent to the Opti-MEM media Incubate the mixture for 5 min at room temperature (*see* **Note 3**).
4. Add 5 μg of plasmid for Rluc-antigen fusion constructs (NiV-N, NiV-M, NiV-F, and NiV-G). Mix by inverting/tapping the tube.
5. Incubate this mixture for 15 min at room temperature.
6. After incubation, transfer the DNA- FuGENE 6-Opti-MEM solution to the cells by distributing evenly in a drop-wise manner onto the media of the COS-1 cells.
7. Incubate transfected plates at 37 °C with 5% CO_2 for 48 h.

Table 1
Primers used for the amplification of Nipah virus genes

No.	Primers	Sequence
1	NiV N forward	5′ ATGCCATGGATCCCGAATGAGTGATATTTTTGAAGAGGCGGCTAG 3′
2	NiV N reverse	5′ CGTAGCACTCGAGGATTCACACATCAGCTCTGACAAAGTCAAG 3′
3	NiV M forward	5′ ATGCCATGGATCCCGAATGGAGCCAGACATCAAGAG 3′
4	NiV M reverse	5′ CGTAGCACTCGAGGATTTAGCCCTTTAGAATTCTCCCTGTATTG 3′
5	NiV F forward	5′ ATGCCATGGATCCCGAATGGCAGTTATACTTAACAAGAG 3′
6	NiV F reverse	5′ CGTAGCAGCGGCCGCGATCTACGTCCCAATGTAATAGAG 3′
7	NiV G forward	5′ ATGCCATAAGCTTCGAATGCCGACAGAAAGCAAGAAAGTTAG 3′
8	NiV G reverse	5′ CGTAGCAGCGGCCGCGATTTATGTACATTGCTCTGGTATC 3′

8. At 48 h post transfection, remove the media and rinse cells with 5–6 mL of cold PBS. Repeat the wash.
9. Add 1.4 mL of cold lysis buffer. Harvest cells with a cell scrapper and quickly transfer the lysate to a 2 mL Eppendorf tube on ice.
10. Keep the tube on ice and sonicate cells using a sonicator with a pulse setting of 5 s on/5 s off at 50% amplitude.
11. Incubate the lysed cells at 4 °C for 20 min (Use an Eppendorf tube rotator).
12. Centrifuge the cell lysate at 16,000 × g for 5 min at 4 °C. Collect the supernatant in a 2 mL Eppendorf tube.
13. Centrifuge the supernatant again at 16,000 × g for 10 min at 4 °C. Collect the supernatant in a 2 mL Eppendorf tube.
14. Measure the luminescence by luciferase assay using manufacturer's protocol (Promega, E2820) using a luminometer.
    (a) Equilibrate coelenterazine substrate, assay buffer, and lysis buffer stored at room temperature and mix by vortexing.
    (b) Calculate the total volume of the substrate solution required (required volume- 50 μL/well).
    (c) To prepare 1 mL of luciferase substrate, mix 10 μL of coelenterazine substrate, 790 μL of Assay buffer, and 200 μL of lysis buffer.
    (d) Add 50 μL of luciferase substrate in each well using a luminescence reader (injector function) and read luminescence.
    (e) Export data in an Excel file.

15. Store the Ruc-antigen lysates at −80 °C in aliquots of 200–500 μL/tube.

3.1.3 Antibody Detection Using LIPS

1. Equilibrate protein A/G beads to room temperature. Mix by inverting to make a uniform solution.
2. Label an Eppendorf tube as 30% slurry beads.
3. To make 1 mL of 30% slurry beads, add 600 μL of beads (stock 50% slurry beads) to 400 μL of PBS (filtered).
4. Wash beads 3–5 times with PBS.
5. Thaw sera on ice.
6. Prepare a 1:10 dilution of sera in Buffer B.
7. 10 μL serum (1:10 diluted) is required per well.
8. Calculate the required volume of the Rluc-antigens corresponding to 5×10^6 light units (LU) according to the luminescence reading observed after expression.
9. Calculate the required volume of Buffer A for a total volume of 84 μL in each well and add accordingly.
10. Pipette the calculated volume (corresponding to 5×10^6 LU) of respective Rluc-antigen in each well. Add the desired volume of the washed protein A/G beads (6 μL/well) and mix with Buffer A containing Rluc-antigens.
11. Mix the solution using a multichannel pipette and distribute 90 μL of the mixture into 96-well plates.
12. Add 10 μL of diluted sera to the respective wells and mix.
13. Seal the plate carefully with BioRAD plate sealer to avoid any leakage or evaporation during incubation.
14. Incubate at 4 °C, with rotation, for 2 h (use a plate rotator).
15. Centrifuge at 2300 × *g* at 4 °C for 3 min.
16. Resuspend samples carefully and transfer to 96-well filter plates. One well of sample will be transferred to one well of 96-well filter plate.
17. Assemble a vacuum manifold platform for 96-well filter plates.
18. Take the 96-well filter plate, cover the lid, and place over the vacuum manifold. Switch on the vacuum to drain the samples.
19. To wash the samples, add 100 μL of Buffer A to each well.
20. Close the lid of the plate and switch on the vacuum to drain out the buffer.
21. Repeat this wash step six times with Buffer A followed by two times with PBS.

22. Take out the filter plate and put it on tissue paper to absorb the remaining buffer.
23. Prepare the substrate and read the plate as described above.

3.2 Luminex

3.2.1 Cloning and Expression of Target Genes

1. Amplify open reading frame of NiV-N, NiV-M, NiV-F, and NiV-G genes from cDNA using forward and reverse primers (*see* **Note 2**).
2. Run 1% agarose gel to confirm the correct size of each DNA fragment.
3. Excise the correct size DNA fragment for each gene by viewing on a UV gel illuminator and purify the DNA using an E.Z.N.A gel extraction kit according to the manufacturer's instructions.
4. Digest the amplicons and pcDNA3.1-C6His vector using *BamHI* and *XhoI* restriction enzymes in 20 μL reaction at 37 °C for 1 h.
5. Purify the digested amplicons and pREN-2 vector DNA.
6. Ligate using T4 DNA ligase with an amplicon to a vector ratio of 3:1 at 4 °C for 16 h.
7. Add 1 μL of the ligation mix to 15 μL NEB 5-alpha competent *E. coli* and incubate on ice for 20 min.
8. Heat-shock the cells at 42 °C for 45 s in a water bath and immediately place on ice for 2 min.
9. Plate the cells on agar containing ampicillin as the selection marker. Incubate at 37 °C overnight.
10. Select the positive clones by colony PCR and extract the plasmid DNA for restriction enzyme analysis and sequencing.
11. Seed HEK 293 T cells into 100 × 20 mm tissue culture dishes at 5×10^6 cells per plate and incubate at 37 °C for 24 h.
12. The HEK 293 T cells should be 70–80% confluent at the time of transfection. Allow the PEI transfection reagent, which is stored at 4 °C, to warm up to room temperature.
13. Add 230 μL of Opti-MEM media to each tube. Add 60 μL of PEI transfection reagent to the Opti-MEM media. Mix and incubate the mixture for 5 min at room temperature (*see* **Note 4**).
14. Add 20 μg of plasmid from NiV-N, NiV-M, NiV-F, and NiV-G separately in each tube. Mix by vortexing the tube.
15. Incubate this mixture for 15 min at room temperature.
16. After incubation, transfer the DNA-PEI-Opti-MEM solution to the cells by distributing evenly in a drop-wise manner onto the media of the HEK 293T cells.
17. Incubate transfected plates at 37 °C with 5% CO_2 for 48 h.
18. At 48 h post transfection, harvest the cells and wash with PBS.

19. Add 800 μL of RIPA lysis buffer.
20. Keep the lysate on ice and sonicate cells using a sonicator with a pulse setting of 5 s on/5 s off at 50% amplitude.
21. Incubate the lysate at 4 °C for 30 min, with rotation.
22. Centrifuge the cell lysate at 12,500 rpm for 5 min at 4 °C. Collect the supernatant in a 2 mL Eppendorf tube.
23. Centrifuge the supernatant at 12,500 rpm for 10 min at 4 °C. Collect the supernatant in a 2 mL Eppendorf tube.
24. Prepare a 12% SDS-PAGE gel and confirm the expression of the proteins by Western blot using anti-His antibody.

3.2.2 Purification of Recombinant Proteins

1. Seed HEK 293T cells into 100 × 20 mm tissue culture dishes (25 dishes) at 5×10^6 per plate and incubate at 37 °C for 24 h.
2. Transfect cells as described in the above protocol (12–17).
3. At 48 h post transfection, harvest the cells and wash with PBS.
4. Add 20 mL of cell lysis buffer.
5. Keep the Falcon tube on ice and sonicate cells using a sonicator with a pulse setting of 5 s on/5 s off at 50% amplitude.
6. Incubate the lysed cells at 4 °C for 30 min, with rotation.
7. Centrifuge the cell lysate at 16,000 × g for 15 min at 4 °C. Collect the supernatant in a 50-mL Falcon tube.
8. Filter the protein lysate through a 0.45 μM filter and collect lysate in a Falcon tube. Remove 250 μL of the filtered protein lysate to confirm protein expression by Western blot.
9. Remove 250 μL of Ni-NTA 6 fast flow resin and wash with 1 mL of water three times.
10. Incubate the Ni-NTA 6 Fast flow beads with 1 mL of cell lysis buffer at 4 °C for 30 min.
11. Centrifuge beads at 300 × g at 4 °C for 3 min.
12. Collect the beads and add the filtered protein lysate. Incubate overnight at 4 °C with rotation.
13. After overnight incubation, centrifuge at 300 × g for 3 min at 4 °C. Transfer the clear supernatant without disturbing the beads to a Falcon tube, leaving 500 μL to 1 mL residual volume in the original Falcon tube.
14. Label the supernatant as 'flow through' and store at −20 °C for further analysis.
15. Collect the beads and load on a C column (GE healthcare) connected to an AKTA smart purifier (GE healthcare). Prepare purification Buffer 1 and purification Buffer 2.
16. Wash the column with 4 mL of purification Buffer 1.

17. Using the AKTA purifier, run a step imidazole gradient with 3 mL steps each of 50 mM imidazole, 100 mM imidazole, 150 mM imidazole, 200 mM imidazole, 300 mM imidazole, and 500 mM imidazole, respectively.
18. Collect the purified protein in 500 μL fractions.
19. Confirm the purity of the protein by resolving on a 12% SDS-PAGE gel and staining with Coomassie blue.
20. Pool the purified fractions and dialyze against PBS.
21. Calculate the protein concentration by measuring the O.D. at 280 nM using a spectrophotometer.

3.2.3 Conjugation of Proteins to Luminex Beads

1. Take 25 μg of the purified protein and couple with 5×10^6 Luminex beads using xMAP Antibody Coupling Kit (AbC, Luminex corporation) using the manufacturer's protocol.
2. Incubate the conjugated beads overnight at 4 °C before using them for the assay.
3. Calculate the number of beads using a hemocytometer.
4. Confirm the presence of the coupled protein by anti-His PE conjugate antibody.

3.2.4 Antibody Detection Using Luminex

1. Thaw sera on ice.
2. Prepare a 1:50 dilution of sera in Luminex assay buffer. The total required volume of each serum is 50 μL/well.
3. Beads required: 1250 beads/antigen/50 μL. If testing one 96-well plate, calculate for 105 wells (required beads for each antigen is $105 \times 1250 = 131{,}250$ beads).
4. Add the required volume of beads (as calculated above) and add Luminex assay buffer to make up the volume to 50 μL/ well. Keep the master bead mix tube in the dark at all times. (*see* **Note 5**).
5. Vortex the master bead mix tube for 30 s and distribute 50 μL of beads per well in a 96-well plate.
6. Transfer the 50 μL diluted serum samples into the aliquoted beads and mix.
7. Carefully seal the plate using BioRad plate sealer and cover with the black plate lid (Luminex).
8. Incubate antigen and serum mixture at 37 °C in an orbitor shaker (set at low to medium speed) for 90 min.
9. Wash the plate three times with Luminex assay buffer using Tecan (hydro speed) plate washer containing 96-well plate magnetic platform adaptor (Use magnetic bead wash protocol, recommended by Luminex).

10. Add 6 μL of the anti-human IgG PE conjugate or anti-human IgM PE conjugate to 12 mL of Luminex assay buffer.
11. Vortex for 30 s and add 100 μL of the diluted antibody (anti-IgG or anti-IgM) into each well and mix.
12. Carefully seal the plate using a BioRad plate seal and cover with the black plate lid (Luminex).
13. Incubate antigen and antibody mixture at 37 °C in an orbitor shaker (set at low to medium speed) for 60 min.
14. Wash the plate three times with Luminex assay buffer using Tecan (hydro speed) plate washer containing 96-well plate magnetic platform (Use magnetic bead wash protocol, Luminex).
15. Add 75 μL of Luminex assay buffer in each well and mix the beads using a 50-μL multichannel pipette (use 100 μL tips).
16. Read the plate using a Luminex reader.

3.3 Pseudotyped Virus

3.3.1 Cloning of Henipavirus G and F Genes into pCAGGS Mammalian Expression Vector

1. Extract NiV RNA using a QIAamp viral RNA mini kit (according to manufacturer's instructions (*see* **Note 2**).
2. Reverse transcribe the RNA into cDNA using random hexamers.
3. Add 1 μL of viral RNA, 1 μL of random hexamer, and 3 μL of nuclease-free water. Incubate the reaction at 70 °C for 5 min. Immediately chill on ice for at least 5 min.
4. Add 4 μL of ImProm-II 5X reaction buffer, 3.7 μL of $MgCl_2$ (25 mM), 1 μL of dNTP (10 mM), 20 units of RNasin ribonuclease inhibitor, and 1 μL of ImProm-II reverse transcriptase. Add H_2O to the reverse transcription reaction to a final volume of 15 μL. Add 15 μL of the reverse transcription reaction to a tube containing 5 μL of viral RNA-primer mix. Incubate the tubes in a thermal cycler at 42 °C for 1 h followed by 70 °C for 15 min to inactivate the reverse transcriptase.
5. Amplify the open reading frame of NiV-G and NiV-F using Q5 high-fidelity DNA polymerase with gene-specific primers containing *Not*I and *Nhe*I restriction sites at the 5′ end and 3′ end, respectively. It is important to include a Kozak sequence (GCC ACC **ATG**) prior to the ATG start codon (underlined).
6. Resolve the PCR amplicon in 1% agarose by gel electrophoresis in 1X TAE buffer and run at 80 V.
7. Excise the desired bands by viewing on a UV gel illuminator and purify the DNA using E.Z.N.A gel extraction kit according to manufacturer's instructions.
8. Perform the digestion on the amplicons and pCAGGS vector using *Not*I and *Nhe*I in 20 μL reaction at 37 °C for 1 h.

9. Perform DNA purification for digested amplicons and pCAGGS vector.
10. Perform ligation using T4 DNA ligase with amplicon to vector ratio of 5:1 at room temperature for 1 h.
11. Add 1 μL of the ligation mix to 15 μL NEB 5-alpha competent *E. coli* and incubate on ice for 20 min.
12. Heat-shock the cells at 42 °C for 45 s in a water bath and immediately place on ice for 2 min.
13. Plate the cells on an agar plate with ampicillin as the section marker. Incubate at 37 °C overnight.
14. Select the positive clones and extract the plasmid for restriction enzyme analysis and sequencing.

3.3.2 Production of Pseudotyped Virus

1. Pre-seed BHK-21 cells at 2×10^6 cells in a 10 cm culture dish and incubate overnight at 37 °C in a CO_2 incubator.
2. Perform transfection of the pCAGGS-NiV-F and pCAGGS-NiV-G into BHK-21 cells using Lipofectamine 3000 and P3000 reagent.
3. Add 250 μL of Opti-MEM with 10 μg of pCAGGS-NiV-F, 10 μg of pCAGGS-NiV-G, and 20 μL of P3000 reagent (Tube A).
4. Prepare 250 μL of Opti-MEM with 60 μL of Lipofectamine 3000 (Tube B).
5. Mix both tubes A and B and incubate at room temperature for 15 min.
6. Add the DNA-Lipofectamine 3000 complexes into BHK-21 cells in a drop-wise manner.
7. At 4 h post-transfection, remove the medium containing Lipofectamine 3000 and replenish with fresh medium containing 10% FBS.
8. At 24 h post-transfection, infect the transfected cells with defective G-VSVΔG-GFP at a MOI of 1.
9. Remove the inoculum at 1 h post-infection, wash the infected cells with Dulbecco's PBS for three times to remove unattached defective G-VSVΔG-GFP viruses (*See* **Note 6**).
10. Replenish the infected cells with DMEM supplemented with 10% FBS and incubate for 24 h.
11. At 24 h post-infection, collect the supernatant containing NiV and HeV pseudotyped viruses and clarify the supernatant by centrifugation at 2000 × g for 10 min.
12. Filter the supernatant using 0.45 μm filter unit and aliquot the supernatant. Store at −80 °C.

3.3.3 Antibody Detection Using Pseudovirus (Virus Neutralization Test)

1. Plate Vero cells in a 96-well plate with 1×10^4 cells/well.
2. Perform two-fold serial dilution of the serum using serum-free DMEM.
3. Dilute the NiV pseudotyped virus to a final concentration of 800 fluorescent forming unit/mL.
4. Add 50 μL of diluted serum to 50 μL of NiV pseudotyped virus and incubate at 37 °C for 1 h.
5. Add the serum-pseudotyped virus mix to Vero cells and incubate at 37 °C for 1 h. Remove the inoculum and wash the cells with DPBS three times to remove unattached viruses. Replenish the cells with 100 μL of medium containing 2% FBS.
6. Incubate the infected cells for 24 h. At 24 h post-infection, image the green fluorescent using a CYTATION 5 imaging reader (BioTek).

4 Notes

1. Although the focus of this chapter is on IgG antibody detection, two of the three platforms (LIPS and Luminex) can be adapted to IgM testing. The bottleneck for the development of the henipavirus IgM test lies in the lack of a positive control serum panel.
2. Here, we have described methods for Nipah virus (NiV) only. The same protocols can be used for Hendra virus (HeV) or other related henipavirus without any significant change.
3. Adjust the volume of Opti-MEM media according to DNA concentration to make the final total volume at 250 μL (Opti-MEM media + FuGENE + DNA).
4. Adjust the volume of Opti-MEM media according to DNA concentration to make the final total volume at 250 μL (Opti MEM media + PEI + DNA).
5. When ready to use, vortex the beads for 30 s and take the required volume immediately before the beads settle down.
6. The washing step after defective G-VSVΔGFP infection is critical to ensure no G-VSVΔGFP contamination.

References

1. Washington JA (1996) Principles of diagnosis: Serodiagnosis. In: Barton S (ed) Baron's medical microbiology. University of Texas Medical Branch
2. Li W, Shi Z, Yu M, Ren W, Smith C, Epstein JH, Wang H, Crameri G, Hu Z, Zhang H (2005) Bats are natural reservoirs of SARS-like coronaviruses. Science 310:676–679
3. Tu C, Crameri G, Kong X, Chen J, Sun Y, Yu M, Xiang H, Xia X, Liu S, Ren T (2004) Antibodies to SARS coronavirus in civets. Emerg Infect Dis 10:2244

4. Young PL, Halpin K, Selleck PW, Field H, Gravel JL, Kelly MA, Mackenzie JS (1996) Serologic evidence for the presence in Pteropus bats of a paramyxovirus related to equine morbillivirus. Emerg Infect Dis 2:239–240
5. Zhou P, Fan H, Lan T, Yang XL, Shi WF, Zhang W, Zhu Y, Zhang YW, Xie QM, Mani S et al (2018) Fatal swine acute diarrhoea syndrome caused by an HKU2-related coronavirus of bat origin. Nature 556:255–258
6. Yob JM, Field H, Rashdi AM, Morrissy C, van der Heide B, Rota P, bin Adzhar A, White J, Daniels P, Jamaluddin A et al (2001) Nipah virus infection in bats (order Chiroptera) in peninsular Malaysia. Emerg Infect Dis 7:439–441
7. Hasebe F, Thuy NT, Inoue S, Yu F, Kaku Y, Watanabe S, Akashi H, Dat DT, Mai le TQ, Morita K (2012) Serologic evidence of nipah virus infection in bats, Vietnam. Emerg Infect Dis 18:536–537
8. Iehle C, Razafitrimo G, Razainirina J, Andriaholinirina N, Goodman SM, Faure C, Georges-Courbot MC, Rousset D, Reynes JM (2007) Henipavirus and Tioman virus antibodies in pteropodid bats, Madagascar. Emerg Infect Dis 13:159–161
9. Hayman DT, Suu-Ire R, Breed AC, McEachern JA, Wang L, Wood JL, Cunningham AA (2008) Evidence of henipavirus infection in west African fruit bats. PLoS One 3:e2739
10. Pernet O, Schneider BS, Beaty SM, LeBreton M, Yun TE, Park A, Zachariah TT, Bowden TA, Hitchens P, Ramirez CM et al (2014) Evidence for henipavirus spillover into human populations in Africa. Nat Commun 5: 5342
11. Li Y, Wang J, Hickey AC, Zhang Y, Li Y, Wu Y, Zhang H, Yuan J, Han Z, McEachern J (2008) Antibodies to Nipah or Nipah-like viruses in bats, China. Emerg Infect Dis:14, 1974
12. Wang LF, Daniels P (2012) Diagnosis of henipavirus infection: current capabilities and future directions. Curr Top Microbiol Immunol 359:179–196
13. Burbelo PD, Ching KH, Klimavicz CM, Iadarola MJ (2009) Antibody profiling by luciferase immunoprecipitation systems (LIPS). J Vis Exp
14. Burbelo PD, Ching KH, Bush ER, Han BL, Iadarola MJ (2010) Antibody-profiling technologies for studying humoral responses to infectious agents. Expert Rev Vaccines 9:567–578
15. Bossart KN, McEachern JA, Hickey AC, Choudhry V, Dimitrov DS, Eaton BT, Wang L-F (2007) Neutralization assays for differential henipavirus serology using bio-Plex protein Array systems. J Virol Methods 142:29–40
16. Kaku Y, Noguchi A, Marsh GA, McEachern JA, Okutani A, Hotta K, Bazartseren B, Fukushi S, Broder CC, Yamada A (2009) A neutralization test for specific detection of Nipah virus antibodies using pseudotyped vesicular stomatitis virus expressing green fluorescent protein. J Virol Methods 160:7–13
17. Kaku Y, Noguchi A, Marsh GA, Barr JA, Okutani A, Hotta K, Bazartseren B, Fukushi S, Broder CC, Yamada A (2012) Second generation of pseudotype-based serum neutralization assay for Nipah virus antibodies: sensitive and high-throughput analysis utilizing secreted alkaline phosphatase. J Virol Methods 179:226–232

Part V

Host Responses to Henipavirus Infection

Chapter 19

Profiling Host MicroRNA Responses to Henipavirus Infection

Ryan J. Farr, Sudeep Dahal, Leon Tribolet, Andrew G. D. Bean, Christopher Cowled, and Cameron R. Stewart

Abstract

Diseases caused by henipaviruses feature incubation periods of up to 16 days, during which infected animals may show no apparent signs of disease yet be capable of transmitting the virus to humans. This risk has prompted research into host-derived biomarkers for early disease detection. Here, we describe a methodology for the assaying of host microRNAs (miRs), small non-coding RNAs that show promise as biomarkers for several human diseases and are responsive during early-stage henipavirus infection. In addition to their potential as disease biomarkers, miRNA profiling of henipavirus infections provides insight into cellular and immune pathways associated with disease pathogenesis.

Key words microRNA, Biomarker, Henipavirus, Diagnostic

1 Introduction

miRs are short (~22 nucleotides) non-coding RNAs that regulate gene expression in eukaryotes at the post-transcriptional level (reviewed in [1]). Base pairing between miRNAs and complementary sequences within messenger RNA (mRNA) targets leads to the inhibition of gene function via RNA silencing, either by transcript degradation or translational inhibition [1]. First discovered in *C. elegans*, miRNAs are abundant and functional in higher organisms and are estimated to regulate between 30% and 60% of protein-coding genes in humans and other mammals [1]. The number of characterized miRs is also growing, due in part to the development of sensitive technologies such as next-generation sequencing (NGS), thereby facilitating the discovery of novel miRs. It is currently estimated that the human genome encodes 2654 mature miRs classified into families based on sequence homology and physiological function (miRBase release 22 [2]).

miRs associated with henipavirus infection were first studied to better understand cellular host factors exploited by these highly pathogenic viruses for replication. Initial studies analyzed the

Alexander N. Freiberg and Barry Rockx (eds.), *Nipah Virus: Methods and Protocols*, Methods in Molecular Biology, vol. 2682, https://doi.org/10.1007/978-1-0716-3283-3_19,

expression levels of select host miRs using qPCR arrays, revealing that Hendra virus (HeV) infection alters the transcription levels of several host miRs, including the NF-κB-responsive miR-146a [3]. Interestingly, miR-146a promotes HeV replication, suggesting that HeV exploits innate immune responses to favor replication. A key finding from this study was that miR-146a up-regulation in the blood of ferrets (an established model for human HeV disease [3, 4]) and horses occurs days before the detection of virus genome, indicating that host miRNA profiling has the potential to detect HeV infection during the incubation period. Knowledge that miR-146a transcription is stimulated by several immune ligands, however, including several viral and bacterial stimuli [5–7], prompted more comprehensive transcriptome-wide studies to define a more HeV-specific disease biomarker. NGS and the MiR-Deep2 algorithm [8] demonstrated that 37 circulating miRNAs in horse blood (approximately 5% of total) are significantly altered by HeV infection [9]. Current efforts are focused on validating these candidates in a larger sample cohort and assessing their specific impact on disease progression.

In this chapter, we describe methodologies for the measurement of host miRs in samples derived from henipavirus infection, both at the transcriptome-wide level (using NGS and bioinformatics) and individual miR level (using TaqMan qPCR). Other methods for high-throughput analysis (microarrays, qPCR arrays) and low-throughput analysis (Northern blotting, Sybr-green based qPCR approaches) of miRNAs are described elsewhere [10–12]. Our justification for using methods described in this chapter is several-fold. Firstly, NGS allows comprehensive miR profiling, yielding both quantitative and structural/qualitative data on the entire genome-wide set of expressed miRs. Secondly, NGS is relatively cost-effective for this broad stage of analysis. Finally, NGS also offers the opportunity to detect novel miRs which are yet to be defined in miRBase. While a detailed procedure for identifying and characterizing novel miRs is beyond the scope of this review, we recommend the use of miRDeep2 as an appropriate tool [9, 13]. In contrast, both microarrays and qPCR arrays require pre-defined targets, thereby limiting their scope to known miRs. Until recently, Northern blotting was routinely used for the confirmation of miR expression but this has largely been surpassed by TaqMan qPCR due to its greater sensitivity.

2 Materials

miRs were purified from tissues and other samples containing cells using the miRNeasy Mini kit (Qiagen, Cat No. 217004), while the miRNeasy Serum/plasma kit (Qiagen, Cat No. 21784) were used for serum, plasma, and other cell-free samples. Ethanol and chloroform should be analytical grade preparations, and ethanol dilutions should be made fresh with nuclease-free water. The quantity and size distribution of small RNA is determined using an Agilent 2100 Bioanalyzer Small RNA kit (Cat No. 5067-1548). Due to the limited yield of RNA from cell-free samples, when using this type of starting material, we recommend that NGS libraries be prepared using the Qiagen QIAseq miRNA Library kit (Cat No. 331505) and the QIAseq miRNA NGS Index IL (Cat No. 331585), which are able to generate functional libraries from 1–500 ng of input total RNA. NGS library clean-up is performed using the Promega MagneSphere® Technology Magnetic Separation Stand (Cat No. Z5342). Library quality control is assessed using the Agilent 2100 Bioanalyzer High-sensitivity DNA kit (Cat No. 5067-4626). Sequencing is conducted using the HiSeq2500 system (Illumina). Quantitative PCR analysis of miR expression is performed using TaqMan MicroRNA assays (Applied Biosystems, Cat No. 4427975) and TaqMan Fast Advanced Master Mix (Applied Biosystems, Cat No. 4352042). Relative quantitation is conducted on a QuantStudio 3 or 6 (Applied Biosystems) real-time PCR machine.

3 Methods

3.1 miR Harvesting and Purification

1. HeV is a biosafety level (BSL)-4 organism and as such all experimental work must be completed following established BSL-4 protocols. When extracting nucleic acids, the ability of the procedure to completely inactivate HeV must be verified (*see* **Note 1**).
2. Gloves should be cleaned of ribonucleases prior to handling samples, and whenever a new pair of gloves is worn (*see* **Note 2**).
3. Working within a biosafety level II cabinet (BSCII) within a BSL-4 laboratory, add 700 μL of Qiazol Lysis Reagent to 2 mL Sarstedt tubes containing 100 μL whole blood or serum. Pipette samples several times and incubate for 10 minutes (min) at room temperature (15–25 °C).
3. After incubation with Qiazol Lysis Reagent, transfer samples to a BSL-2 laboratory. Transfers must be completed following established procedures with respect to local legislation.
4. Working in a fume cabinet, add 140 μL chloroform to each tube, cap securely, and shake vigorously for 15 seconds (s). Place tubes at room temperature for 5 min and centrifuge for 15 min at 12,000 × g_{max} at 4 °C.
5. After centrifugation, samples will separate into three phases (upper, colorless, and aqueous phase containing RNA; a

white interphase containing DNA; and a lower, red, organic phase containing proteins). Transfer approximately 350 μL of upper aqueous phase (being careful to avoid any interphase) to a 1.5 mL collection tube.

6. Add 525 μL of 100% ethanol and mix by pipetting up and down several times.
7. Transfer 700 μL of the sample into an RNeasy mini spin column in a 2 mL collection tube and centrifuge at 8000 × g_{max} for 15 s at room temperature. Discard the flow-through.
8. Add 700 μL of buffer RWT to the RNeasy mini spin column and centrifuge at 8000 × g_{max} for 15 s to wash the column. Discard the flow-through.
9. Add 500 μL of buffer RPE to the RNeasy mini spin column and centrifuged at 8000 × g_{max} for 15 s; discard the flow-through. Repeat this process.
10. Centrifuge the column at 8000 × g_{max} for 2 min to dry the column membrane; the flow-through being discarded along with the tube.
11. Place the RNeasy mini spin column into a new 2 mL collection tube, centrifuge at full speed in a microcentrifuge for 1 min; discard the flow-through and the collection tube. Transfer the RNeasy mini spin column to a new 1.5 mL collection tube.
12. Add between 30 μL and 50 μL of RNase-free water to the RNeasy mini spin column membrane. Centrifuge at 8000 × g_{max} for 1 min to elute the RNA.
13. Determine the concentration and quality of eluted RNA using microfluidic gel electrophoresis (Bioanalyzer Small RNA kit).
14. Store samples at −80 °C until required.

3.2 cDNA Library Preparation

3.2.1 3′ Ligation

1. Thaw template RNA on ice. Mix and briefly centrifuge at ≤10,000 × g_{max} for 5 s to collect residual liquid.
2. Thaw QIAseq miRNA NGS 3′ Adapter, QIAseq miRNA NGS 3′ Buffer, QIAseq miRNA NGS Ligation Activator, and Nuclease-Free Water at room temperature. Mix each solution by flicking the tubes and briefly centrifuge at ≤10,000 × g_{max} for 5 s.
3. QIAseq miRNA NGS RI and QIAseq miRNA NGS 3′ RNA Ligase should be removed from the −20 °C freezer just before use, and place on ice or inside a freezer block. Both enzymes should be returned to the freezer immediately after use.
4. If working with low RNA inputs or serum/plasma samples, dilute the QIAseq miRNA NGS 3′ Adapter in nuclease-free water as per Table 1.

Table 1
3′ adaptor dilutions

Input Total RNA	3′ Adaptor Dilution
500 ng	Undiluted
100 ng	Undiluted
10 ng	Dilute 1:5
1 ng	Dilute 1:10
Serum/plasma	Dilute 1:5

Table 2
3′ ligation reagents

Reagent	Volume (μL) per reaction
Nuclease-free water	Variable depending on input RNA
QIAseq miRNA NGS 3′ adapter[a]	1
QIAseq miRNA NGS RI	1
QIAseq miRNA NGS 3′ ligase	1
QIAseq miRNA NGS 3′ buffer	2
QIAseq miRNA NGS ligation activator	10
Template RNA	Variable
Total	**20**

[a] Diluted as per Table 1, if necessary

5. On ice, prepare the 3′ ligation reaction according to Table 2, in the order listed. If preparing more than one reaction, create a mastermix with 10% extra volume to account for pipetting errors. Mix by pipetting up and down 20 times and then briefly centrifuge at ≤10,000 × g_{max} for 5 s. It is important to pipette slowly as many of the reagents are extremely viscous.
6. Add the template RNA to the 3′ ligation reaction in a 0.2 μL tube. Although this method can produce libraries from 1 ng of input total RNA, it is recommended to use 100 ng for cell/tissue samples, and 5 μL of eluted RNA from cell-free samples. Mix by pipetting up and down 20 times. Briefly centrifuge at ≤10,000 × g_{max} for 5 s.
7. Place the tubes into a thermocycler and run the following parameters:

Table 3
5′ adaptor dilutions

Input Total RNA	5′ Adaptor Dilution
500 ng	Undiluted
100 ng	Undiluted
10 ng	Dilute 1:2.5
1 ng	Dilute 1:5
Serum/plasma	Dilute 1:2.5

   (a) Incubate at 28 °C for 1 hour (h).
   (b) Incubate at 65 °C for 20 min.
   (c) Hold at 4 °C for at least 5 min.
8. Proceed immediately to 3.2.2. 5′ ligation.

3.2.2 5′ Ligation

1. Thaw QIAseq miRNA NGS5′ Adapter and QIAseq miRNA NGS 5′ Buffer at room temperature. Mix by agitating the tube. Briefly centrifuge at ≤10,000 × g_{max} for 5 s.
2. QIAseq miRNA NGS RI and QIAseq miRNA NGS 5′ RNA Ligase should be removed from the −20 °C freezer just before use, and place on ice or inside a freezer block. Both enzymes should be returned to the freezer immediately after use.
3. If working with low RNA inputs or serum/plasma samples, dilute the QIAseq miRNA NGS 5′ Adapter in nuclease-free water as per Table 3.
4. On ice, prepare the 5′ ligation reaction according to Table 4, in the order listed. If preparing more than one reaction, create a mastermix with 10% extra volume to account for pipetting errors. Mix by pipetting up and down 10–15 times and then briefly centrifuge at ≤10,000 × g_{max} for 5 s. It is important to pipette slowly as many of the reagents are extremely viscous
5. Place the tubes into a thermocycler and run the following parameters:
   (a) Incubate at 28 °C for 30 min.
   (b) Incubate at 65 °C for 20 min.
   (c) Hold at 4 °C for at least 5 min.
6. Proceed immediately to 3.2.3. Reverse transcription.

Table 4
5′ ligation reagents

Reagent	Volume (μL) per reaction
3′ ligation reaction (from 3.2.1.)	20
Nuclease-free water	15
QIAseq miRNA NGS 5′ buffer	2
QIAseq miRNA NGS RI	1
QIAseq miRNA NGS 5′ ligase	1
QIAseq miRNA NGS 5′ adaptor[a]	1
Total	**40**

[a] Diluted as per Table 3, if necessary

Table 5
RT initiator incubation parameters

Temperature (°C)	Time (min)
75	2
70	2
65	2
60	2
55	2
37	5
25	5
4	Hold

3.2.3 Reverse Transcription (RT)

1. Thaw QIAseq miRNA NGS RT Initiator, QIAseq miRNA NGS RT Buffer, and QIAseq miRNA NGS RT Primer at room temperature. Mix by flicking the tube. Briefly centrifuge at ≤10,000 × g_{max} for 5 sec.
2. QIAseq miRNA NGS RI and QIAseq miRNA NGS RT enzyme should be removed from the −20 °C freezer just before use, and place on ice or inside a freezer block. Both enzymes should be returned to the freezer immediately after use.
3. Add 2 μL QIAseq miRNA NGS RT Initiator to each tube. Mix by pipetting up and down 15 to 20 times and briefly centrifuge at ≤10,000 × g_{max} for 5 s.
4. Incubate the tubes as per Table 5.

Table 6
RT primer dilutions

Input Total RNA	RT Primer Dilution
500 ng	Undiluted
100 ng	Undiluted
10 ng	Dilute 1: 5
1 ng	Dilute 1: 10
Serum/plasma	Dilute 1: 5

Table 7
RT reagents

Reagent	Volume (μL) per reaction
5′ ligation reaction and RT initiator	42
QIAseq miRNA NGS RT primer[a]	2
Nuclease-free water	2
QIAseq miRNA NGS RT buffer	12
QIAseq miRNA NGS RI	1
QIAseq miRNA NGS RT enzyme	1
Total	**60**

[a] Diluted as per Table 6, if necessary

5. If working with low RNA inputs or serum/plasma samples, dilute the QIAseq miRNA NGS RT Primer in nuclease-free water as per Table 6.
6. On ice, prepare the RT reaction according to Table 7, in the order listed. If preparing more than one reaction, create a mastermix with 10% extra volume to account for pipetting errors. Mix by pipetting up and down 10 times and then briefly centrifuge at ≤10,000 × g_{max} for 5 s. It is important to pipette slowly as many of the reagents are extremely viscous.
7. Place the tubes into a thermocycler and run the following parameters:
   (a) Incubate at 50 °C for 1 h.
   (b) Incubate at 70 °C for 15 min.
   (c) Hold at 4 °C for at least 5 min.

8. While the reverse transcription reaction is taking place, prepare the QIAseq miRNA NGS beads (QMN beads). Thoroughly vortex the QIAseq beads and QIAseq miRNA NGS Bead Binding Buffer. Do not centrifuge. Both solutions need to be homogenous; if there is a delay or the beads start to settle, vortex again.
9. Carefully add 400 μL of the QIAseq beads to a 2-mL microfuge tube. It is important to pipette slowly as the buffer is extremely viscous. This volume of beads is sufficient to process one sample. Simply scale up the reagent volumes for >1 sample to be processed. Up to four samples worth of beads (1.6 mL) can fit into a tube. Briefly centrifuge at ≤10,000 × g_{max} for 5 s and then place on the magnetic stand.
10. Once the beads have fully migrated, carefully remove and discard the supernatant. Do not disturb the beads; a small amount of liquid (5–10 μL) can be left behind at this stage.
11. Remove the tube from the magnetic stand and carefully pipette 150 μL of binding buffer onto the beads. It is important to pipette slowly as the buffer is extremely viscous. Vortex thoroughly, briefly centrifuge at ≤10,000 × g_{max} for 5 s, and then immediately place back onto the magnetic stand.
12. Once the beads have fully migrated, carefully remove and discard the supernatant. Remove as much liquid as possible without disturbing the beads.
13. Remove the tube from the magnetic stand and carefully pipette 400 μL of binding buffer onto the beads. It is important to pipette slowly as the buffer is extremely viscous. Vortex thoroughly.
14. Prepared beads should be stored at 4 °C, if they are not to be used immediately. Beads can be stored at 4 °C for up to 1 week.
15. Once the RT reaction is complete, combine 143 μL of the prepared QMN beads with the entire cDNA solutions in a new 1.5-mL tube. Vortex for 3 s and then centrifuge briefly at ≤10,000 × g_{max} for 5 s.
16. Incubate for 5 min at room temperature.
17. Place the tubes on the magnetic stand. Leave for ~4 min, or until the beads have fully migrated. Remove and discard the supernatant.
18. With the tubes still on the magnetic stand, add 200 μL of 80% ethanol and then immediately remove and discard. Repeat this wash. After the second ethanol wash, it is important to remove as much liquid as possible. Use a 10 or 20 μL pipette to remove any residual ethanol.

19. Let the tubes air dry for 10 min on the magnetic stand by opening their lids. Placing the tubes in a laminar flow cabinet can assist with this process.
20. With the tubes still on the magnetic stand, add 17 μL of nuclease-free water to the beads. Immediately remove from the stand and pipette to resuspend the beads. Close the lid and briefly centrifuge at ≤10,000 × g_{max} for 5 s.
21. Incubate at room temperature for 2 min.
22. Return the tubes to the magnetic stand for ~2 min or until the beads have migrated.
23. Transfer 15 μL of the eluted cDNA to new 0.2 mL tubes. Discard the beads.
24. Proceed to 3.2.4. Library amplification or store the cDNA product at −20 °C in a constant-temperature freezer.

3.2.4 Library Amplification

1. Thaw QIAseq miRNA NGS Library Buffer, QIAseq miRNA NGS ILM Library Forward Primer, and required index primers (QIAseq miRNA NGS ILM IDP1 – IDP48). To pool samples together during sequencing, each sample requires a unique index. Mix by flicking and then briefly centrifuge at ≤10,000 × g_{max} for 5 s.
2. HotStarTaq DNA Polymerase should be removed from the − 20 °C freezer just before use, and place on ice or inside a freezer block. This enzyme should be returned to the freezer immediately after use.
3. On ice, prepare the amplification reaction according to Table 8, in the order listed. If preparing more than one reaction, create a mastermix with 10% extra volume to account for pipetting errors. Mix by pipetting up and down 10 times and then briefly centrifuge at ≤10,000 × g_{max} for 5 s. It is important to pipette slowly as some of the reagents are extremely viscous.

Table 8
Library amplification reagents

Reagent	Volume (μL) per reaction
cDNA product from 3.2.3 reverse transcription	15
QIAseq miRNA NGS library buffer	16
HotStarTaq DNA polymerase	3
QIAseq miRNA NGS ILM library forward primer	2
QIAseq miRNA NGS ILM IDP1 through IDP48 index primer[a]	2
Nuclease-free water	42
Total	**80**

[a]Where possible, use a different index for each sample

Table 9
Amplification cycling parameters

Step	Time	Temperature
Hold	15 min	95 °C
Amplification cycle[a]		
Denaturation	15 s	95 °C
Annealing	30 s	60 °C
Extension	15 s	72 °C
Hold	2 min	72 °C
Hold	At least 5 min	4 °C

[a] Number of cycles dependent on RNA input, please see Table 10

Table 10
Number of amplification cycles

Input Total RNA	Amplification Cycle Number
500 ng	13
100 ng	16
10 ng	19
1 ng	22
Serum/plasma	22

4. Place the tubes in a thermocycler and run the cycling parameters outlined in Table 9. The number of amplification cycles needed are dependent on the original RNA input and is outlined in Table 10.

5. Add 75 μL of QMN Beads to new 1.5 mL tubes. Ensure the QMN Beads are thoroughly mixed at all times. If a delay in the protocol occurs or the beads begin to settle, simply vortex.
6. Briefly centrifuge the 80 μL library amplification reactions at ≤10,000 × g_{max} for 5 s, and then transfer 75 μL to the tubes containing the QMN Beads. Vortex for 3 s and briefly centrifuge at ≤10,000 × g_{max} for 5 s.
7. Incubate for 5 min at room temperature.
8. Place tubes on a magnet stand for ~4 min or until beads have fully migrated.
9. Transfer 145 μL of the supernatant to new tubes. Discard the tubes containing the beads. Do not discard the supernatant at this step.

10. Add 130 μL of QMN Beads to the 145 μL supernatant. Vortex for 3 s and briefly centrifuge at ≤10,000 × g_{max} for 5 s.
11. Incubate at room temperature for 5 min.
12. Place the tubes on the magnetic stand until beads have fully migrated. Discard the supernatant and keep the beads.
13. With the tubes still on the magnetic stand, add 200 μL of 80% ethanol and then immediately remove and discard. Repeat this wash. After the second ethanol wash, it is important to remove as much liquid as possible. Use a 10 or 20 μL pipette to remove any residual ethanol.
14. Let the tubes air dry for 10 min on the magnetic stand by opening their lids. Placing the tubes in a laminar flow cabinet can assist with this process.
15. With the tubes still on the magnetic stand, add 17 μL of nuclease-free water to the beads. Immediately remove from the stand and pipette to resuspend the beads. Close the lid and briefly centrifuge at ≤10,000 × g_{max} for 5 s.
16. Incubate at room temperature for 2 min.
17. Return the tubes to the magnetic stand for ~2 min or until the beads have migrated.
18. Transfer 15 μL of the eluted cDNA to a new tube. Discard the beads.
19. Run 1 μL of the generated library on the Agilent 2100 Bioanalyzer High-sensitivity DNA kit as per the manufacturer's instructions, or store the library at −20 °C in a constant-temperature freezer. A miRNA library should have a significant peak at approximately 180 bp (Fig. 1). A large peak at 157 bp indicates the presence of adapter dimers. If this, or any other unwanted bands are seen, gel excision is recommended.

3.3 Next-Generation Sequencing

1. All samples should be sequenced using the same platform and underlying chemistry to reduce control any variation introduced during the sequencing process (*see* **Note 3**). Here, we recommend the Illumina HiSeq 2500 using high throughput chemistry. Ultimately, to produce robust data for biomarker discovery, the following parameters should be met:
   (a) 100 bp single end reads
   (b) 5–10 million usable reads per sample, which translates to 15–25 samples pooled in each lane of the HiSeq 2500.

3.4 MicroRNA Identification via Bioinformatics

There are numerous software packages that are able to process, align, and quantify miRNA NGS data, however, we recommend using command-line tools for their power, flexibility, and open-source nature. The following analyses can be completed on a standard computer (2–4 CPU cores, 4–8 GB RAM, LINUX operating

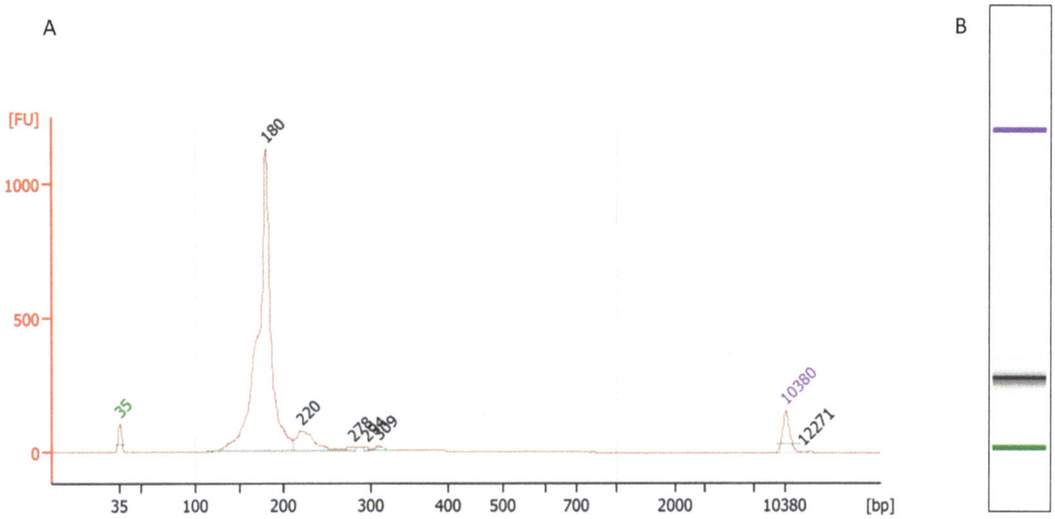

Fig. 1 This Agilent Bioanalyzer profile of an amplified miRNA cDNA library is typical of samples yielding high-quality miRNA-Seq data. (**a**) Electropherogram obtained following library preparation described in Subheading 3.2. (**b**) The corresponding simulated gel image

system) once you have downloaded and installed FastQC, FastX, cutadapt, miRDeep2, and Python 3. If you wish to conduct this workflow on a cluster computing system, you will need to load the required modules (our current pipeline uses the following software versions), e.g.:

```
module load fastqc/0.11.8    module load fastx/0.0.14
   module load mirdeep/2.0.0.8
   module load python/3.6.1
```

1. Run quality control (QC) on your files. This can be completed using the unzipped .gz file. The output will give you an overview of the base and sequence quality scores (ideally ≥30), sequence length distribution, and many other metrics

```
fastqc <sample1.fastq.gz>
```

2. Trim the NGS adaptor from the reads. You do not need to unzip the file to complete this step; it is good practice to avoid changing the original zipped file. The adaptor sequence listed in the command below is the QIAseq miRNA NGS 3′ Adaptor

```
gunzip -c <sample1.fastq.gz> | cutadapt -a
AACTGTAGGCACCATCAAT -m 18 -M 26 –o <sample1.
trimmed.fastq>
```

Options:

-c	Write the output to standard output while keeping the original file unchanged.
-a	Specify the adaptor sequence.
-m	Minimum read length after trimming.
-M	Maximum read length after trimming.
-o	Output file. If no file is specified, it will be sent to the standard output.

3. Rerun QC analyses on the trimmed files. The read length distribution should peak around 22 nucleotides (Figure 2). Note: FASTQC was designed to assess conventional mRNA-Seq data, and while it works very well on small RNA-Seq data, several apparent 'problems' will be auto-detected, some of which can be safely ignored. In particular, the "Per base sequence content," "Per sequence GC content," "Sequence Duplication Levels," and "Overrepresented sequences" can show warnings due to the composition of many small RNA samples. In contrast, warnings in "Per base sequence quality," "Per sequence quality scores," "Per base N content," or "Adapter Content" can reflect poor sequencing results or incorrect adaptor sequences used for trimming.

```
fastqc <sample1.trimmed.fastq>
```

4. Assemble the mature and hairpin reference files from miRBase. MirBase allows you to download all of these sequences for a particular species by using the "Browse" function (http://www.mirbase.org/cgi-bin/browse.pl). The hairpin and mature sequences must be saved as different FASTA files. These files must be properly formatted and converted from RNA to DNA. The FastX toolkit contains FASTA_Formatter and FASTA_Nucleotide_Changer that will complete these steps.
5. Map and quantify reads using miRDeep2.

```
mapper.pl <sample1.reads.fasta> -e -h -m -s <sample1.collapsed.fasta>    quantifier.pl –d –j –W –y <sample1> -p <mirbase_hairpin.fasta> -m <mirbase_mature.fasta> -r <sample1.collapsed.fasta>
```

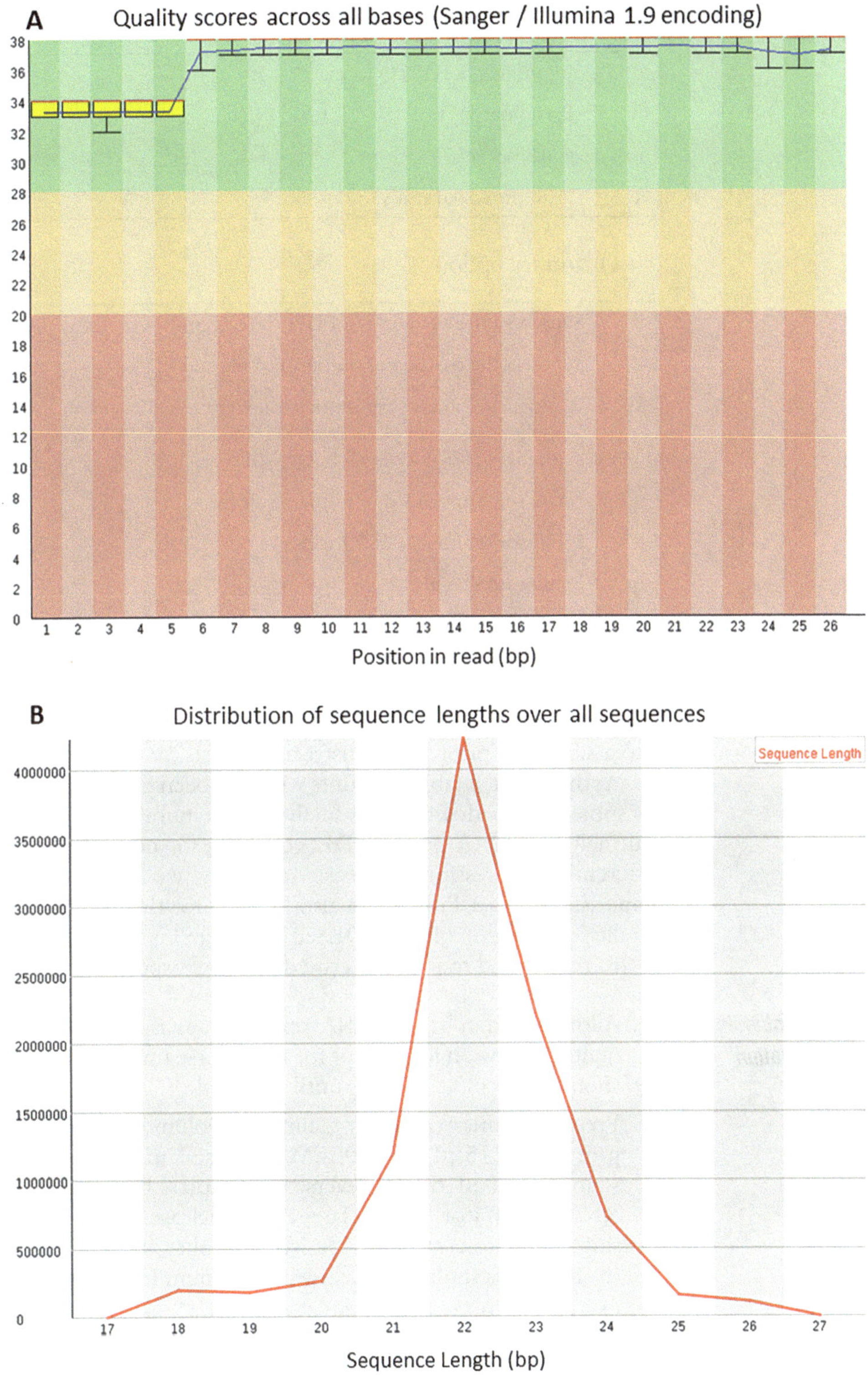

Fig. 2 (**a**) A representative example of per-base sequence quality for miRNA-Seq data following trimming and filtering as described in Subheading 3.4. (**b**) Size distribution of trimmed reads. Both plots were generated using the program FastQC

Mapper options:

-e	Input file is a FASTQ format
-h	Parses output to FASTA format
-m	Collapses reads
-s	Print processed reads to this file

Quantifier options:

-d	Suppress the generation of PDFs for each miRNA.
-j	Suppress the creation of output.mrd file and PDFs.
-W	If a sequence maps to more than one location, a fractional count is applied. For example, if one read is mapped to two different locations, 0.5 count will be applied to each.
-y	Name to be appended onto the result file.
-p	Precursor (hairpin) FASTA file.
-m	Mature FASTA file.
-r	Read sequences.

The output of quantifier.pl is a series of .csv files containing count data for each individual sample. These need to be merged into a single file prior to downstream analysis.

At this point, a table of counts will have been generated that can be subjected to downstream analysis in a number of ways. We routinely use the R package DESeq2 [14] for normalization and differential expression analysis, however, we have previously demonstrated that EdgeR can also be used for this task [9, 15]. A detailed description of using DESeq2 or EdgeR is beyond the scope of this review and requires intermediate level experience using R.

3.5 cDNA Synthesis for qPCR Validation

1. Allow TaqMan® microRNA reverse transcription kit components to thaw on ice, except for the reverse transcriptase, which should be kept at −20 °C until required.
2. Prepare RT master mix by scaling the volumes as stated by the protocol (0.15 μL of 100 mM dNTPs, 1 μL of reverse transcriptase, 1.5 μL of 10X reverse transcriptase buffer, 0.19 μL of RNAse inhibitor, and 4.16 μL of nuclease-free water for a single reaction) to the desired number of RT reactions (5–10% extra should be included to account for pipette errors).
3. Gently mix this master mix and centrifuge at ≤10,000 × g_{max} for 5 s to bring the solution to the bottom of the tube. Place master mix on ice until the RNA template is prepared.
4. Dilute RNA samples to the desired concentration i.e. 2 ng/μL using nuclease-free water.

5. Add 7 μL of RT master mix to each of the tube, followed by 5 μL each of diluted RNA samples. Add 3 μL of RT primer from each assay set (specific to each miRNA) so that the total volume is 15 μL.
6. Centrifuge samples at ≤10,000 × g_{max} for 5 s to mix the solution.
7. Incubate samples on ice for 5 min and then loaded on a thermal cycler. The thermal cycling parameters are 30 min at 16 °C, 30 min at 42 °C, 5 min at 85 °C, and on hold at 4 °C.
8. cDNA samples may be stored at −20 °C until further use.
9. When ready to prepare a qPCR reaction, thaw samples on ice, gently vortex then briefly centrifuge cDNA samples and TaqMan assays at ≤10,000 × g_{max} for 5 s.
10. To prepare the qPCR reaction mix, pipette 10 μL of TaqMan universal fast PCR master mix, 1 μL of TaqMan small RNA assay, and 7.67 μL of nuclease-free water for a single reaction. Adjust volumes according to the number of reactions required and compensate for losses that occur during pipetting.
11. Cap and invert tubes several times to mix and centrifuge at ≤10,000 × g_{max} for 5 s. Add 18.67 μL of respective qRT-PCR reaction mix into corresponding wells of a 96-well plate. Add 1.33 μL of each of cDNA to the respective wells for a total volume of 20 μL.
12. Seal the plate with a qPCR compatible cover and centrifuge at 12,000 × g_{max} for 1 min.
13. Load the plate into qPCR machine using cycling conditions of system using the following parameters: a standard run mode with 20 μL sample volume and thermal cycling conditions of 10 min at 95 °C, followed by 40 cycles of 15 s at 95 °C and 60 s at 60 °C (*see* **Notes 4, 5**, and **6**).

4 Notes

1. CRITICALLY IMPORTANT: Methods used for nucleic acid extraction from henipavirus-infected samples must be proven to inactivate the virus prior to removal from a BSL-4 laboratory. Guanidium thiocyanate-based extraction buffer used in this method has been shown to inactivate a range of viruses including Nipah virus [16].
2. It is recommended to remove endogenous ribonucleases from gloves prior to commencing miR extraction by applying a decontamination solution, such as RNaseZap (Invitrogen, Cat No. AM9780). This avoids degradation of the extracted miRNA.

3. There are many sequencing technologies available, each with their own strengths and weaknesses. It is important to utilize the same sequencing method for all samples within a study, and to adhere to the parameters to read length and depth. Too little read depth will not produce any meaningful data, while too high wastes resources without giving any additional information.
4. Observe the qPCR amplification curves to confirm that they demonstrate the expected exponential amplification. If the cycle threshold (CT) value is ≥40, then it is unlikely to be true amplification.
5. When reporting qPCR results, it is beneficial to adhere to the MIQE guidelines [17].
6. Several kits for miRNA isolation, cDNA synthesis, and qPCR are commercially available and may be used in place of the kits described in this chapter.

References

1. Bartel DP (2009) MicroRNAs: target recognition and regulatory functions. Cell 136(2): 215–233. https://doi.org/10.1016/j.cell.2009.01.002
2. Kozomara A, Birgaoanu M, Griffiths-Jones S (2019) miRBase: from microRNA sequences to function. Nucleic Acids Res 47(D1):D155–D162. https://doi.org/10.1093/nar/gky1141
3. Stewart CR, Marsh GA, Jenkins KA, Gantier MP, Tizard ML, Middleton D, Lowenthal JW, Haining J, Izzard L, Gough TJ, Deffrasnes C, Stambas J, Robinson R, Heine HG, Pallister JA, Foord AJ, Bean AG, Wang LF (2013) Promotion of Hendra virus replication by microRNA 146a. J Virol 87(7):3782–3791. https://doi.org/10.1128/JVI.01342-12
4. Pallister J, Middleton D, Wang LF, Klein R, Haining J, Robinson R, Yamada M, White J, Payne J, Feng YR, Chan YP, Broder CC (2011) A recombinant Hendra virus G glycoprotein-based subunit vaccine protects ferrets from lethal Hendra virus challenge. Vaccine 29(34): 5623–5630. https://doi.org/10.1016/j.vaccine.2011.06.015
5. Taganov KD, Boldin MP, Chang KJ, Baltimore D (2006) NF-kappaB-dependent induction of microRNA miR-146, an inhibitor targeted to signaling proteins of innate immune responses. Proc Natl Acad Sci U S A 103(33): 12481–12486. https://doi.org/10.1073/pnas.0605298103
6. Cameron JE, Yin Q, Fewell C, Lacey M, McBride J, Wang X, Lin Z, Schaefer BC, Flemington EK (2008) Epstein-Barr virus latent membrane protein 1 induces cellular MicroRNA miR-146a, a modulator of lymphocyte signaling pathways. J Virol 82(4):1946–1958. https://doi.org/10.1128/JVI.02136-07
7. Hou J, Wang P, Lin L, Liu X, Ma F, An H, Wang Z, Cao X (2009) MicroRNA-146a feedback inhibits RIG-I-dependent type I IFN production in macrophages by targeting TRAF6, IRAK1, and IRAK2. J Immunol 183(3): 2150–2158. https://doi.org/10.4049/jimmunol.0900707
8. Friedlander MR, Mackowiak SD, Li N, Chen W, Rajewsky N (2012) miRDeep2 accurately identifies known and hundreds of novel microRNA genes in seven animal clades. Nucleic Acids Res 40(1):37–52. https://doi.org/10.1093/nar/gkr688
9. Cowled C, Foo CH, Deffrasnes C, Rootes CL, Williams DT, Middleton D, Wang LF, Bean AGD, Stewart CR (2017) Circulating microRNA profiles of Hendra virus infection in horses. Sci Rep 7(1):7431. https://doi.org/10.1038/s41598-017-06939-w
10. Wong W, Farr R, Joglekar M, Januszewski A, Hardikar A (2015) Probe-based real-time PCR approaches for quantitative measurement of microRNAs. J Vis Exp 98. https://doi.org/10.3791/52586
11. Blevins T (2017) Northern blotting techniques for small RNAs. Methods Mol Biol 1456:141–162. https://doi.org/10.1007/978-1-4899-7708-3_12
12. Androvic P, Valihrach L, Elling J, Sjoback R, Kubista M (2017) Two-tailed RT-qPCR: a novel method for highly accurate miRNA

quantification. Nucleic Acids Res 45(15):e144. https://doi.org/10.1093/nar/gkx588

13. Cowled C, Stewart CR, Likic VA, Friedlander MR, Tachedjian M, Jenkins KA, Tizard ML, Cottee P, Marsh GA, Zhou P, Baker ML, Bean AG, Wang LF (2014) Characterisation of novel microRNAs in the black flying fox (Pteropus alecto) by deep sequencing. BMC Genomics 15:682. https://doi.org/10.1186/1471-2164-15-682
14. Love MI, Huber W, Anders S (2014) Moderated estimation of fold change and dispersion for RNA-seq data with DESeq2. Genome Biol 15(12):550. https://doi.org/10.1186/s13059-014-0550-8
15. Robinson MD, McCarthy DJ, Smyth GK (2010) edgeR: a Bioconductor package for differential expression analysis of digital gene expression data. Bioinformatics 26(1): 139–140. https://doi.org/10.1093/bioinformatics/btp616
16. Kochel TJ, Kocher GA, Ksiazek TG, Burans JP (2017) Evaluation of TRIzol LS inactivation of viruses. Appl Biosaf 22(2):52–55. https://doi.org/10.1177/1535676017713739
17. Bustin SA, Benes V, Garson JA, Hellemans J, Huggett J, Kubista M, Mueller R, Nolan T, Pfaffl MW, Shipley GL, Vandesompele J, Wittwer CT (2009) The MIQE guidelines: minimum information for publication of quantitative real-time PCR experiments. Clin Chem 55(4):611–622. https://doi.org/10.1373/clinchem.2008.112797

Chapter 20

Host Transcriptome Analysis of Ferret Tissues Following Henipavirus Infection

Tian S. Zeng, D. S. Yang, A. A. Kelvin, and David J. Kelvin

Abstract

Ferrets are commonly used as experimental models of infection for a variety of viruses due to their susceptibility to human respiratory viruses and the close resemblance of pathological outcomes found in human infections. Even though ferret-specific reagents are limited, the use of ferrets as a preclinical experimental model of infection has gained considerable interest since the publication of the ferret transcriptome and draft ferret genome. These advances have made it feasible to easily perform whole-genome gene expression analysis in the ferret infection model. Here, we describe methods for genome-wide gene expression analysis using RNA sequence (RNAseq) data obtained from the lung and brain tissues obtained from experimental infections of Hendra (HeV) and Nipah (NiV) viruses in ferrets. We provide detailed methods for RNAseq and representative data for host gene expression profiles of the lung tissues that show early activation of interferon pathways and later activation of inflammation-related pathways.

Key words Transcriptome, RNA analysis, Henipavirus, Host Immunity, Interferon

1 Introduction

High-throughput sequencing of RNA (RNAseq) has become the main choice to measure expression levels and the identification of differentially expressed genes (DEGs) between specific conditions, and is an important tool for the understanding of host responses to infection over time [1, 2]. However, high-throughput sequencing of RNA (RNAseq) for gene expression in the ferret model previously relied on non-parametric methods which required de-novo assembly of the transcriptome and resulted in taxing sequencing and computing resources. The publishing of the ferret transcriptome and draft genome provided the framework for easily conducting high-throughput RNAseq to study changes in the gene expression analysis of ferrets infected with various pathogens [1, 3, 4]. Ferrets are susceptible to a variety of human respiratory viruses including influenza and RSV. When infected with influenza viruses, ferrets display sneezing, coughing, fever, become lethargic,

Alexander N. Freiberg and Barry Rockx (eds.), *Nipah Virus: Methods and Protocols*, Methods in Molecular Biology, vol. 2682, https://doi.org/10.1007/978-1-0716-3283-3_20,

and often develop upper respiratory pathology [5, 6]. These clinical and pathological features closely resemble the clinical and pathological features found in human influenza infections [5, 7]. Furthermore, ferrets are a good model for studying clinical and pathological diseases caused by emerging zoonotic infections including the development of severe respiratory and neurological diseases caused by henipavirus infections [4, 8].

Here, we describe methods for performing RNAseq to determine host gene expression profiles of lung tissues from experimental infections of Hendra (HeV) and Nipah (NiV) viruses in ferrets. We also provide a pipeline for data analysis. Representative data show the infection leads to early activation of interferon pathways and later activation of inflammation-related pathways.

2 Materials

All infections and animal work should be performed as previously described [1, 4] in a class II BSC in a biosafety level 4 laboratory (BSL4). Animal housing, care, and experimental protocols should be in accordance with the NIH guidelines of the Office of Laboratory Animal Welfare. All tissues should be collected under BSL4 conditions and placed in TRIzol reagent.

2.1 RNA Extraction, Library, and Sequencing

2.1.1 TRIzol reagent.

2.1.2 Qiagen RNeasy mini kit.

2.1.3 TruSeq RNA prep kit v2.

2.1.4 qPCR using the Kappa Illumina quantification kit).

2.1.5 Illumina HiSeq2500 (50 bp single end, Illumina).

2.2 Sequencing Analysis

2.2.1 fastqcversion 0.11.8. This can be found at:

https://www.bioinformatics.babraham.ac.uk/projects/fastqc/

2.2.2 Trimmomaticversion 0.38. This can be found at:

http://www.usadellab.org/cms/?page=trimmomatic

2.2.3 TopHat 2.1.1 This can be found at:

https://ccb.jhu.edu/software/tophat/index.shtml

2.2.4 Cufflinks 2.2.1. This can be found at:

http://cole-trapnell-lab.github.io/cufflinks/

2.2.5 R packages: edgeRversion3.24.3, limma version3.38.3, clusterProfilerversion 3.10.1, Glimma version3.8, ggplot2 version3.1.0, gplots version3.0.1.1, org.Hs.eg.db version3.8. These packages can be downloaded at: http://bioconductor.org/, https://cran.r-project.org

2.2.6 metascapeversion 3.0. http://metascape.org/gp/index.html

3 Methods

3.1 RNA extraction was performed on lung tissue samples from Days 3 and 5 post-infection with HeV and NiV-B. Infections were carried out as previously described [4].

3.1.1 100 mg of each tissue is collected in 1 ml of TRIzol reagent. (*See* **Note 1**).

3.1.1.2 TRIzol reagent and tissue are homogenized and placed at −70 °C until extraction of RNA. (*See* **Note 2**).

3.1.1.3 RNA is isolated according to the TRIzol instructions. (*See* **Note 3**).

3.1.1.4 A cleanup step is then performed using a Qiagen RNeasy kit.

3.1.1.5 The resulting RNA samples are analyzed in an Agilent Bioanalyzer 2100 to ensure that each sample meets minimal quality requirements for library construction and sequencing (RIN ≥ 7.5). (*See* **Note 4**).

3.2 Library Construction

3.2.1 The cDNA sequencing libraries are prepared according to the manufacturer's recommendations using the TruSeq RNA prep kit v2. (*See* **Note 3**).

3.2.2 The resulting libraries are quantified by qPCR using the Kappa Illumina quantification kit.

3.2.3 Libraries are pooled at equimolar concentrations.

3.2.4 Libraries are sequenced according to the manufacturer's instructions in an Illumina HiSeq2500.

3.2.5 Fastq files are obtained for each sample.

3.3 Data Analysis

3.3.1 Quality Control and Adapter Removal

3.3.1.1 To determine sequence quality, the Fastq file for each sample is used as input into FastQC to check for Basic Statistics, per base sequence quality, per tile sequence quality, per sequence quality scores, per base sequence content, per sequence GC content, per base N content, sequence length distribution, sequence duplication levels, overrepresented sequences, and adapter content. Samples are excluded from further analysis if more than three warnings arise in the fastq file [9]

3.3.1.2 Removal of the single-end TruSeq adapters is then performed [10].

3.3.2 Reads Mapping to the Reference Genome

3.3.2.1 The reference genome (fa) and gene model annotation files (GFF) of Mustela putorius furor can be downloaded [3] from the following:

(a) Website: https://www.ncbi.nlm.nih.gov/genome/?term=AEYP00000000.1

3.3.2.2 The reference genome is indexed using bowtie2 found in TopHat2.1.1.

3.3.2.3 The single-end clean reads are aligned to the reference genome using TopHat2.1.1 resulting in output Aligned.bam files for each sample [11].

3.3.3 Quantification of Gene Expression Levels

3.3.3.1 Gene expression profiles are calculated using cufflinks by inputting the Aligned.bam file from 3.3.2.2 and saved in abundances.cxb [12].

3.3.3.2 All abundances.cxb (raw read counts) from all samples are loaded into cuffnorm outputting the readscount.cxb abundance file for each sample and each gene. Readscount.tst is input into cuffnormal to generate the normal reads count files for all the samples, resulting in output files readcounts.tst.

3.3.4 Differential Gene Expression Analysis

3.3.4.1 To determine what genes are differentially expressed following Henipavirus infection the following pipeline is performed.

3.3.4.2 An edgeR object of DEGlist with readcount.tst files is created [13]. The readcount.tst files consist of files for 15 lung tissue samples, the control group, and the two viruses' infection groups. These include three files for both viruses at 5 d.p.i, three files for each virus at 3d.p.i., and three files for the control samples. (*See* **Note 5**, **Note 6** & **Note 7**).

3.3.4.3 Counts per million (CPM) are then calculated (log2-counts per million (log-CPM) with the edgeR function "cpm". (*See* **Note 8** & **Note 9**).

3.3.4.4 "Low expression genes" which have less than 10 reads across all the samples are filtered out with the edgeR function "filterByExpr".

3.3.4.5 Normalized gene expression distributions are generated by the edgeR function "calcNormFactors", the "TMM" [14] method is selected in "calcNormFactors". (*See* **Note 10**).

3.3.4.6 Unsupervised clustering of samples with normalized expression data is performed using the R package, limma version3.38.3, and then limma:plotMDS [15] (Figs. 1 and 2). (*See* **Note 10** & **Note 11**).

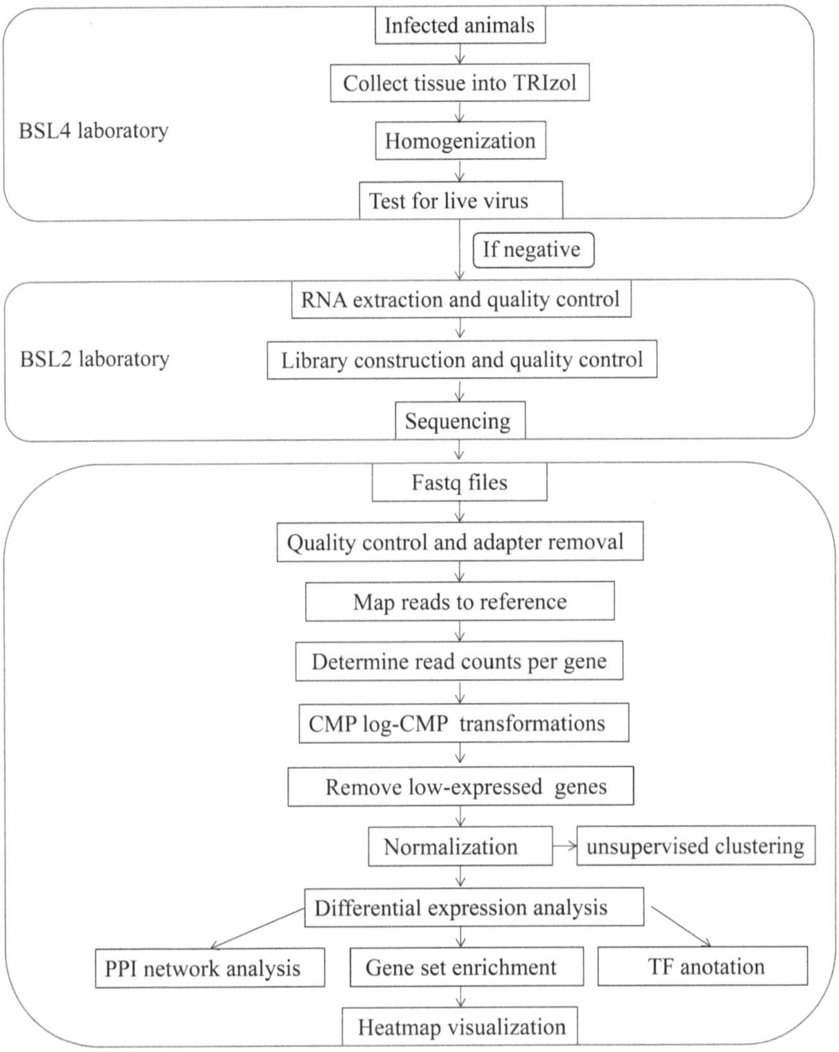

Fig. 1 *Flow chart of work procedures.* Animal infection, tissue collection, and homogenization are performed under BSL4 laboratory conditions. Inactivated homogenates are processed further using approved methods for inactivation, and tested for the presence of live virus. If negative, RNA is extracted, purified, and libraries are constructed under BSL2 conditions

3.3.4.7 A design matrix and contrasts group are created with R package limma version3.38.3 with the function model. matrix and limma: makeContrasts. (*See* **Note 12** & **Note 13**).

3.3.4.8 Heteroscedasticity is removed from the data counts using glimma:voom (Fig. 3) [16]. (*See* **Note 14** & **Note 15**).

3.3.4.9 Linear models are fitted for comparisons of interest with limma:lmFit and contrasts.fit. (*See* **Note 16 & Note 17**).

3.3.4.10 Empirical Bayes moderation in Edge R is carried out to obtain more precise estimates of gene-wise variability.

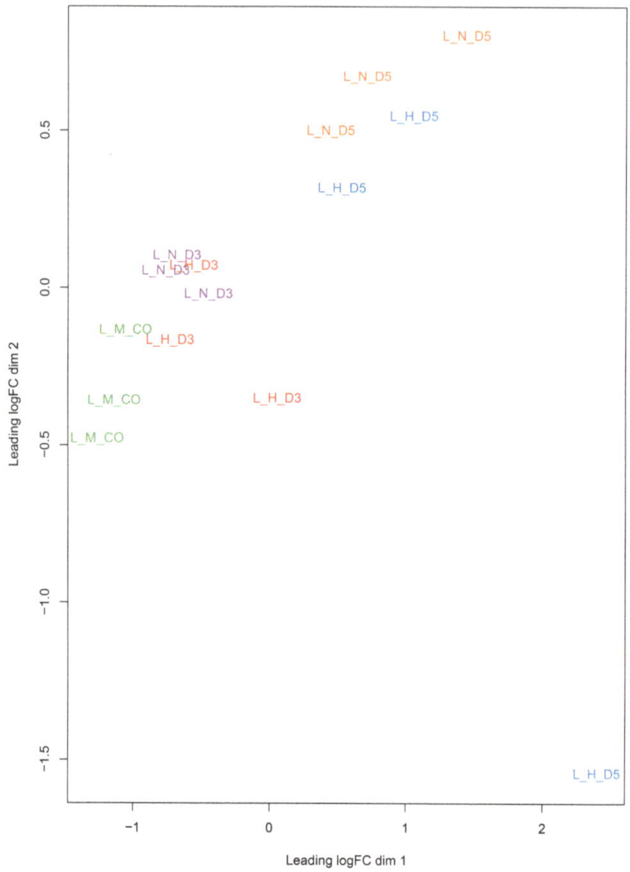

Fig. 2 *MDS plots of Nipah and Hendra virus-infected and control samples*. MDS plots of log-CPM values over dimensions 1 and 2 with samples colored and labeled by sample groups. The label L represents tissue type lung; the labels H or N represents virus type NiV (Nipah) or HeV (Hendra); D3 or D5 represents days post infections. The L_M_CO represents the control groups. Distances on the plot correspond to the leading fold-change, which is the average (root-mean-square) log2-fold-change for the 500 genes most divergent between each pair of samples. The plot indicates that Day3 and Day 5 virus samples cluster in a similar pattern, while Day 5 viral samples show considerable divergence. Control samples are very close to baseline values

3.3.4.11 The treat method [17] in Edge R is used to calculate p-values from empirical Bayes moderated t-statistics with a minimum log-FC requirement: adjusting P values and a 1.2-fold difference. (*See* **Note 18**).

3.3.4.12 Differentially expressed genes for Day 5 post-infection are shown for L_H_D5 vs L_M_CO in Fig. 4. (*See* **Note 18**) To generate differentially expressed genes use edgR:decideTests(logFC>1.2 & P value <0.05). Visualize the number of up-regulated and down-regulated genes using ggplot2:ggplot.

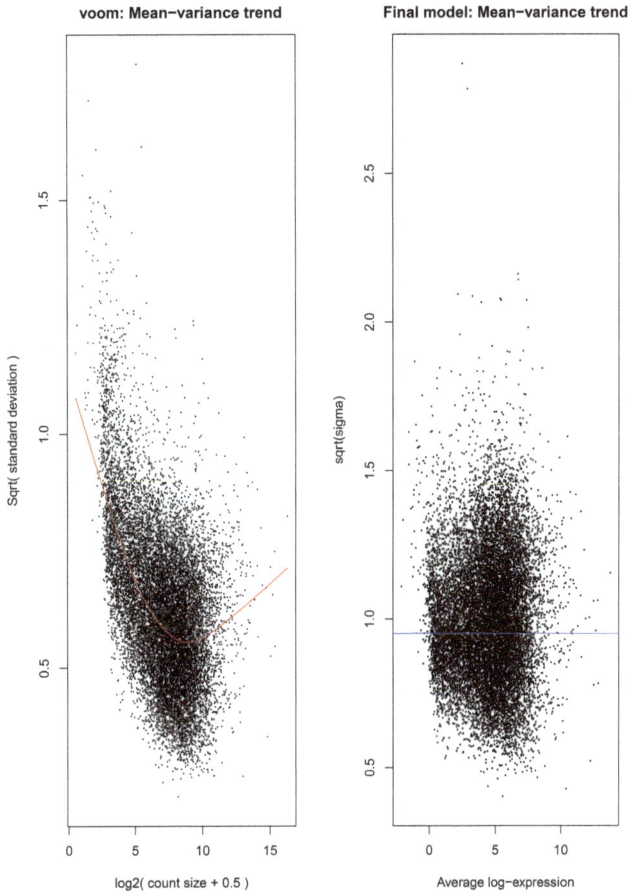

Fig. 3 *Voom correction of data.* Before voom precision weights are applied, a decreasing trend between the means and variances is evident due to a combination of technical variation in the sequencing step. A flatter trend is observed after applying the voom function

3.3.4.13 List all the genes by using Toptreat from Edge R. Adjust P value and logFC for desired statistical significance. (*See* **Note 19**).

3.3.5 KEGG Gene Set Enrichment Analysis. (See Note 20)

3.3.5.1 Extract the Gene symbol and logFC columns from the previous toptreat to geneList, and convert the Gene symbol to ENTREZID by using ClusterProfiler:bitr.

3.3.5.2 Sort the geneList by logFC in the decreasing order.

3.3.5.3 Perform the gene set enrichment analysis on the geneList file with ClusterProfiler:gseKEGG [18, 19]. Results show that cytokine–cytokine receptor interaction and an additional five pathways are enriched in the top or bottom of the geneList for L_H_D5 vs L_M_CO (Fig. 5). (*See* **Note 21**).

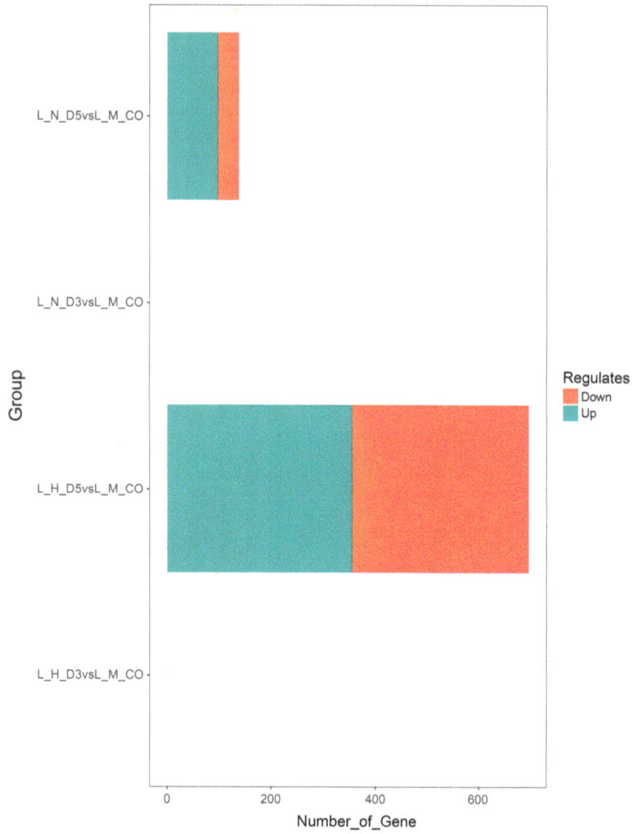

Fig. 4 *Gene expression profiles in the lungs of ferrets infected with HeV and NiV-B.* Ferrets are infected with 5000 TCID50 of HeV and NiV-B and euthanized at 3 and 5 d.p.i. (n = 3 per group, except for HeV_D5 with n = 3). Expression analysis reveals a number of significantly up- and down-regulated genes with respect to each comparison group

3.3.5.4 The gseplot of the cytokine–cytokine receptor interaction pathway is illustrated in **Fig. 6**. (The gseplots of additional significant pathways are not shown.) (*See* **Note 21**).

3.3.6 Determination of Transcription Factor Target Enrichment

To determine the enrichment of transcription factor target motifs in the set of differentially expressed genes, we utilize the C3 TFT dataset from the Molecular Signatures Database (MSigDb). Genes with shared upstream cis-regulatory motifs which can function as potential transcription factor binding sites are used as the basis for the determination of transcription factor target enrichment. The following steps are undertaken to determine the enrichment of transcription factor target motifs. (*See* **Note 22**).

(a) Download the gmt file of C3 TFT dataset from the MSigDb database [20].

(b) Read the gmt files with R clusterProfiler.

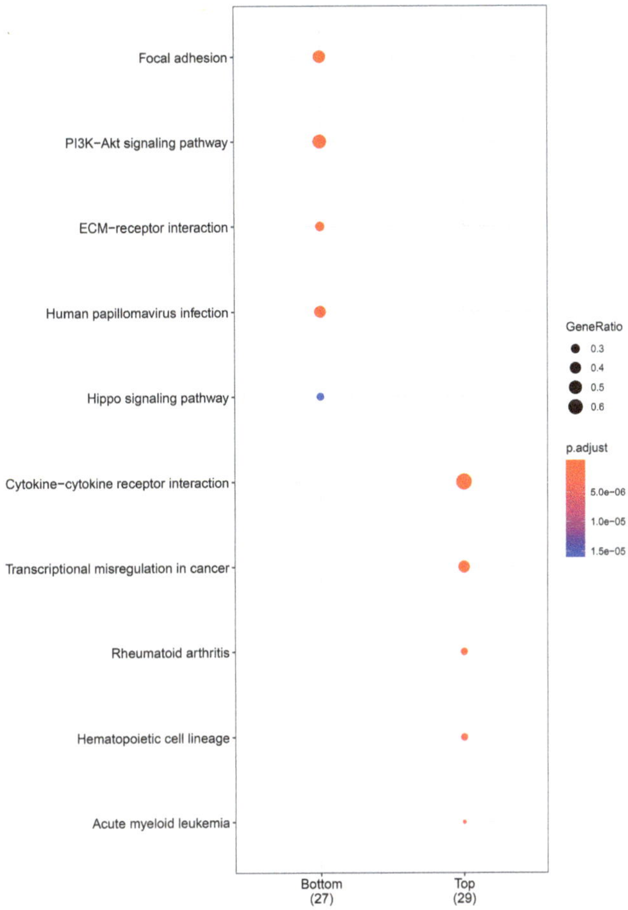

Fig. 5 *KEGG enrichment of differentially expressed genes.* KEGG enrichment of differentially expressed genes showed that cytokine–cytokine receptor interactions (including an additional five pathways) are enriched in the top or bottom of the genelist. The gene list is constructed by decreasing order (log fold change) by comparing 5 d.p.i. of HeV infection with the control group

(c) To identify potentially common transcription factor motifs and transcription factors that could coordinately regulate genes identified in the above enrichment analysis, transcription factor enrichment analysis of differentially expressed genes is performed with C3 TFT: transcription factor target motif using clusterprofiler: enricher. IRF_Q6 and 3 additional transcription factor target motifs are found to be enriched in our differentially expressed gene data sets (Fig. 7).

3.3.7 Transcription factor annotation based on GO ontology. (See Note 23).

3.3.7.1 Annotated the differentially expressed genes by cluster Profiler enrichGO by Biology Process and Molecular Function. Set the pvalue Cutoff and qvalue Cutoff as 1.

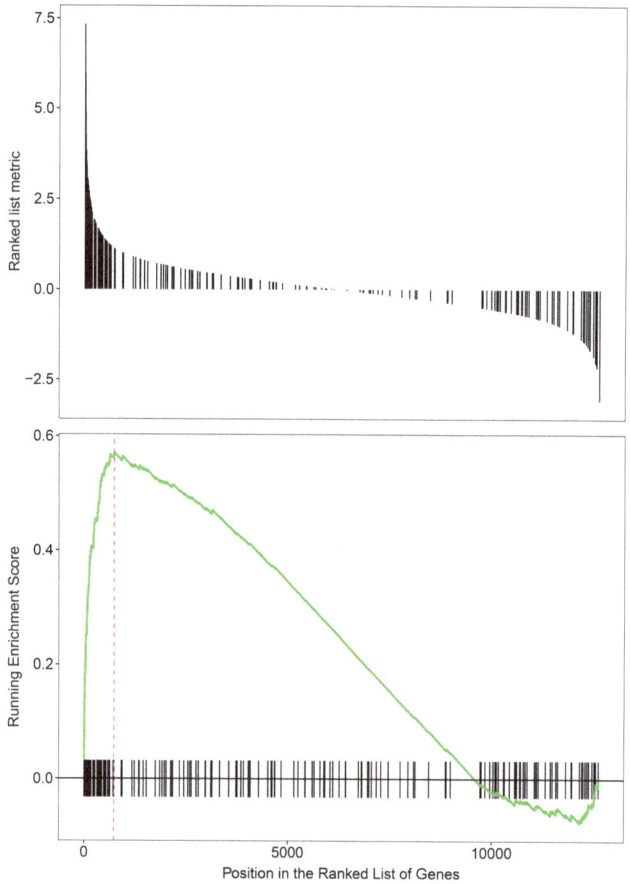

Fig. 6 *gseplot of cytokine–cytokine receptor interaction pathways.* Each line in the x-axis indicates the position in the genelist (decreasing order by log fold change when comparing 5 d.p.i.HeV infection and control groups). In the upper panel, the y-axis of the bar plot is the log fold change; in the lower panel, the curve is the enrichment score change across the gene list

3.3.7.2 Extracted the genes that are found in GO:0001228, GO:0001077,GO:0001205, GO:0001190, GO:0001227,GO:0001078,GO:0001206, GO:0001191,GO:0001228,GO:0001077, GO:0001205,GO:0001190,GO:0001227, GO:0001078,GO:0001206,GO:0000981, GO:0000982,GO:0003705,GO:0001076, GO:0006357,GO:0045944,GO:0000122, GO:0043565,GO:0000976,GO:0000977, GO:0000978,GO:0000980,GO:00008134, GO:0001805 [21]. (*See* **Note 24**).

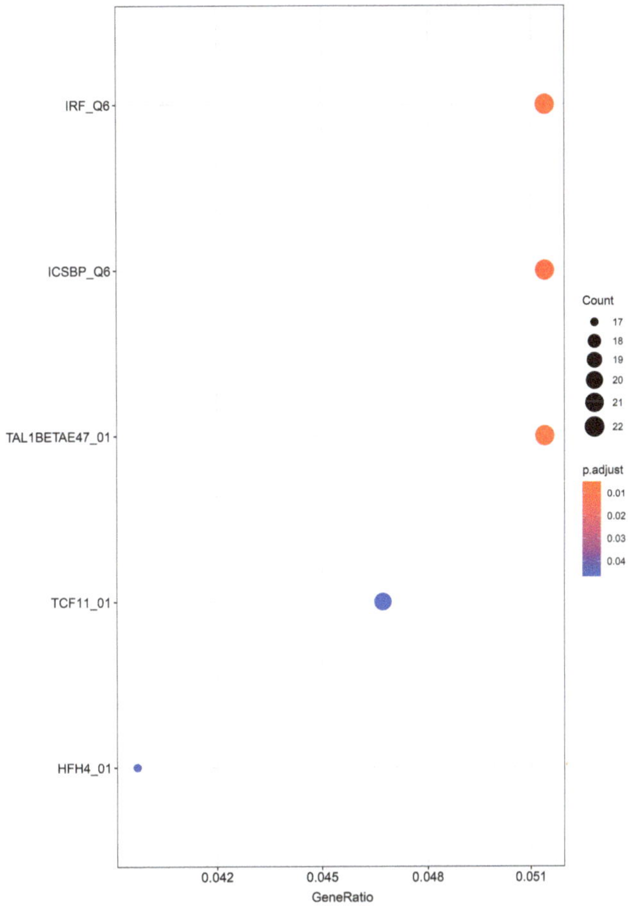

Fig. 7 *Transcription factor target enrichment.* To better understand the regulation of networks of genes, Transcription factor target enrichment is undertaken. First, all differentially expressed genes are examined for transcription factor binding sites found in the UTR of each gene. Common transcription factor binding sites in the UTR region among different differentially expressed genes are determined. The number of genes with common transcription factor binding sites is shown as circles in Fig. 7. The larger the circle, the higher the number of different differentially regulated genes containing a binding motif(s) for a specific transcription factor. There are more than 20 differentially expressed genes containing IRF binding motif(s). This represents enrichment for the IRF transcription factor target(s). The associated p-value for the enrichment of IRF is less than $p < 0.01$ (bright red color). IRF1, Interferon Regulatory Factor 1, is a well-known transcription factor that binds to the IRF binding motif and regulates multiple transcription pathways during host defense. Other enriched transcription factor target motifs are for ICSBP, TAL1BETAE47, TCF11, and HFH4.Enrichment was performed using the C3 TFT: transcription factor targets database

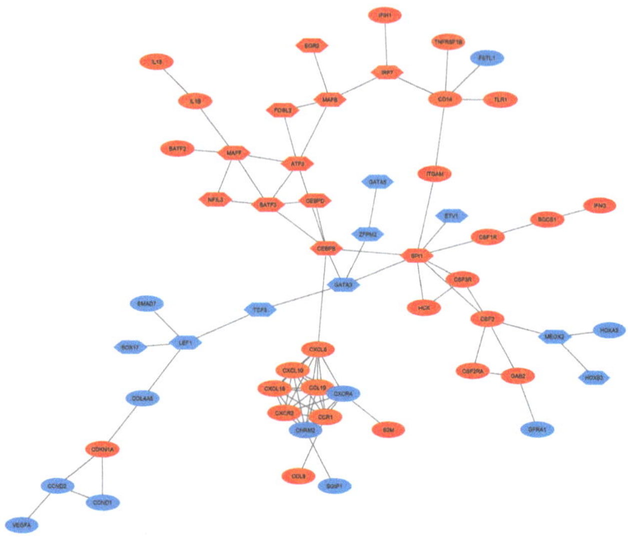

Fig. 8 *Protein–Protein interaction networks*. This figure represents a summary of the differentially expressed genes and potential protein–protein interactions. Nodes that are annotated as transcript factors are represented in a polygonal shape. Red color indicates up-regulated nodes; blue color indicates down-regulated nodes

3.3.8 PPI Network Analysis

3.3.8.1 All the differentially expressed genes that are enriched in the gseKEGG,C3 target motif or annotated as transcript factors are extracted and input into Metacape to obtain protein–protein interactions. Networks are based on databases: BioGrid6, InWeb_IM7, OmniPath8 [22–24].

3.3.8.2 Input the network into Cytoscapeas to obtain regulation and transcript information [25].

3.3.8.3 The resulting networks in our study are visualized in Fig. 8. All the nodes that are annotated as transcript factors are represented as Polygonsin shape. Red highlights represent up-regulated nodes; blue highlight represents down-regulated nodes (Fig. 8).

3.3.9 Identification of Cytokine–Cytokine Receptor Interaction Pathways

To determine cytokine–cytokine receptor interaction pathways, the following steps are followed. A Heatmap is generated (log-CPM values) for genes in cytokine–cytokine receptor interaction pathways in L_H_D5 vs L_M_CO. (*See* **Note 25**).

(a) Core genes that are enriched in KEGG cytokine–cytokine receptor interaction pathways are extracted from the gseKEGG enrichment file.

(b) The subset of the log CMP(lcmp) fit file by gene ID is extracted from the first step.

(c) A heatmap for visualization is created with the heatmap function from the ComplexHeatmap: package (Fig. 9) (*See* **Note 25**).

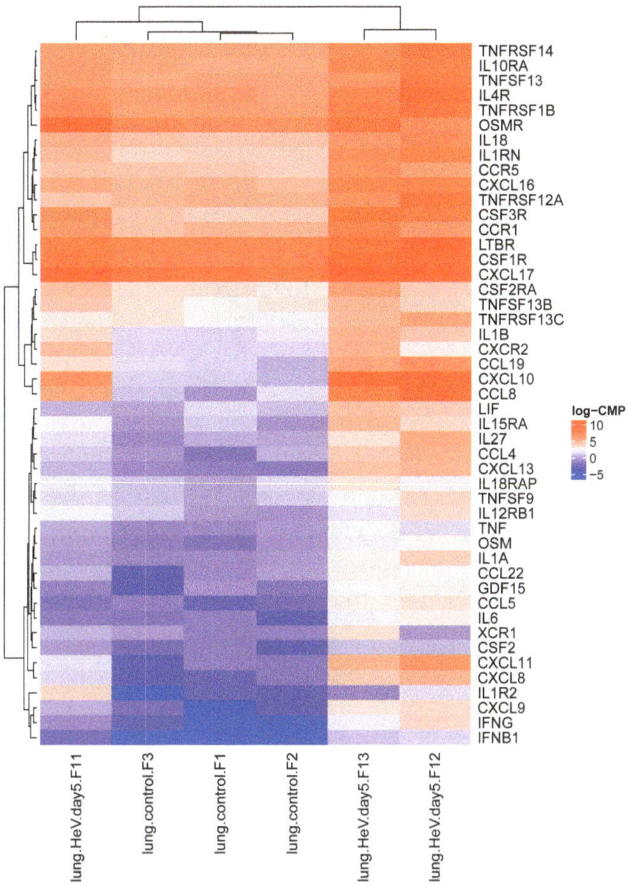

Fig. 9 *Heatmap of differentially expressed genes (Cytokines and Cytokine Receptors).* To better visualize up-regulated and down-regulated genes, a heat map of log-CPM values of differential expression patterns for cytokine–cytokine receptor pathways was constructed. Samples with relatively high expression within a gene are marked in red; samples with relatively low expression are marked in blue. CCL8 and CXCL10 are highly expressed in infected lungs. Interestingly, IFNB has reduced expression in the control tissues

4 Notes

1. Ferret lungs are quite large, and pathology is not uniform for many viral diseases. It is recommended that gross pathology be used as a guide in collecting samples. Side-by-side tissue sampling for histopathology and RNA extraction should be carried out to correlate histopathology to gene expression. The protocol for which tissue samples are selected for RNA should be determined prior to initiating the experiment; for example, tissue selection will be based on gross pathology, or tissue selection will be random, or tissue selection will be based on imaging data, or tissue selection will be based on a defined lobe and an anatomical position of the lung determined prior to necropsy.

2. Homogenization was performed in these studies with a bead-based homogenizer (TissueLyser LT, Qiagen, Toronto, Canada). This type of homogenizer increases efficiency by allowing multiple samples to be homogenized simultaneously. An alternate method uses a TissueRuptor II homogenizer (Qiagen, Toronto, Canada) for 1–3 minutes. This style of homogenizer comes with disposable probes reducing cross-contamination and possible introduction of RNAses.
3. All downstream methods are dependent on RNA quality. Because of the abundance of RNAses, it is highly recommended that a dedicated RNA room be used for isolating RNA. All surfaces should be cleaned to remove RNAse, and all glassware and plasticware should be cleaned to remove RNAse. Several vendors sell RNAse inhibitors and RNAse-free water. Wear gloves at all times.
4. The amount of RNA input varies with different RNA library kits. It is highly recommended to use a high RIN value greater than or equal to 7.5.
5. edgeR utilizes the read_count directly for differential gene expression analysis. FPKM value is not necessary for the analysis.
6. ##Reading in count data.

```
read_count<-read.table("read_counts.txt",header=T,
    sep="\t")
count_matrix<-as.matrix(read_count[,2:10])
```

7. ##Organizing sample information.

```
library(edgeR)
row.names(count_matix)<-read_count[1,]
group<-as.factor(substr(colnames(count_matrix),1,6))
y<-DGEList(count=,group=group)
```

8. In this analysis, CPM and log-CPM are used although they do not take into account the gene length, which RPKM and FPKM values do. However, RPKM and FPKM values can be used (in this case gene length must be added).
9. Transformations from the raw-scale to counts per million:

```
cpm<- cpm(y)
lcpm<- cpm(y, log=TRUE, prior.count=2)
keep.exprs<- filterByExpr(y, group=group)
y <- y[keep.exprs,, keep.lib.sizes=FALSE][Should these be
    separate bullets?]
```

10. ##Normalizing gene expression distributions.

```
y <- calcNormFactors(y, method = "TMM")
Figure2<-plotMDS(lcpm, labels=group)
```

11. The Glimma package enables interactive exploration of differential gene expression analysis results, allowing individual samples and genes to be examined by the user [26].
12. In this analysis, experimental or technical effects have been modeled using a random effect. Limma's linear modeling approach is able to handle more complicated experimental factorial designs.
13. Creating a design matrix and contrasts.

```
design <- model.matrix(~0+group)
colnames(design) <- gsub("group", "", colnames(design))
contr.matrix<- makeContrasts(
L_H_D5vsL_M_CO=L_H_D5-L_M_CO,
levels = colnames(design)))
```

14. The voom-plot provides a visual check on the level of lowly-expressed genefiltering. If a drop in variance levels can be observed at the low end of the expression scale, return to the earlier filtering step and increase the expression threshold applied to the dataset.
15. ##Removing heteroscedascity from count data.

```
library(limma)
y <- voom(y, design, plot=TRUE)
vfit<- lmFit(v, design)
Figure3<-plotSA(vfit, main="Final model: Mean-variance
   trend")
```

16. It has been shown that when the raw counts of RNA-seq transformed to log-CPM values, the variance is not independent of the mean. In limma, linear modeling is carried out on the log-CPM values, which are assumed to be normally distributed and a quadratic mean-variance relationship is accommodated using precision weights calculated by the voom function [16].
17. Fitting linear models for the comparisons of interest.

```
vfit<- lmFit(v, design)
vfit<- contrasts.fit(vfit, contrasts=contr.matrix)
efit<- eBayes(vfit)
```

18. ##Examining the number of DE genes.

```
tfit<- treat(vfit, lfc=log(1.2,base=2)
DEG<- decideTests(tfit)
DEG<-as.data.frame(summary(decideTests(tfit)))
names(DEG)<-c("regulates","Group","Number_of_Gene")
DEG<-subset(DEG,regulates!="NotSig")
```

```
Figure4<-ggplot(DEG,aes(x=Group,y=Number_of_Gene,
    fill=regulates))+geom_bar(stat="identity")+coord_flip()
    +theme_bw()
```

19. ##Creating a gene List with genes ranked by a decreasing logFC.

```
library(clusterProfiler)
library(org.Hs.eg.db)
L_H_D5 vs L_M_CO <- topTreat(tfit, coef=1, n=Inf)
geneID1<-bitr(L_H_D5vsL_M_CO$ID,fromType="SYM-
    BOL", toType="UNIPROT", OrgDb="org.Hs.eg.db")
geneID2<- bitr_kegg(geneID1$UNIPROT, fromType='u-
    niprot', toType='kegg', organism='hsa')
names(geneID2)[1]<-"UNIPROT"
geneID<-merge(geneID1,geneID2,by="UNIPROT")
names(L_H_D5vsL_M_CO)[1]<-"SYMBOL"
L_H_D5vsL_M_CO<-merge(L_H_D5-L_M_CO,geneID,
    by="SYMBOL")
L_H_D5vsL_M_CO<-L_H_D5vsL_M_CO[order
    (L_H_D5vsL_M_CO$logFC,decreasing=T),]
geneList<- as.vector(L_H_D5vsL_M_CO$logFC)
attr(geneList,"names")<-as.character(L_H_D5vsL_M_CO
    $kegg)
```

20. The species was set for *H. Sapiens* (not *Mustela putorius furo*) in the enrichment analysis, such as KEGG, GO, and protein–protein interaction network analysis because of the lack of accumulated data on *Mustela putorius furo*.

21. KEGG gene set enrichment analysis gene <- names(geneList)[-abs(geneList) > 2].

```
kk <- enrichKEGG(gene = gene, organism= 'hsa', pvalue-
    Cutoff = 0.05)
Figure5<-dotplot(kk)
kk2 <- gseKEGG(geneList geneList,organism= 'hsa',
    nPerm=1000, minGSSize= 120, pvalueCutoff = 0.05,
    verbose= FALSE)
Figure6<-gseaplot(kk2, geneSetID = "hsa04060")
```

22. Transcript factor target motif enrichment analysis.

```
C3<-readgmt("c3.tft.v6.2.entrez.gmt")
DEGs<-subset((L_H_D5vsL_M_CO, adj.p.value<0.05&|
    logFC|>log(1.2,base=2)
DEGs<- DEGs$ ENTREZID
C3enrich<- enricher (DEGs, TERM2GENE=c5)
Figure7<-dotplot(C3enrich)
```

23. Transcript factor annotation.

```
Ego1 <- enrichGO(gene =DEGs,ont = "MF",pAdjustMethod = "BH", pvalueCutoff = 1, qvalueCutoff = 1)
Ego2 <- enrichGO(gene =DEGs,ont = "BP",pAdjustMethod = "BH", pvalueCutoff = 1, qvalueCutoff = 1)
Ego<-rbind(Ego1,Ego2)
TFs<-subset(Ego,Ego$ID%in%c
  ("GO:0001228","GO:0001077","GO:0001205",
  "GO:0001190","GO:0001227","GO:0001078",
  "GO:0001206","GO:0001191","GO:0001228",
  "GO:0001077","GO:0001205","GO:0001190",
  "GO:0001227","GO:0001078","GO:0001206",
  "GO:0000981","GO:0000982","GO:0003705",
  "GO:0001076","GO:0006357","GO:0045944",
  "GO:0000122","GO:0043565","GO:0000976",
  "GO:0000977","GO:0000978","GO:0000980",
  "GO:00008134","GO:0001805"))
```

24. The transcription factor annotation can be obtained from TFcatdatabase, http://cisreg.ca/tfcat/as well, instead of the GO terms.

25. ##Creating log-CMP heatmap for differentially expressed genes in cytokine–cytokine interaction pathway.

```
p<-which(kk$Description=="Cytokine–cytokine receptor interaction")
cytogenes<-strsplit(kk$geneID[p],"/")
cytogenes<-cytogenes[[1]]
cytogenes<-subset(geneID,geneID$kegg%in%cytogenes)$SYMBOL
pos<-which(row.names(lcpm)%in%cytogenes)
library(ComplexHeatmap)
Figure9<-Heatmap(lcpm[pos,],name="log-CMP")
```

Acknowledgements

This work was supported by the Li Ka-Shing Foundation (DJK), Canada Research Chairs (DJK), Dalhousie Medical Research Foundation (DJK), and Nova Scotia Health Research Foundation (AAK). DJK is the Canada Research Chair in Translational Vaccinology and Inflammation.

References

1. Leon AJ, Banner D, Xu L, Ran L, Peng Z, Yi K, Chen C, Xu F, Huang J, Zhao Z, Lin Z, Huang SHS, Fang Y, Kelvin AA, Ross TM, Farooqui A, Kelvin DJ (2013) Sequencing, annotation, and characterization of the influenza ferret Infectome. J Virol 87(4): 1957–1966. https://doi.org/10.1128/jvi.02476-12
2. Bruder CE, Yao S, Larson F, Camp JV, Tapp R, McBrayer A, Powers N, Granda WV, Jonsson CB (2010) Transcriptome sequencing and development of an expression microarray platform for the domestic ferret. BMC Genomics 11:251. https://doi.org/10.1186/1471-2164-11-251
3. Peng X, Alfoeldi J, Gori K, Eisfeld AJ, Tyler SR, Tisoncik-Go J, Brawand D, Law GL, Skunca N, Hatta M, Gasper DJ, Kelly SM, Chang J, Thomas MJ, Johnson J, Berlin AM, Lara M, Russell P, Swofford R, Turner-Maier J, Young S, Hourlier T, Aken B, Searle S, Sun X, Yi Y, Suresh M, Tumpey TM, Siepel A, Wisely SM, Dessimoz C, Kawaoka Y, Birren BW, Lindblad-Toh K, Di Palma F, Engelhardt JF, Palermo RE, Katze MG (2014) The draft genome sequence of the ferret (Mustela putorius furo) facilitates study of human respiratory disease. Nat Biotechnol 32(12):1250–U1114. https://doi.org/10.1038/nbt.3079
4. Leon AJ, Borisevich V, Boroumand N, Seymour R, Nusbaum R, Escaffre O, Xu L, Kelvin DJ, Rockx B (2018) Host gene expression profiles in ferrets infected with genetically distinct henipavirus strains. PLoS Negl Trop Dis 12(3):e0006343. https://doi.org/10.1371/journal.pntd.0006343
5. Belser JA, Katz JM, Tumpey TM (2011) The ferret as a model organism to study influenza a virus infection. Dis Model Mech 4(5): 575–579. https://doi.org/10.1242/dmm.007823
6. Banner D, Kelvin AA (2012) The current state of H5N1 vaccines and the use of the ferret model for influenza therapeutic and prophylactic development. J Infect Dev Ctries 6(6): 465–469
7. Rowe T, Leon AJ, Crevar CJ, Carter DM, Xu L, Ran L, Fang Y, Cameron CM, Cameron MJ, Banner D, Ng DCK, Ran R, Weirback HK, Wiley CA, Kelvin DJ, Ross TM (2010) Modeling host responses in ferrets during a/California/07/2009 influenza infection. Virology 401(2):257–265. https://doi.org/10.1016/j.virol.2010.02.020
8. Bossart KN, Zhu Z, Middleton D, Klippel J, Crameri G, Bingham J, McEachern JA, Green D, Hancock TJ, Chan Y-P, Hickey AC, Dimitrov DS, Wang L-F, Broder CC (2009) A neutralizing human monoclonal antibody protects against lethal disease in a new ferret model of acute Nipah virus infection. PLoS Pathog 5(10). https://doi.org/10.1371/journal.ppat.1000642
9. Brown J, Pirrung M, McCue LA (2017) FQC dashboard: integrates FastQC results into a web-based, interactive, and extensible FASTQ quality control tool. Bioinformatics 33:3137. https://doi.org/10.1093/bioinformatics/btx373
10. Bolger AM, Lohse M, Usadel B (2014) Trimmomatic: a flexible trimmer for Illumina sequence data. Bioinformatics 30(15): 2114–2120. https://doi.org/10.1093/bioinformatics/btu170
11. Ghosh S, Chan CK (2016) Analysis of RNA-Seq data using TopHat and cufflinks. Methods Mol Biol 1374:339–361. https://doi.org/10.1007/978-1-4939-3167-5_18
12. Pollier J, Rombauts S, Goossens A (2013) Analysis of RNA-Seq data with TopHat and cufflinks for genome-wide expression analysis of jasmonate-treated plants and plant cultures. Methods Mol Biol 1011:305–315. https://doi.org/10.1007/978-1-62703-414-2_24
13. Robinson MD, McCarthy DJ, Smyth GK (2010) edgeR: a Bioconductor package for differential expression analysis of digital gene expression data. Bioinformatics 26(1): 139–140. https://doi.org/10.1093/bioinformatics/btp616
14. Robinson MD, Oshlack A (2010) A scaling normalization method for differential expression analysis of RNA-seq data. Genome Biol 11(3):R25. https://doi.org/10.1186/gb-2010-11-3-r25
15. Ritchie ME, Phipson B, Wu D, Hu Y, Law CW, Shi W, Smyth GK (2015) Limma powers differential expression analyses for RNA-sequencing and microarray studies. Nucl Acids Res 43(7):e47. https://doi.org/10.1093/nar/gkv007
16. Law CW, Chen Y, Shi W, Smyth GK (2014) Voom: precision weights unlock linear model analysis tools for RNA-seq read counts. Genome Biol 15(2):R29. https://doi.org/10.1186/gb-2014-15-2-r29
17. McCarthy DJ, Smyth GK (2009) Testing significance relative to a fold-change threshold is a TREAT. Bioinformatics 25(6):765–771. https://doi.org/10.1093/bioinformatics/btp053

18. Yu G, Wang LG, Han Y, He QY (2012) clusterProfiler: an R package for comparing biological themes among gene clusters. OMICS 16(5):284–287. https://doi.org/10.1089/omi.2011.0118
19. Subramanian A, Tamayo P, Mootha VK, Mukherjee S, Ebert BL, Gillette MA, Paulovich A, Pomeroy SL, Golub TR, Lander ES, Mesirov JP (2005) Gene set enrichment analysis: a knowledge-based approach for interpreting genome-wide expression profiles. Proc Natl Acad Sci U S A 102(43):15545–15550. https://doi.org/10.1073/pnas.0506580102
20. Liberzon A, Subramanian A, Pinchback R, Thorvaldsdottir H, Tamayo P, Mesirov JP (2011) Molecular signatures database (MSigDB) 3.0. Bioinformatics 27(12): 1739–1740. https://doi.org/10.1093/bioinformatics/btr260
21. Tripathi S, Christie KR, Balakrishnan R, Huntley R, Hill DP, Thommesen L, Blake JA, Kuiper M, Laegreid A (2013) Gene ontology annotation of sequence-specific DNA binding transcription factors: setting the stage for a large-scale curation effort. Database (Oxford) 2013:bat062. https://doi.org/10.1093/database/bat062
22. Li T, Wernersson R, Hansen RB, Horn H, Mercer J, Slodkowicz G, Workman CT, Rigina O, Rapacki K, Staerfeldt HH, Brunak S, Jensen TS, Lage K (2017) A scored human protein-protein interaction network to catalyze genomic interpretation. Nat Methods 14(1):61–64. https://doi.org/10.1038/nmeth.4083
23. Chatr-Aryamontri A, Breitkreutz BJ, Oughtred R, Boucher L, Heinicke S, Chen D, Stark C, Breitkreutz A, Kolas N, O'Donnell L, Reguly T, Nixon J, Ramage L, Winter A, Sellam A, Chang C, Hirschman J, Theesfeld C, Rust J, Livstone MS, Dolinski K, Tyers M (2015) The BioGRID interaction database: 2015 update. Nucleic Acids Res 43 (Database issue):D470–D478. https://doi.org/10.1093/nar/gku1204
24. Turei D, Korcsmaros T, Saez-Rodriguez J (2016) OmniPath: guidelines and gateway for literature-curated signaling pathway resources. Nat Methods 13(12):966–967. https://doi.org/10.1038/nmeth.4077
25. Shannon P, Markiel A, Ozier O, Baliga NS, Wang JT, Ramage D, Amin N, Schwikowski B, Ideker T (2003) Cytoscape: a software environment for integrated models of biomolecular interaction networks. Genome Res 13(11):2498–2504. https://doi.org/10.1101/gr.1239303
26. Su S, Law CW, Ah-Cann C, Asselin-Labat ML, Blewitt ME, Ritchie ME (2017) Glimma: interactive graphics for gene expression analysis. Bioinformatics 33(13):2050–2052. https://doi.org/10.1093/bioinformatics/btx094

Index

Alexander N. Freiberg and Barry Rockx (eds.), *Nipah Virus: Methods and Protocols*, Methods in Molecular Biology, vol. 2682, https://doi.org/10.1007/978-1-0716-3283-3,

FSC
www.fsc.org
MIX
Papier | Fördert gute Waldnutzung
FSC® C083411

Kolibri 360 GmbH
Ferdinand-Jühlke-Straße 7
99095 Erfurt, Deutschland
produktsicherheit@kolibri360.de